Social Anxiety Disorder

Medical Psychiatry

ADDITIONAL VOLUMES IN PREPARATION

Social Anxiety Disorder

edited by
Borwin Bandelow
University of Göttingen
Göttingen, Germany

Dan J. Stein
University of Stellenbosch
Cape Town, South Africa
and
University of Florida
Gainesville, Florida, U.S.A.

MARCEL DEKKER, INC.   NEW YORK • BASEL

Library of Congress Cataloging-in-Publication Data
A catalog record for this book is available from the Library of Congress.

ISBN: 0-8247-5454-9

This book is printed on acid-free paper.

Headquarters
Marcel Dekker, Inc., 270 Madison Avenue, New York, NY 10016, U.S.A.
tel: 212-696-9000; fax: 212-685-4540

Distribution and Customer Service
Marcel Dekker, Inc., Cimarron Road, Monticello, New York 12701, U.S.A.
tel: 800-228-1160; fax: 845-796-1772

Eastern Hemisphere Distribution
Marcel Dekker AG, Hutgasse 4, Postfach 812, CH-4001 Basel, Switzerland
tel: 41-61-260-6300; fax: 41-61-260-6333

World Wide Web
http://www.dekker.com

The publisher offers discounts on this book when ordered in bulk quantities. For more information, write to Special Sales/Professional Marketing at the headquarters address above.

Preface

*"But that isn't right. The King of Beasts shouldn't
be a coward," said the Scarecrow.*

*"I know it," returned the Lion, wiping a tear
from his eye with the tip of his paw. "It is my
great sorrow, and makes my life very unhappy.
But whenever there is danger, my heart begins to
beat fast."*

*"Perhaps you have a heart disease," said the Tin
Woodsman.*

"It may be," said the Lion.
— L. Frank Baum, *The Wizard of Oz*

Man is the only animal that blushes. Or needs to.
— Mark Twain

The idea that people who suffer from social anxiety can be diagnosed with a medical disorder remains a controversial one. Whereas depression may be increasingly accepted by laypeople, primary care practitioners, and health-care policy-makers as a valid entity, there continues to be profound skepticism about many of the anxiety disorders. Indeed, prominent critics have charged that "social anxiety disorder" is merely a label that has been hyped by the pharmaceutical industry, in an attempt to extend product lines and improve profits. To justify a volume devoted to social anxiety disorder, a few paragraphs are needed to air such criticisms, and to provide an appropriate rejoinder.

Several observations provide ammunition for the suggestion that a diagnosis of "social anxiety disorder" is merely an artifact of Western society in the 21st century. Variations in normal personality such as shyness have arguably long been accepted as normal. Indeed, in some cultures, shyness and modesty are perceived as virtues, and rewarded accordingly. The notion that self-confidence and extraversion are outcomes of treatment seems peculiarly Western. Certainly, before the industry sponsored direct-to-consumer marketing campaigns around social anxiety disorder, it was rare for patients to present to primary practitioners or mental health clinicians with complaints of social fears.

Furthermore, the technologies of the modern world have led to significant changes in our social interactions, and so perhaps to peculiar forms of social anxiety. With radio and television we do not need to talk to our neighbors to hear the news, with electronic cash registers we do not have to ask a shopkeeper for milk and bread, with car navigation systems we don't have to ask for directions, with mobile phones we do not have to look someone in the eye when conversing, and with the Internet a whole world opens up without our needing to leave home and meet real people. It is not surprising, therefore, that people have difficulties in social situations and are tempted to seek medical solutions.

Nevertheless, the distress and dysfunction that can accompany social anxiety have long been recognized. The Bible describes several cases of social anxiety, including those of Moses and Saul. Saul's case is particularly interesting insofar as he went on to develop a severe depression, an early illustration of the high comorbidity and morbidity associated with this condition. Classical literature also provides depictions of anxiety in general and social anxiety in particular. The Greek poet Sappho (610–580 B.C.) wrote:

He is a god in my eyes
the man who is allowed
to sit beside you–he

who listens intimately
to the sweet murmur of
your voice, the enticing

laughter that makes my own
heart beat fast. If I meet
you suddenly, I can't

speak–my tongue is broken;
a thin flame runs under
my skin; seeing nothing,

hearing only my own ears
drumming, I drip with sweat;
trembling shakes my body

and I turn paler than
dry grass. At such times
death isn't far from me

Here is a detailed account of a panic attack occurring in a social situation. A young girl admires a young man and is glad that she can speak to him. But suddenly, to her surprise, she realizes that feelings of anxiety overwhelm her. Her symptoms are similar to those enumerated in modern nomenclatures— tachycardia, dry mouth, blushing, blurred vision, tinnitus, sweating, trembling, turning pale, and fear of dying. What is particularly useful about the depiction here is the way in which distress and suffering are conveyed; people suffering from social anxiety disorder may deeply want social contact, but at the same time their symptoms lead to social avoidance.

The early medical literature also describes the phenomenon of social phobia. In 1621, Robert Burton described symptoms of anxiety attacks in social anxious men in *Anatomy of Melancholy*:

Many lamentable effects this fear causeth in man, as to be red, pale, tremble, sweat; it makes sudden cold and heat come over all the body, palpitation of the heart, syncope, etc. It amazeth many men that are to speak or show themselves in public.

In the same book, Burton cited Hippocrates writing on one of his patients, who apparently suffered from social anxiety disorder:

He dare not come into company for fear he should be misused, disgraced, overshoot himself in gestures or speeches, or be sick; he thinks every man observeth him.

The term "social phobia" dates back only to 1966, when Marks and Gelder described "a condition in which the individual becomes very anxious in situations where he or she may be subject to scrutiny by others while performing a specific task." The provision of reliable diagnostic criteria in DSM-III in 1980 encouraged detailed epidemiological surveys. The Epidemiological Catchment Area study in the United States established that social anxiety disorder was prevalent and chronic, and that it was associated with significant comorbidity and morbidity. Furthermore, a cross-national study undertaken in a range of different countries confirmed many of the findings of the ECA, establishing the universal importance of the condition. Subsequent community surveys and clinical studies in the United States and elsewhere have provided clear evidence of the prevalence and morbidity of social anxiety disorder.

Why then do primary care practitioners and the lay public continue to believe that social anxiety disorder is better understood as "shyness"? Perhaps the universality of normal social anxiety prevents people from recognizing the less common—but extremely disabling—phenomena of excessive social anxiety. Symptoms of social anxiety may themselves prevent people from seeking help. Cultural mores have perhaps contributed to the normalization of social anxiety. In their volume on social phobia, Schneier and Wolkowitz recall the case of a famous female actor who was advised not to seek treatment for social anxiety, because this was seen as an attractive trait. Such a view ignores the suffering associated with social anxiety, and consequences such as comorbid depression and suicide.

Fortunately, the data on the prevalence and morbidity of social anxiety disorder are beginning to persuade primary care practitioners and the lay public that this is a valid diagnostic entity that deserves to be taken seriously, and to be treated rigorously. This view has been strengthened by advances in understanding the psychobiology of animal anxiety and of human social anxiety disorder, and by the discovery of effective and safe pharmacotherapies and psychotherapies. Such work culminated in the registration of the first medications for social anxiety disorder; this work has helped relieve symptoms and disability in many patients with this condition.

There is growing awareness of the importance of increasing mental health literacy in the community and in primary care practitioners. Certainly, increased awareness of social anxiety disorder might increase early diagnosis and rigorous intervention. As part of this campaign, it might be useful to portray the battle that prominent people have fought with their social anxiety. Sir Lawrence Olivier was always frightened to forget his text and once did a play with his back mostly turned toward the audience because of stage fright. Robert Falcon Scott, the intrepid explorer, was noted by his companion and physician, William Wilson, to suffer from social anxiety:

> Yet back at home he found normal social intercourse so difficult that he confided his diary that he took sedatives before going to parties, and one of his biographers wrote that it required far more courage for him to face an audience than to cross a crevasse.

The purpose of this book is to provide an authoritative and up-to-date review of social anxiety disorder, covering psychopathology (including symptomatology, epidemiology, comorbidity, disability, and spectrum disorders), assessment (including diagnosis in adults and in children, and rating scales) pathogenesis (including animal models, neurobiology, genetics, brain imaging, cognitive models, environmental and cross-cultural factors), and treatment (including pharmacotherapy, cognitive-behavioral psychotherapy, psychodynamic psychotherapy, integrated management, treatment of children). Bringing together leading authorities from seven countries from all over the world, the book provides state-of-the-art analyses of the research, and evidence-based guidelines for clinical treatment. We wish to thank the contributing authors for their hard work, and also to thank our editor at Marcel Dekker for her constant encouragement. We hope this effort will enhance readers' ability to improve the lives of their patients.

Borwin Bandelow
Dan J. Stein

Contents

Section II: Pathogenesis

Section III: Management

Contributors

Candice Alfano Department of Psychology, University of Maryland, College Park, Maryland, U.S.A.

David S. Baldwin Mental Health Group, Department of Psychiatry, University of Southampton, Southampton, United Kingdom

Borwin Bandelow Department of Psychiatry and Psychotherapy, University of Göttingen, Göttingen, Germany

Deborah C. Beidel Department of Psychology, University of Maryland, College Park, Maryland, U.S.A.

Robert M. Berman New York State Psychiatric Institute, Columbia University College of Physicians and Surgeons, New York, New York, U.S.A.

Carlos Blanco New York State Psychiatric Institute, Columbia University College of Physicians and Surgeons, New York, New York, U.S.A.

Christel Buis Mental Health Group, Department of Psychiatry, University of Southampton, Southampton, United Kingdom

Fredric Busch Department of Psychiatry, Weill Medical College of Cornell University, and Columbia University Center for Psychoanalytic Training and Research, New York, New York, U.S.A.

Aicha Charimo Torrente Department of Psychiatry and Psychotherapy, University of Göttingen, Göttingen, Germany

Jeremy D. Coplan Division of Neuropsychopharmacology and Primate Behavioral Laboratory, State University of New York, Downstate, Brooklyn, and New York State Psychiatric Institute, New York, U.S.A.

Lydia Fehm   Clinical Psychology and Psychotherapy, Dresden University of Technology, Dresden, Germany

Courtney Ferrell   Department of Psychology, University of Maryland, College Park, Maryland, U.S.A.

Mats Fredrikson   Department of Psychology, Uppsala University, Uppsala, Sweden

Tomas Furmark   Department of Psychology, Uppsala University, Uppsala, Sweden

Carolina Garcia   New York State Psychiatric Institute, Columbia University College of Physicians and Surgeons, New York, New York, U.S.A.

Joel Gelernter   Department of Psychiatry, Yale University School of Medicine, New Haven, Connecticut, U.S.A.

Robert M. Holaway   Adult Anxiety Clinic, Department of Psychology, Temple University, Philadelphia, Pennsylvania, U.S.A.

Richard G. Heimberg   Adult Anxiety Clinic, Department of Psychology, Temple University, Philadelphia, Pennsylvania, U.S.A.

Liezl Koen   Stikland Hospital, Department of Psychiatry, University of Stellenbosch, Cape Town, South Africa

Michael R. Liebowitz   New York State Psychiatric Institute, Columbia University College of Physicians and Surgeons, New York, New York, U.S.A.

Joshua D. Lipsitz   New York State Psychiatric Institute, Columbia University College of Physicians and Surgeons, New York, New York, U.S.A.

Catherine Mancini   Department of Psychiatry and Behavioural Neurosciences, McMaster University, Hamilton, Ontario, Canada

Sanjay J. Mathew   New York State Psychiatric Institute and Department of Psychiatry, Columbia University College of Physicians and Surgeons, New York, New York, U.S.A.

Barbara L. Milrod   Weill Medical College of Cornell University, and New York Psychoanalytic Institute, New York, New York, U.S.A.

Tracy L. Morris   Department of Psychology, West Virginia University, Morgantown, West Virginia, U.S.A.

Jacqueline E. Muller   Medical Research Council's Unit on Anxiety Disorders, Department of Psychiatry, University of Stellenbosch, Cape Town, South Africa

Toshihiko Nagata   Department of Neuropsychiatry, Osaka City University Medical School, Osaka, Japan

Deborah A. Roth   Center for the Treatment and Study of Anxiety, Department of Psychiatry, University of Pennsylvania, Philadelphia, Pennsylvania, U.S.A.

Eckart Rüther   Department of Psychiatry and Psychotherapy, University of Göttingen, Göttingen, Germany

Franklin R. Schneier   New York State Psychiatric Institute, Columbia University College of Physicians and Surgeons, New York, New York, U.S.A.

Soraya Seedat   Department of Psychiatry, University of Stellenbosch, Cape Town, South Africa

Jordan W. Smoller   Department of Psychiatry, Massachusetts General Hospital, Boston, Massachusetts, U.S.A.

Dan J. Stein   Department of Psychiatry, University of Stellenbosch, Cape Town, South Africa, and University of Florida, Gainesville, Florida, U.S.A.

Murray B. Stein   Department of Psychiatry, University of California San Diego, San Diego, California, U.S.A.

Michael Van Ameringen   Department of Psychiatry and Behavioural Neurosciences, McMaster University, Hamilton, Ontario, Canada

Hans-Ulrich Wittchen   Clinical Psychology and Psychotherapy, Dresden University of Technology, Dresden, Germany

Robin Yeganeh   Department of Psychology, University of Maryland, College Park, Maryland, U.S.A.

Talia I. Zaider   Adult Anxiety Clinic, Department of Psychology, Temple University, Philadelphia, Pennsylvania, U.S.A.

1

Symptomatology and Diagnosis of Social Anxiety Disorder

Robert M. Berman and Franklin R. Schneier

New York State Psychiatric Institute, Columbia University
College of Physicians and Surgeons,
New York, New York, U.S.A.

I. PHENOMENOLOGY/SYMPTOMATOLOGY

A. History of Diagnostic Criteria

Social anxiety disorder (SAD), also known as social phobia, was first recognized as a specific diagnostic entity in the late 1960s and was incorporated into the diagnostic nomenclature in the 1980s in the third edition of the *Diagnostic and Statistical Manual of Mental Disorders* (DSM-III) (1). The term *social phobia* itself, however, has been in use since the early 1900s to characterize people with performance anxiety (2). In earlier editions (3,4) of the DSM, social phobia had been subsumed under broader categories of phobic reaction or phobic neurosis. Specific diagnostic criteria for social phobia were established after research revealed that social phobia differed from other phobias in respect to such clinical features as age of onset and course (5). DSM-III criteria emphasized fear of performance situations such as speaking, writing, or eating in public or using public restrooms.

DSM-III-R (6) and DSM-IV (7) subsequently broadened the definition to include fear and distress in most social situations.

B. Symptoms and Characteristics

A core feature of SAD is excessive fear of social or performance situations involving unfamiliar people or scrutiny. The individual fears embarrassment and negative evaluation. Beyond this central fear of embarrassment, however, is a diversity of presenting complaints and associated symptoms. The symptoms, in turn, may relate to a variety of social or performance situations. Public speaking is one of the most common anxiety-provoking situations for people in general, and it is the single situation most commonly feared by SAD patients as well (8). Other situations feared by a majority of SAD patients include informal interactions such as going to a party, meeting strangers or initiating a date, assertive behaviors such as talking to people in authority or expressing a disagreement, and situations involving scrutiny, such as working while being observed. Less commonly feared are other discrete situations such as taking tests, eating in front of others, using a public telephone, working or writing while being observed, or urinating in a public restroom (9). In the generalized subtype of SAD, fear or avoidance is elicited by most situations involving contact with other people.

Symptoms of SAD can be categorized as somatic, cognitive, and behavioral. Blushing and perspiration are among the most common somatic symptoms, with palpitations, trembling, abdominal distress, and muscular tension being somewhat less frequent (10). Anxiety symptoms may take the form of a panic attack. Common cognitive and emotional symptoms include unpleasant thoughts about the situation, blocked thoughts, and difficulty thinking or concentrating. Persons with SAD often fear that others will notice their nervousness, discomfort, blushing, sweating, or trembling. They also fear that others will question or criticize them and judge them to be stupid or ignorant. Behavioral symptoms include attempts to hide the reaction, difficulty speaking, becoming silent, avoiding eye contact, fumbling, restlessness, and immobility (10). The most impairing behavioral symptom is often avoidance of feared situations, which in addition to directly interfering with function prevents persons with SAD from opportunities to gain experience and social confidence.

In addition to symptoms experienced within the feared social situation, persons with SAD often experience troubling symptoms both before and afterwards. Anticipatory anxiety may commence weeks before a scheduled event, such as a speech or meeting, and may rise to a crescendo as a social situation is entered. After avoiding or leaving a feared social situation, persons with SAD are often highly self-critical and experience ruminations, decreased self-esteem and depressed mood (10).

C. Diagnostic Criteria

1. DSM-IV Criteria

DSM-IV categorizes *Social Phobia (Social Anxiety Disorder)* under the heading of *Anxiety Disorders*, which include panic, obsessive-compulsive, posttraumatic stress, and generalized anxiety disorders as well as agoraphobia and specific phobias. DSM-IV requires a patient to meet eight criteria in order to be diagnosed with SAD (Table 1). The first four regard symptomatology, the fifth addresses functional impairment, the sixth requires a duration of at least 6 months in children under 18 years, and the last two include relevant exclusions. In most categories, criteria specific to children are provided.

Necessary symptoms include a marked, persistent, and intensely distressing fear and/or avoidance of at least one social or performance situation involving scrutiny by others or exposure to unfamiliar people; fear of acting in an embarrassing or humiliating way, including exhibiting anxiety symptoms; anxiety nearly always provoked by the feared situation; and recognition of the fear as excessive or unreasonable. In children, age-appropriate social function must have been established before the onset of symptoms, the fear must occur with peers as well as adults, and the criterion of recognition of excessiveness or irrationality is waived.

As a threshold for caseness, the symptoms must result in a degree of functional impairment, including relationships with others, or there must be marked distress caused by the symptoms. Additionally, symptoms must not be caused by drugs of abuse or medications, general medical conditions, or other primary psychiatric disorders, especially including the related diagnoses of panic disorder, separation anxiety, pervasive developmental disorder, body dysmorphic disorder, or schizoid personality disorder. Fear of scrutiny caused by medical conditions or disorders—for example, stuttering, Parkinsonian tremor, or abnormal eating behaviors, as in eating disorders—must not be the primary cause of social anxiety symptoms.

The DSM-IV also allows for specification of subtype (generalized) if symptoms involve most social situations. The additional diagnosis of avoidant personality disorder is to be considered for persons with the generalized subtype.

2. ICD-10 Criteria and Comparison

While the DSM system was conceived by the American Psychiatric Association with both clinical and research applications in mind, the *International*

TABLE 1   DSM-IV Diagnostic Criteria for Social Phobia

A. A marked and persistent fear of one or more social or performance situations in which the person in exposed to unfamiliar people or to possible scrutiny by others. The individual fears that he or she will act in a way (or show anxiety symptoms) that will be humiliating or embarrassing. Note: In children, there must be evidence of the capacity for age-appropriate social relationships with familiar people and the anxiety must occur in peer settings, not just in interactions with adults.

B. Exposure to the feared situation almost invariably provokes anxiety, which may take the form of a situationally bound or situationally predisposed Panic Attack. Note: In children, the anxiety may be expressed by crying, tantrums, freezing, or shrinking from social situations with unfamiliar people.

C. The person recognizes that the fear is excessive or unreasonable. Note: In children, this feature may be absent.

D. The feared social or performance situations are avoided or else are endured with intense anxiety or distress.

E. The avoidance, anxious anticipation, or distress in the feared social or performance situation(s) interferes significantly with the person's normal routine, occupational (academic) functioning, or social activities or relationships, or there is marked distress about having the phobia.

F. In individuals under age 18 years, the duration is at least 6 months.

G. The fear or avoidance is not due to the direct physiological effects of a substance (e.g., a drug of abuse, a medication) or a general medical condition and is not better accounted for by another mental disorder (e.g., Panic Disorder With or Without Agoraphobia, Separation Anxiety Disorder, Body Dysmorphic Disorder, a Pervasive Developmental Disorder, or Schizoid Personality Disorder).

H. If a general medical condition or another mental disorder is present, the fear in Criterion A is unrelated to it; e.g., the fear is not of Stuttering, trembling in Parkinson's disease, or exhibiting abnormal eating behavior in Anorexia Nervosa or Bulimia Nervosa.

Specify if:

Generalized: if the fears included most social situations (also consider the additional diagnosis of Avoidant Personality Disorder).

Classification of Diseases (ICD) system (11) was designed by the World Health Organization as a research-oriented manual, with the aim of codifying diagnostic categories that would represent an international norm for interpreting research results from very different sources. The ICD-10 manual contains striking dissimilarities with the DSM-IV in respect to SAD.

The category of *Social Phobias* is subsumed under the major division of *Neurotic, Stress-related, and Somatoform Disorders*, in the subcategory of *Phobic Anxiety Disorders*, which includes agoraphobia, social phobias, and specific (isolated) phobias, as well as other phobic anxiety disorders and unspecified phobic anxiety disorder. Another subcategory entitled *Other Anxiety Disorders* includes panic disorder, generalized anxiety disorder, and mixed anxiety and depressive disorder.

In the ICD-10 system, social phobia shares with all other phobias a common set of criteria. To meet phobia criteria, a patient must have at least one symptom of autonomic arousal and at least one symptom—from a list of 13 others—occurring together on at least one occasion since the onset of the disorder. The symptoms are grouped into four categories: 1) autonomic arousal symptoms, including palpitations or increased heart rate, sweating, trembling or shaking, and dry mouth; 2) chest and abdominal symptoms, including shortness of breath, choking sensation, chest pain or discomfort, and nausea or other abdominal distress; 3) mental state symptoms, including feeling dizzy, light-headed, unsteady, or faint, derealization or depersonalization, fear of fainting or "going crazy," and fear of dying; and 4) general symptoms, including hot flushes or cold chills and numbness or tingling. In addition, the patient must also manifest at least one of the following symptoms in the setting of a feared social situation: blushing or shaking, fear of vomiting, or urgency or fear of micturition or defecation.

For social phobia specifically, one must experience either a marked fear of being the focus of attention or of behaving in an embarrassing or humiliating way or marked avoidance of situations in which these fears are stimulated. These fears must occur in social situations, such as small group encounters or speaking, eating, or meeting a known person in public. As with the DSM-IV, there must be significant emotional distress and a recognition that such fears are excessive or unreasonable; symptoms should be restricted to or predominate while contemplating or being in feared situations; and the usual rule-outs apply, i.e., symptoms are not caused by primary mood, psychotic, or organic disorders, obsessive-compulsive disorder (OCD), or cultural beliefs.

What is most distinct about the ICD-10 criteria in comparison to the DSM-IV system is the marked focus on somatic symptoms. While the DSM-IV alludes to the possibility of panic symptoms in criterion B, physiological symptoms are not otherwise mentioned and are certainly not required. The ICD-10, however, requires at least one autonomic symptom, one of 13 other mostly somatic symptoms, and the presence or fear of at least one of three other somatic symptoms. In this regard, the ICD-10 system would appear to focus on the more acute phobic response, whereas the DSM-IV, especially in respect to the generalized subtype, describes a more pervasive entity. In fact, the lack of resemblance of DSM-IV–defined generalized SAD to a typical discrete phobia may partially explain why the term *social phobia* has given way in recent years to the more descriptive designation *social anxiety disorder*.

While the DSM-IV distinguishes between adult and childhood forms of the disorder, the ICD-10 has no specific childhood qualifiers, including the presence of a pervasive developmental disorder. The ICD-10 refers to anxiety around known individuals, whereas the DSM-IV considers encounters with unfamiliar people to be relevant. Functionality is not addressed in the ICD-10, but degree of distress is shared by both criteria sets. Time frame is not considered in the ICD-10, while persistence and, in children, duration of symptoms is noted in the DSM-IV. Minor differences include reference to the fear of exhibiting one's anxiety, allusion to substance abuse and medication effects as important rule-outs, and reference to subtypes in the DSM-IV but not in the ICD-10.

D. Subtypes of Social Anxiety Disorder

The generalized subtype of SAD, defined by fear of most social situations, was first introduced in the DSM-III-R. Whereas fear of many or most social interactions had been subsumed previously under the diagnosis of avoidant personality disorder and was specifically excluded from the diagnosis of social phobia in the DSM-III, subsequent studies had shown avoidant personality disorder to be quite similar to severe SAD (12). As a result, the generalized subtype was defined under the rubric of SAD and retained in the current DSM-IV criteria. SAD patients with fears limited to fewer than most social interactions, typically performance fears, have been referred to as nongeneralized, specific, circumscribed, or discrete.

Generalized SAD represents about half of the SAD in the community (13) but has comprised the great majority of patients entering research studies and clinical treatment due to its greater severity and resultant functional impairment and distress. Patients with generalized SAD tend to view themselves as severely shy and inhibited in social interactions, and they also fear scrutiny and performance situations. Persons with the generalized subtype tend to have more comorbidity and a more extensive family history of SAD (14). Laboratory investigations suggest that despite experiencing greater anxiety symptoms, fear, and impairment than patients with nongeneralized SAD, patients with the generalized subtype manifest less physiological reactivity (15). It remains debatable, however, whether these differences are best described by a qualitative, categorical distinction or a continuum of severity (16). Some community studies have supported the notion of a continuum based on continuity in number of social situations feared (17).

II. CLINICAL DIAGNOSIS

A. The Diagnostic Interview for SAD

Persons with SAD often present for treatment only after many years of suffering. They may not have recognized their symptoms as a treatable problem due to relative lack of public awareness of SAD and its treatments. The early onset and chronicity of SAD contribute to a tendency to view symptoms as intrinsic personality features rather than a treatable disorder. Finally, the symptoms of shame and social avoidance themselves may contribute to a sense of intense stigma and reluctance to seek treatment.

Signs of social anxiety may be present in the first clinical interactions with the patient. Patients with SAD may avoid eye contact, introduce themselves awkwardly or self-consciously, and offer weak handshakes. Patients may be excessively deferential in conversation and may display nervous mannerisms such as touching their faces or wringing their hands. Initiating a chief complaint or acknowledging symptoms may seem difficult or embarrassing. Other patients may be well related and comfortable, however, in the presence of an accepting and empathic clinician and relieved to be able to unburden themselves of secret fears.

Some patients will present in a crisis related to an impending interview, presentation, or social gathering or related to functional consequences of the illness, such as a lost job or relationship. Often, the patient will not present with the chief complaint of social anxiety, either because the patient has not formulated particular symptoms around that concept, or because associated symptoms—such as fatigue, depression, or loneliness—are most prominent. Somatic complaints, such as sweating, blushing, trembling, or panic attacks, may predominate.

A diagnosis of nongeneralized or discrete social anxiety disorder may appear relatively straightforward if the patient's concerns and functional deficits are related solely to performance-related events. It is important, however, to take a thorough inventory of performance and interpersonal situations around which anxiety and avoidance may occur. A chief complaint of performance anxiety will often grow into a fuller picture of generalized social difficulties upon further investigation. We find it useful also to try to delineate situations in which the patient feels socially comfortable. This can counteract what is sometimes a demoralizing excavation of pathology and helps identify a foundation of social competence upon which treatment can build.

A thorough evaluation of SAD should investigate physical symptoms, cognitions, and avoidance related to feared social situations. Symptoms occurring during, in anticipation of, and in the aftermath of these situations should be considered. The impact of SAD on friendships, romantic relationships, sexual functioning, school or work performance, mood, and substance use should be routinely explored. Similarly, it is essential to determine what areas of social functioning are most important to the patient, so that treatment goals can take into account the patient's goals rather than some generic concept of normal social function.

B. Laboratory Tests and Clinical Rating Scales

Patients presenting with complaints of SAD, particularly if significant physical manifestations are prominent (tremor, sweating, shortness of breath, palpitations, etc.), should receive a thorough physical evaluation to rule out medical conditions that may produce similar symptoms. Depending on the nature of symptoms and treatment under consideration, this may include a physical exam, vital signs, electrocardiogram (ECG), and routine laboratory tests including complete blood count, chemistry panel, liver function tests, and especially thyroid function tests. While SAD has been associated with abnormalities in some neuropsychological tests, measures of serotonin, dopamine, and GABA system functions, and positron emission tomography (PET) and functional magnetic resonance imaging (fMRI) measures of central nervous system (CNS) blood flow, no laboratory tests have proven to be clinically useful to date in positively establishing or confirming a diagnosis (18–21).

   Numerous diagnostic and severity rating scales for social anxiety disorder have been devised over the past three decades. While a detailed discussion of assessment tools appears elsewhere (this volume, chapter by Lipsitz and Liebowitz), a brief summary of some diagnostic instruments is presented here. Due to the self-consciousness inherent in a face-to-face interview for many with SAD, self-report scales may be particularly helpful in eliciting additional information. Rating instruments may supplement but cannot substitute for a careful psychiatric history.

   The Structured Clinical Interview for DSM-IV (SCID) (22) and the Anxiety Disorders Interview Schedule (ADIS) (23) are structured diagnostic interviews commonly employed in research settings to confirm the clinical diagnosis of SAD in a uniform and reproducible manner. Additionally, the Social Phobia and Anxiety Inventory (24) has been used in research to differentiate systematically between panic disorder and SAD. Recently, attempts to quantify severity thresholds for meeting diagnostic criteria have suggested that a total score of over 30 on the Liebowitz Social Anxiety Scale may best identify patients meeting DSM-IV diagnostic criteria for SAD, and a score of over 60 may best identify patients with the generalized subtype (25). A three-item screening tool, the Mini-SPIN, has also been reported to have good sensitivity (88.7%) and specificity (90.0%) for the diagnosis of generalized SAD in a nonclinical sample (26).

C. Differential Diagnosis

SAD includes a broad range of symptoms that frequently overlap with other diagnostic entities. There are several likely reasons for such overlap. One factor is the high prevalence of SAD; moderate social anxiety is a universal human experience, and SAD itself is one of the most common psychiatric disorders. Additionally, SAD and other internalizing disorders may share some common underlying genetic predisposition. Especially given its early age of onset and pervasive quality, SAD may contribute to the development of secondary conditions. Finally, a variety of other physical conditions and most forms of mental illness carry great stigma that can lead to secondary social anxiety.

Frequencies of other psychiatric disorders (primary, secondary, or comorbid) associated with SAD were assessed in the community by the Epidemiologic Catchment Area (ECA) study and include simple phobia (59%), agoraphobia (45%), alcohol abuse (19%), major depression (17%), and abuse of other drugs (13%) (8). Patient samples show similar patterns but tend to have higher rates of comorbidity as well. While comorbid disorders associated with SAD are discussed elsewhere (this volume, chapter by Fehm and Wittchen), this chapter focuses on clinical issues in the differentiation of some of these conditions from primary SAD. A discussion of some of the more common issues in differential diagnoses follows.

1. Generalized Anxiety Disorder

Generalized anxiety disorder (GAD) and SAD share symptoms of excessive, usually chronic, worry that is difficult to control and is often accompanied by physical symptoms. The generalized subtype of SAD may be so pervasive as to appear to encompass most aspects of daily life. The key to differentiating between GAD and SAD diagnoses is to determine carefully whether other sources of anxiety for the patient have a social component. For example, a patient who also reports anxiety over accomplishing certain tasks may reveal fear of negative judgment as the motivating factor for the anxiety. A diagnosis of GAD should be considered only if the patient has excessive worry about a number of events and the focus of the anxiety is not confined to fears related to embarrassment or humiliation. These nonsocial worries may include concerns about work or school, the welfare of oneself or family or friends, finances, etc., which may have social connotations; however, the anxiety is not predominantly focused on the social aspects of these concerns.

GAD also commonly occurs comorbidly with social anxiety disorder (8). Undetected comorbid GAD may complicate treatment of SAD, particularly if the treatment is specifically directed only to social anxiety symptoms (e.g., in some forms of behavioral or cognitive-behavioral treatment) or is known to be effective only for one of the disorders (e.g., pharmacotherapy with monoamine oxidase inhibitors for SAD) (27).

2.   Panic Disorder With/Without Agoraphobia

Panic disorder, especially with agoraphobia, may resemble SAD or present comorbidly with it. Physical symptoms of panic—including palpitations, hyperhydrosis, dyspnea, tremor, dizziness or light-headedness, or a sense of being trapped—may accompany SAD when induced by a highly feared social situation (28–30). Subjects with SAD may avoid certain situations also avoided by agoraphobic subjects, such as crowds or gatherings. Additionally, patients with panic disorder may develop a significant social anxiety component secondary to fear of being embarrassed should a panic attack occur in public.

Aspects of panic disorder not present in SAD include spontaneous or nocturnal attacks (i.e., attacks not cued by feared stimuli). These patients are more likely to experience fears of impending doom, death, or losing control during an attack. They are also more likely to experience certain physical symptoms, including chest pain and blurry vision. In SAD, physical symptoms such as blushing and muscular twitching are more highly characteristic (28). And, as always, anxiety associated with SAD is uniformly associated with fear of humiliation or embarrassment, whereas panic and anxiety attacks in panic disorder may occur with a wide variety of stimuli or with no apparent stimulus at all.

It is therefore clinically important in evaluating a patient with panic attacks to determine whether such attacks are limited to situations associated with fear of embarrassment. A panic disorder patient, for example, will report fear of riding the train because it is a confined space where help will not be readily available in the event of a panic attack. The panic patient likely would feel worse in an empty train and better if accompanied by a trusted companion. A patient with SAD, on the other hand, will fear primarily feelings of self-consciousness, embarrassment, and negative evaluation by others. An empty train would be preferable to such an individual, and being accompanied by a companion is unlikely to provide the same relief as it might for the panic patient. Panic disorder is more likely than SAD to have an episodic course, and the disorders are differentially responsive to some forms of treatment (e.g., specific cognitive-behavioral techniques for each, tricyclic antidepressant activity in panic disorder but not SAD) (31).

3.   Major Depression and Dysthymia

The diagnostic evaluation of depressive symptomatology in a patient with apparent SAD is sometimes challenging. Social avoidance may occur secondary to fears of embarrassment in SAD or secondary to the social disinterest or anhedonia of major depression. Atypical depression in particular, with its characteristic interpersonal rejection sensitivity, often overlaps with SAD symptoms of fear of embarrassment and related forms of negative evaluation (12,32). On the other hand, depression may result from the social isolation and functional impairment that are sequelae of primary social anxiety. Sometimes chronic social anxiety is accompanied by chronic low-level depressive symptoms bordering on dysthymia, and major depression and SAD may also be comorbid conditions (this volume, chapter by Fehm and Wittchen). Distinguishing between these possibilities may have a significant impact on treatment strategies.

As with other diagnostic dilemmas, the character and chronology of symptoms are key factors. It is important to determine the relative onset of symptoms associated social anxiety and depression. SAD, unlike depression, generally does not involve significant mood or neurovegetative symptoms such as sadness or crying, sleep or appetite disturbance, low energy, or anhedonia, although demoralization may follow an extended period of social dysfunction as a result of SAD. Social avoidance in depression is usually due to low energy, disinterest, or anticipated insults to self-esteem due to rejection sensitivity. In contrast, patients with primary social anxiety generally desire and might expect to enjoy contact with others but are inhibited specifically by fear of scrutiny or judgment by others.

Depression secondary to SAD represents a comorbid condition that must be fully evaluated, complete with assessment of suicidality, and specifically treated. Generalized SAD, with its characteristic earlier onset, has been shown to increase the risk of development of major depression, with an odds ratio of 3.5 in a prospective community study (33). Similarly, in clinical samples, more than 25% of depressed patients have been found to have a comorbid diagnosis of SAD (34). While SAD occurs first in most comorbid cases, SAD occurring secondary to major depressive disorder (MDD) may be associated with seasonal features of MDD (35).

4. Eating Disorders

Fear of eating in public is a symptom mentioned in the diagnostic criteria for both SAD and eating disorders. Social anxiety symptoms may also occur secondary to a primary eating disorder, and both disorders frequently co-occur in the same patients. In order to evaluate eating fears, the specific characteristics of the behavior and its motivation must be considered. In eating disorders, the primary concern is body image, and the fear of scrutiny or judgment is related particularly to the concern that others will judge the individual to be overeating or overweight. In addition, patients with eating disorder often develop peculiar eating patterns or rituals that may draw attention and lead to embarrassment. In SAD, however, the focus of the anxiety is not on the results of eating or on unusual aspects of eating behavior. Patients with SAD may fear that others will notice them trembling, spilling food, or chewing, resulting in negative evaluation from others, or they may simply report anxiety over the scrutiny, possibly related to the perceived intimate nature of the act of eating.

While in SAD fear of eating is relatively uncommon and is usually just one of a broader range of social fears, eating disorder patients may report few if any other social concerns. Many eating disorder patients, however, do report social fears beyond the realm of eating, consistent with the considerable comorbidity between anorexia/bulimia and SAD. In one sample, a majority (55 to 59%) of patients with eating disorder met criteria for SAD as a comorbid diagnosis (36). In over 75% of these subjects, social anxiety symptoms predated the eating disorder. Treatment of eating disorders with comorbid generalized SAD may need to target not only cognitive and behavioral aspects of the food/weight/body image issues but also general social anxiety as well. While selective serotonin reuptake inhibitors (SSRIs) have emerged as a first-line treatment in SAD, they have not proved to be especially efficacious in the treatment of eating disorders (37).

5. Body Dysmorphic Disorder

In body dysmorphic disorder (BDD), preoccupation with a perceived physical defect or excessive concern over a slight physical anomaly frequently leads to social avoidance and considerable anxiety in social situations; however, this preoccupation may also occur without a focus on embarrassment. Patients with SAD are typically concerned about others judging their behaviors rather than perceived physical anomalies. Clearly, however, symptoms sometimes may overlap. Two studies have shown that 20 to 50% of BDD patients to have comorbid SAD (38,39).

6. Substance Abuse and Dependence

While substance abuse issues should be considered in the diagnosis of any psychiatric disorder, substance abuse may be particularly confounding in SAD. For the purposes of differential diagnosis, it is important to consider whether symptoms of social anxiety, particularly social withdrawal and avoidance, might be secondary to a primary substance abuse problem. Alcohol, marijuana, opioids, and sedatives can be associated with social withdrawal, and a patient may complain of discomfort in social situations without necessarily relating this to substance abuse patterns.

Substance abuse also occurs comorbidly with SAD, and the relationship between the disorders may be quite complex. Preexisting social anxiety has been shown to predispose to substance abuse and/or dependence, often in an attempt at self-medication (40). Occasionally, a person with severe SAD will discover that alcohol or other substances may provide dramatic initial relief of symptoms, leading to patterns of drinking (or using) before attending social gatherings or even prior to public speaking. This relief is seldom persistent, but secondary substance abuse and dependence may continue even in the absence of social stressors. Conversely, substance abuse and dependence can lead to secondary shame and guilt, leading to self-consciousness and anxiety in social situations. Popular group treatment modalities, such as Alcoholics Anonymous, may present special difficulties for persons with primary SAD, who are especially uncomfortable speaking in groups. Nevertheless, ongoing substance abuse is very likely to interfere with efforts to treat SAD and often requires specific intervention.

7. Schizophrenia and Associated Conditions

Fear and anxiety in social situations, and social withdrawal or avoidance, are features common to a number of psychotic conditions. Paranoia, whether part of overt psychosis or of Cluster A personality disorders, is usually easily distinguished from SAD, in that the paranoid individual is concerned more with fear of harm than with embarrassment or shame. Excessive fear of judgment by others may be common to both, but in SAD there is a recognition that the fear is excessive, unreasonable, or unrealistic. Fears may be overvalued in SAD, but they do not take on the quality of fixed delusions. In schizophrenia, social withdrawal may also present as a result of disturbing auditory or visual hallucinations, other anxiety-provoking delusions, or negative symptoms such as flatness of affect or social disengagement. Schizotypal personality disorder presents with bizarre beliefs or behaviors in addition to social anxiety. Social anxiety in schizotypal and paranoid patients tends to be accompanied by mistrust and does not diminish with familiarity.

Of greater concern is prodromal, or premorbid, psychosis. Social withdrawal is a hallmark of the earliest stages of schizophrenia and related disorders (41). Especially in younger patients or in patients who are brought in by family or friends for decreased social function, a careful assessment should be undertaken to determine the cause of the avoidant behavior. Again, disinterest, lack of desire for contact, and failure either to recognize the behavior or to complain of the consequences of social isolation would suggest a diagnosis other than SAD. SAD also has been suggested as a risk factor for the later onset of schizophrenia (42); however, this may reflect limitations in distinguishing premorbid decline in social function from social phobic symptoms and requires further analysis. Only a small minority of SAD cases deteriorate in such a fashion.

8. Childhood and Developmental Disorders

The nomenclature for childhood anxiety disorders was revised in the DSM-IV to better align these conditions with corresponding adult disorders. The childhood anxiety disorders historically have been considered relatively difficult to assess, however, and may be less clearly differentiated from each other than the adult syndromes (43). Children with separation anxiety differ in being comforted by the presence of a familiar adult or when in a familiar environment, whereas in SAD, feared situations are more likely to generate symptoms regardless of the venue or the presence of known and trusted supports.

Pervasive developmental disorders (PDDs) such as autism and Asperger's disorder are present from an early age, result in significant social dysfunction, and generally persist into adulthood. In these patients, however, normal social function is rarely established. The presence of numerous additional and often striking abnormalities of behavior or function, such as repetitive patterns of interests in Asperger's disorder or delays in acquisition of language skills in autism, aid in making the differential diagnosis. Where these are subtle, however, the clinician can distinguish the disorders based on the character of the social impairment. In PDDs, social interaction is limited by lack of interest, lack of skills, or lack of ability to appreciate reciprocity as opposed to intense fear of scrutiny or embarrassment.

9. Personality Disorders

As discussed above and elsewhere (this volume, chapter by Muller, Koen, and Stein), SAD, especially in the generalized form with its early onset and pervasive quality, has many characteristics of a personality trait or disorder. A social anxiety spectrum may be defined by a continuum with mild trait social anxiety or shyness at one end and extreme avoidant personality disorder at the other (16). Diagnostic criteria for avoidant personality disorder closely resemble those of SAD, patients with more severe forms of generalized SAD are more likely to meet criteria for avoidant personality disorder, and comparisons of SAD with and without avoidant personality disorder have suggested that group differences are mainly a matter of severity.

Other personality disorders (PDs), such as dependent and narcissistic personality disorders, share certain features with SAD as well (44). In dependent PD, low self-esteem and associated self-doubt may lead to self-consciousness and sensitivity to criticism. Social contacts may be limited to a few trusted individuals upon whom the patient relies. Individuals with narcissistic personality disorder, particularly those with predominantly low self-esteem and vulnerability to criticism, may also display characteristics of social anxiety disorder. Extreme sensitivity to negative evaluation and fear of humiliation may lead to social withdrawal, depressed mood, fractured interpersonal relationships, and impaired functioning. Cluster A personality disorders, as discussed above, may lead to social withdrawal due to lack of interest (particularly in schizoid PD), excessive social anxiety (in schizotypal PD), or paranoia (any Cluster A PD). In schizoid PD, however, social avoidance is accompanied by indifference to criticism or praise.

10. General Medical Conditions

A number of physical disorders may produce symptoms that mimic the physical or even psychological symptoms of SAD. One such common condition is hyperthyroidism, and thyroid function tests should be considered in any patient presenting with anxiety or panic symptoms. Excessive sweating may be due to primary hyperhydrosis; neurological causes of tremor include essential tremor and Parkinson's disease; and speech hesitancy may be due to stuttering. In addition to disorders that mimic anxiety symptoms (see above), medical disorders such as skin conditions, obesity, and strabismus may lead to secondary social anxiety (12), depending on the severity of the symptoms and the individual's predisposition toward embarrassment and social anxiety (45).

According to DSM-IV decision rules, a diagnosis of SAD is not made when social anxiety is directly related to a general medical condition. In practice, however, cause and effect in respect to physical symptom and anxiety are often difficult to disentangle, although it can be useful to inquire about severity of social anxiety unrelated to the medical condition (e.g., fears of telephoning strangers in a patient with essential tremor). Consultation with the clinician treating the general medical condition may help determine if the patient's social anxiety seems out of proportion to the severity of the physical condition. In treating social anxiety in this population, attention should first be given to the underlying medical condition and associated symptoms; however, concurrent psychotherapy and/or pharmacotherapy targeting the secondary social anxiety may well be beneficial.

III. SUMMARY

In summary, SAD is a common disorder, characterized by excessive fear and avoidance of embarrassment in social and performance situations. The generalized subtype is diagnosed when fear of most social situations is present. A variety of physical, cognitive, and behavioral symptoms may occur, and the disorder often encompasses anticipatory anxiety, anxiety, or panic symptoms in the feared situation and subsequent self-criticism and demoralization. A careful evaluation should investigate each of these realms of symptomatology and consider common comorbid conditions, including depression, substance abuse, and other anxiety disorders.

REFERENCES

1. American Psychiatric Association. Diagnostic and Statistical Manual of Mental Disorders (DSM-III). 3d ed. Washington, DC: APA, 1980.
2. Janet P. Les obsessions et la psychasthénie. Paris: F. Alcan, 1903.
3. American Psychiatric Association. Diagnostic and Statistical Manual of Mental Disorders (DSM-I). 1st ed. Washington, DC: APA, 1952.
4. American Psychiatric Association. Diagnostic and Statistical Manual of Mental Disorders (DSM-II). 2d ed text rev. Washington, DC: APA, 1968.
5. Marks IM, Gelder MG. Different ages of onset in varieties of phobia. Am J Psychiatry 1966; 123:218–221.
6. American Psychiatric Association. Diagnostic and Statistical Manual of Mental Disorders (DSM-III-R). 3d ed rev. Washington, DC: APA, 1987.
7. American Psychiatric Association. Diagnostic and Statistical Manual of Mental Disorders (DSM-IV-TR). 4th ed text rev. Washington, DC: APA, 2000.
8. Schneier FR, Johnson J, Hornig CD, Liebowitz MR, Weissman M. Social phobia: comorbidity and morbidity in an epidemiologic sample. Arch Gen Psychiatry 1992; 49:282–288.
9. Holt CS, Heimberg RG, Hope DA, Liebowitz MR. Situational domains of social phobia. J Anxiety Disord 1992; 6:63–77.
10. Fahlén T. Core symptom pattern of social phobia. Depression Anxiety 1996–1997; 4:223–232.
11. World Health Organization. The International Classification of Diseases and Related Health Problems (ICD-10). 10th ed. Geneva: WHO, Division of Mental Health, 1992.
12. Liebowitz MR, Gorman JM, Fyer AJ, Klein AF. Social phobia: review of a neglected anxiety disorder. Arch Gen Psychiatry 1985; 42:729–736.
13. Kessler RC, McGonagle KA, Zhao S, Nelson CB, Hughes M, Eshelman S, Wittchen H, Kendler KS. Lifetime and 12-month prevalence of DSM-III-R psychiatric disorders in the United States. Arch Gen Psychiatry 1994; 51:8–19.
14. Mannuzza S, Schneier FR, Chapman TF, Liebowitz MR, Klein DF, Fyer AJ. Generalized social phobia: reliability and validity. Arch Gen Psychiatry 1995; 52:230–237.
15. Hoffman SG, Newman MG, Ehlers A, Roth WT. Psychophysiological differences between subgroups of social phobia. J Abnorm Psychol 1995; 104:224–231.
16. Schneier FR, Blanco C, Antia SX, Liebowitz MR. The social anxiety spectrum. Psychiatr Clin North Am 2000; 25:757–774.
17. Stein MB, Torgrud LJ, Walker JR. Social phobia symptoms, subtypes, and severity: findings from a community survey. Arch Gen Psychiatry 2000; 57:1046–1052.

18. Amundson GJ, Stein MB, Larsen DK, Walker JR. Neurocognitive function in panic disorder and social phobia patients. Anxiety 1994–1995; 1:201–207.
19. Stein DJ, Westenberg HG, Liebowitz MR. Social anxiety disorder and generalized anxiety disorder: serotonergic and dopaminergic neurocircuitry. J Clin Psychiatry 2002; 63(suppl 6):12–19.
20. Jefferson JW. Benzodiazepines and anticonvulsants for social phobia (social anxiety disorder). J Clin Psychiatry 2001; 62(suppl 1):50–53.
21. Tillfors M, Furmark T, Marteinsdottir I, Fischer H, Pissiota A, Langstrom B, Frederikson M. Cerebral blood flow in subjects with social phobia during stressful speaking tasks: a PET study. Am J Psychiatry 2001; 158:1220–1226.
22. First M, Spitzer RL, Williams JBW, Gibbon M. Structured Clinical Interview for DSM-IV—Patient edition. Washington, DC: American Psychiatric Press, 1995.
23. DiNardo PA, Barlow DH. Anxiety Disorders Interview Schedule—Revised. Albany NY: Graywind Publications, 1988.
24. Beidel DC, Borden JW, Turner SM, Jacob RG. The Social Phobia and Anxiety Inventory: concurrent validity with a clinical sample. Behav Res Therapy 1989; 27:573–576.
25. Mennin DS, Fresco DM, Heimberg RG, Schneier FR, Davies SO, Liebowitz MR. Screening for social anxiety disorder in the clinical setting: using the Liebowitz Social Anxiety Scale. J Anxiety Disord 2002; 16:661–673.
26. Connor KM, Kobak KA, Churchill LE, Katzelnick D, Davidson JR. Mini-SPIN: A brief screening assessment for generalized social anxiety disorder. Depression Anxiety 2001; 14:137–140.
27. Blanco C, Antia SX, Liebowitz MR. Pharmacotherapy of social anxiety disorder. Biol Psychiatry 2002, 51:109–120.
28. Amies PL, Gelder MG, Shaw PM. Social phobia: a comparative clinical study. Br J Psychiatry 1983; 142:174–179.
29. Cameron O, Thyer B, Nesse R, Curtis G. Symptom profiles of patients with DSM-III anxiety disorders. Am J Psychiatry 1983; 143:1132–1137.
30. Reich J, Noyes R, Yates W. Anxiety symptoms distinguishing social phobia from panic and generalized anxiety disorders. J Nerv Mental Dis 1988; 176: 510–513.
31. Stein MB. Medication treatments for panic disorder and social phobia. Depression Anxiety 1998; 7:134–138.
32. Schneier FR, Blanco C, Campeas R, Lewis-Fernandez R, Lin S-H, Marshall R, Schmidt AB, Sanchez-Lacay JA, Simpson HB, Liebowitz MR. Citalopram treatment of social anxiety disorder and comorbid major depression. Depression Anxiety 2003; 17:191–196.
33. Stein MB, Feutsch M, Muller N. Social anxiety disorder and the risk of depression: a prospective community study of adolescents and young adults. Arch Gen Psychiatry 2001; 58:251–256.
34. Fava M, Rankin MA, Wright EC, Alpert JE, Nierenberg AA, Pava J, Rosenbaum JF. Anxiety disorders in major depression. Compr Psychiatry 2000; 41:97–102.

35. Dilsaver SC, Qamar AB, DelMedico VJ. Secondary social phobia in patients with major depression. Psychiatry Res 1992; 44:33–40.
36. Godart NT, Flament MF, Lecrubier Y, Jeammet P. Anxiety disorders in anorexia nervosa and bulimia nervosa: co-morbidity and chronology of appearance. Eur Psychiatry 2000; 15:38–45.
37. Mayer LE, Walsh BT. The use of selective serotonin reuptake inhibitors in eating disorders. J Clin Psychiatry 1998; 59(suppl 15):28–34.
38. Phillips KA, McElroy SL, Keck PE Jr, Pope HG Jr, Hudson JI. Body dysmorphic disorder: 30 cases of imagined ugliness. Am J Psychiatry 1993; 150:302–308.
39. Altamura C, Paluello MM, Mundo E, Medda S, Mannu P. Clinical and subclinical body dysmorphic disorder. Eur Arch Psychiatry Clin Neurosci 2001; 251:105–108.
40. Randall CL, Thomas S, Thevos AK. Concurrent alcoholism and social anxiety disorder: a first step toward developing effective treatments. Alcohol Clin Exp Res 2001; 25:210–220.
41. Kwapil TR. Social anhedonia as a predictor of the development of schizophrenia-spectrum disorders. J Abnorm Psychol 1998; 107:558–565.
42. Tien AY, Eaton WW. Psychopathologic precursors and sociodemographic risk factors for the schizophrenia syndrome. Arch Gen Psychiatry 1992; 49:37–46.
43. Greenhill L, Pine D, March J, Birmaher B, Riddle M. Assessment issues in treatment research of pediatric anxiety disorders: what is working, what is not working, what is missing, and what needs improvement. Psychopharm Bull 1998; 34:155–164.
44. Fahlén T. Personality traits in social phobia, I: comparison with healthy controls. J Clin Psychiatry 1995; 56:560–568.
45. Oberlander EL, Schneier FR, Liebowitz MR. Physical disability and social phobia. J Clin Psychopharmacol 1994; 14:136–143.

2

The Spectrum of Social Anxiety Disorders

**Jacqueline E. Muller, Liezl Koen,
and Dan J. Stein***
University of Stellenbosch,
Cape Town, South Africa

I. INTRODUCTION

The reliance of current psychiatric nomenclatures on categorical constructs has certainly contributed to the reliability of psychiatric diagnosis. Nevertheless, given that the phenomenology of psychiatric disorders and symptoms often appears continuous, it is also necessary to consider whether dimensional approaches can increase the validity of nosological constructs. The notion of spectrum disorders has received increasing attention in the literature (1,2) and may also prove useful in understanding social anxiety disorders (SAD) and symptoms.

Several approaches to a putative spectrum of social anxiety can be considered. Some researchers have proposed that SAD lies on a spectrum of social discomfort, with shyness representing a nonpathological form but then progressing on to discrete SAD, generalized SAD, and ultimately to avoidant personality disorder (APD) as an extreme form of social discomfort (3,4). There may also be overlaps between SAD and a range of conditions characterized by social fears related to body image concerns, including body dysmorphic disorder (5), olfactory reference syndrome (6),

---

*Also affiliated with University of Florida, Gainesville.

and taijin kyofusho (7). Another approach is the proposed social anxiety/
deficit spectrum, where SAD is placed on a spectrum with disorders (e.g.,
Asperger's syndrome) characterized by deficits in social interaction (8). Core
SAD components such as anxiety, fear of negative evaluation, and avoidant
behavior (each of which possibly has distinctive neurobiological underpinnings) may prove valuable when considering different approaches to the
spectrum of social anxiety symptoms (2).

In this chapter we explore various approaches to defining the spectrum
of social anxiety disorders and symptoms.

II. SPECTRUM OF SOCIAL DISCOMFORT

There is increasing interest in exploring the boundaries between SAD and
constructs from the literature on temperament and personality. Stein and
Chavira propose a spectrum (Fig. 1) of social discomfort with shyness at one
end (transitory with low levels of interference and avoidance) and APD at
the other (more chronic with high interference and avoidance) (3,4). However, questions remain as to the exact relationship between shyness and
SAD and the threshold of symptoms and functional impairment needed to
make a diagnosis of SAD.

A. Shyness

Both shyness and SAD may be characterized by fears of negative social
evaluation, social skills deficits, avoidant behavior (9), and physiological
symptoms of anxiety in social situations (4,10). However, although the majority of people experience periods of shyness (with nearly 90% of individuals
self-reporting feeling shy at some time in their lives), only a minority suffer
from SAD (11,12).

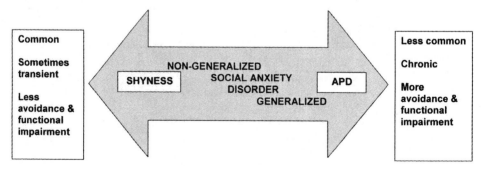

FIGURE 1   Spectrum of social discomfort (based on Refs. 3 and 4).

It has been suggested that social anxiety is necessary for survival and has been evolutionarily selected in a number of animal species, particularly humans. A curvilinear relationship between the level of arousal (anxiety) and efficiency of performance (as described by the Yerkes-Dodson curve) suggests that some anticipation and anxiety enhances performance but that at a certain level of arousal performance starts to decline, leading to functional impairment (13). Indeed, though some performance anxiety and shyness is common in normal individuals, it is usually short-lived, with little functional impairment and avoidant behavior when compared to SAD (14).

To clarify the relationship between shyness and SAD, a study of the rates of SAD in individuals scoring above the 90th percentile on a shyness scale (highly shy) and those scoring within the 40th to 60th percentiles (normatively shy) was undertaken (10). In the highly shy group, approximately 49% of subjects were diagnosed with SAD, with significantly higher rates of generalized SAD (36%) and APD (14%) compared to the normatively shy group (with 18% SAD, 4% generalized SAD, and 4% APD). Results also suggested that high shyness is more associated with interactional fears (as in generalized SAD) than performance fears (as frequently seen in nongeneralized SAD). Moreover, highly shy individuals with SAD were more functionally impaired than those who did not meet criteria for this disorder. The authors concluded that shyness and SAD seem to be related constructs but that they are not synonymous, and an individual can be extremely shy without suffering from SAD.

A developmental perspective sheds further light on the construct of shyness. The emergence of a fear of strangers in infants from around 7 to 10 months old seems to be common (15), although this usually diminishes with time. However, behavioral inhibition, defined as a consistent tendency to withdraw and display fear in unfamiliar situations, appears to be an important predictor of later SAD and other anxiety disorders (16). Indeed, there is growing evidence of some similarities in the neurobiology of behavioral disinhibition and SAD: hemispheric asymmetry on electroencephalographic (EEG) measures has been demonstrated in both behaviorally inhibited children and adults with SAD (17), and there is evidence that on follow-up in adulthood, people with childhood behavioral inhibition show increased activation of the amygdala in response to unfamiliar faces (18).

Selective mutism may represent another form of severe social anxiety in children (19–21), the possibility being that children with this condition are avoiding social interaction by withholding speech (20). Studies have shown that almost 100% of children with selective mutism meet the criteria for SAD (22), and high rates of SAD (70%) are found in their first-degree relatives (19). Small open trials have indicated that children with selective mutism may respond to treatment with phenelzine or selective serotonin re-uptake inhibitors (SSRIs) (22,23), supporting the overlap with SAD. Rather than being a separate disorder, selective mutism may thus be conceptualized as the severe end of a spectrum of social anxiety and speech inhibition in children (20).

B. Social Anxiety Disorder (SAD)

If SAD lies on a spectrum of shyness and social fears, then the question arises as to the optimal threshold of symptoms, distress, and functional impairment required to warrant a diagnosis of SAD. Altering the diagnostic threshold of SAD had a significant impact on reported prevalence, with rates of 18.7% if patients with "moderate interference or distress" are included, compared to only 1.9% prevalence for those reporting "marked interference" (24). When Davidson et al. compared healthy nonanxious controls to individuals with subthreshold social anxiety, the subthreshold group was more impaired regarding level of education, income, school and work performance, social support, and reported more chronic medical problems, mental health visits, use of psychotropic drugs and negative life events (25). Similarly, findings from a community survey supported that SAD seems to exist on a continuum of severity and that patients admitting to a greater number of feared situations suffered more disability (26).

Conversely, if SAD lies on a spectrum of shyness and social fears, then within SAD, it may be possible to delineate subtypes characterized by differences in severity of such symptoms. Two subtypes of SAD have been defined by the fourth edition of the *Diagnostic and Statistical Manual of Mental Disorders* (DSM-IV), nongeneralized and generalized (27). Nongeneralized SAD, also called discrete or specific SAD, is limited to specific social situations such as public speaking or performance, whereas generalized SAD is associated with a wide range of social interactions. Epidemiological and clinical data supports this distinction; with generalized SAD being the most common (approximately 75%) and most severe form of SAD (28). Compared to nongeneralized SAD, generalized SAD has been associated with an earlier onset, more fears of social interaction, a family history of SAD or other anxiety disorders, a higher incidence of comorbidity (especially atypical depression and alcohol abuse disorders), greater functional impairment, and a more persistent course (3,28,29). Furthermore, in a clinical sample of individuals with SAD, three patient subgroups were identified based on their pattern of feared social situations (pervasive social anxiety, moderate social interaction anxiety, dominant public speaking anxiety). With significant subgroup differences in both age and age of onset of SAD, depressive symptomatology, general anxiety, and measures of social anxiety, this adds to growing support for the idea of a spectrum of social fears within SAD (30).

The idea that social anxiety should be conceived of as a dimensional construct rather than a unitary category is arguably supported by family, twin, and adoption studies showing that the etiology of SAD is multifactorial, with genetic and environmental variables contributing to its emergence (31–33). Although it is true that single gene disorders such as fragile X syndrome (resulting from a mutation in the FMRI gene that causes a fragile site on the X chromosome) can be associated with increased social anxiety (34,35) and SAD (36), multiple factors may be at play in the vast majority of SAD cases, contributing to its multidimensional character.

C. Avoidant Personality Disorder (APD)

APD was introduced in DSM-III, which required all five criteria to be fulfilled in order to make a diagnosis and ruled that in the presence of this axis II disorder, SAD could not be diagnosed (37). Furthermore DSM-III stated that APD was apparently common but that it could be complicated by the development of SAD. In subsequent revisions, however, there has been increasing overlap between APD and SAD, with DSM-IV raising the possibility that SAD and APD are the same entity (with APD being more severe). Indeed, most patients with APD also meet the criteria for generalized SAD (38). Six of the seven DSM-IV criteria for APD address social interaction, and the DSM-IV manual prompts the clinician to consider an additional diagnosis of APD in individuals with generalized SAD (27).

Lifetime prevalence rates of APD of between 1.1 and 1.3% (39) have been reported, in comparison to the 13.3% of SAD (28). Compared to those with SAD alone, individuals diagnosed with both SAD and APD have been shown to be more functionally impaired, to have higher rates of comorbidity, and to experience more severe anxiety (40,41). Many authors have therefore suggested that the generalized subtypes of SAD and APD are best understood as similar phenomena but falling along a continuum of severity (3,4,42). The difficulty in separating SAD and APD is particularly acute given that the onset of SAD symptoms typically occurs in early adolescence and the course tends to be enduring, thereby sharing certain features with personality disorders (21). SAD symptoms may therefore take on a trait-like quality, resulting in difficulty distinguishing between state and trait (43).

Family studies have shown that patients with both SAD and APD have more first-degree relatives with SAD (33), although a high incidence of APD has also been shown in individuals with panic disorder (44). In samples of patients with SAD and comorbid APD, both cognitive-behavioral therapy and pharmacotherapy resulted in such a significant reduction of the number of positive diagnostic criteria that, after treatment, patients ceased to meet the criteria of APD (45–47). Such findings support the idea that

APD should be conceptualized as a more severe form of generalized SAD (42), representing a quantitative rather than a qualitative variant (21,43).

In conclusion, a range of data supports the concept of a continuum between shyness, nongeneralized SAD, generalized SAD, and APD (2–4, 9,29,43). Although there is a range of work on the phenomenology of this spectrum, understanding of the underlying psychobiology remains at a preliminary stage. Nevertheless, given rapid advances in this field, we can expect better delineation of this putative spectrum of social discomfort, including more precise neurobiological validation in the future (12).

III. SPECTRUM OF SOCIAL FEARS RELATED TO BODY IMAGE CONCERNS

Social fears often arise in relation to body image concerns. Although concern with body image is normal, particularly at certain life stages (e.g., adolescence), a number of psychiatric conditions may lie on this particular spectrum of social fears (Fig. 2).

Body dysmorphic disorder (BDD) is classified as a somatoform disorder in DSM-IV and is characterized by a preoccupation with an imagined or slight defect in physical appearance (27). Social avoidance can stem from

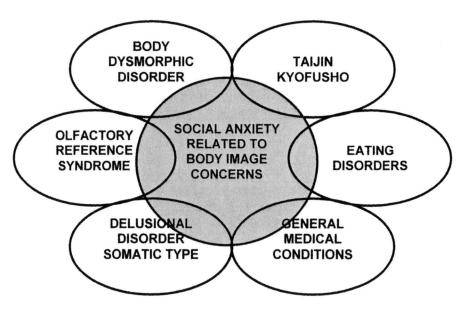

FIGURE 2 Spectrum of body image–related social concerns.

concerns over perceived ugliness (5), and it has been noted that patients with BDD may develop comorbid SAD secondary to preoccupations with physical appearance (48). According to DSM-IV, in BDD the focus lies in an awareness of body image that may result in negative social evaluation rather than their performance in a social situation (42,49). Nevertheless, there are also patients where BDD symptoms seem to lead to awareness of social evaluation and of social performance in equal measure.

Some studies have found BDD to be the fourth most common comorbid disorder in SAD, with prevalence rates between 10 to 11% compared to 1% in patients without SAD (48). Increased rates of SAD (20%) and a family history of SAD were found in a sample of patients diagnosed with BDD, although SAD was less prevalent in this group than obsessive-compulsive disorder (OCD), eating disorders, and somatoform disorders (50). A relatively high rate (57%) of personality disorders has also been reported in subjects with BDD, of which APD was most common (5). Furthermore, there is growing evidence that behavioral techniques (exposure) and classes of medication (SSRIs) useful in SAD are also useful in BDD (51,52). These comorbidity and treatment findings support the suggested phenomenological overlap between SAD and BDD.

Olfactory reference syndrome (ORS) is characterized by a persistent preoccupation with imagined body odor (including halitosis) that persists despite reassurance (53). Symptoms often include marked shame, distress, avoidant behavior, and social isolation, with the degree of insight varying. In ORS, social distress and avoidance result primarily from fears of rejection and humiliation due to a perceived offensive body odor and not anxiety caused by social interaction, as seen in SAD. ORS also does not meet DSM-IV BDD criteria, as the preoccupation is with body odor rather than a defect in appearance. Indeed, the fact the ORS does not quite fit any particular DSM-IV disorder arguably emphasizes the relative failure of this categorical system to recognize the various dimensions of social anxiety. Nevertheless, case reports support the idea that treatments useful in SAD are also effective in ORS (6).

A significant overlap has been described between SAD and taijin kyofusho (TKS) (literally, fear of personal relations), a condition primarily described in the East. Individuals with TKS believe they offend others by their gaze, body odor, and/or imagined ugliness, leading to marked distress, interpersonal sensitivity, and avoidance of social situations. Suggestions have therefore been made that TKS may be best conceptualized as a form of SAD, with the emphasis of the social fears reflecting cultural concerns (in TKS the fear is of offending others, whereas in SAD the fear is of embarrassing oneself) (7,54). Interestingly, SAD patients at times also admit concerns about offending others. TKS has been shown to respond to clomipramine and fluvoxamine (54,55), and some patients with TKS symptoms treated in Western settings improved on monoamine oxidase inhibitors (MAOIs) (56).

An understanding of the universal and local features of social anxiety is clearly important in our increasingly multicultural world (7,57). In Western societies, fear of maintaining gaze may be a symptom of social anxiety, whereas in Eastern and African cultures gaze aversion is often considered polite. Similarly, timidity may be a symptom of SAD but may be viewed as a positive attribute, perhaps particularly in women, in certain cultures (7). Such considerations must be borne in mind during the clinical assessment of patients from nonfamiliar cultures. Better appreciation of the sociocultural mechanisms that underlie such differences may also lead to a more thorough understanding of the spectrum of social fears, including those relating to body image.

Cultural pressures have also been implicated as a risk factor for the development of eating disorders, and body image disturbances in these disorders may also contribute to social fears (58). Both anorexia nervosa and bulimia nervosa are disorders involving a preoccupation with body image, with self-evaluation being overly influenced by body shape and weight (27). These patients commonly have comorbid SAD, with the onset of SAD reported first in more than 75% of subjects (59). However, if the fear in social/performance situations is primarily related to preoccupation with body shape and weight, DSM-IV specifically prohibits the diagnosis of SAD.

General medical conditions leading to disfigurement or visible physical symptoms may also result in fears of negative evaluation and social avoidance, resembling SAD (49). In patients with Parkinson's disease, awareness of physical symptoms such as tremors may contribute to SAD, although the shared dopamine hypoactivity found in both disorders may also play a role in accounting for this comorbidity (60). Interestingly, in a clinical case series of individuals suffering from severe social anxiety symptoms secondary to disfiguring or disabling medical conditions, all had good response to MAOIs (61). Again, it is possible to question the utility of some features of the DSM-IV SAD criteria, which specifically exclude the diagnosis of SAD if the patient's fear or embarrassment is generated by the presence of symptoms caused by a medical condition (e.g., stuttering). A more dimensional approach to the spectrum of disorders characterized by social fear in relation to body image may be useful (21).

Delusional disorder of the somatic type may be viewed as an extreme end of the spectrum of social fears in relation to body image. In such cases, there are fixed false beliefs of having a physical defect. Nevertheless, the boundary between this condition and BDD without insight is not always clear, and it is worth noting that the latter category of patients responds to SSRIs without necessarily requiring antipsychotics (5). In this context it is perhaps worth noting that some types of TKS are characterized by a loss of insight (62). Perhaps further investigation is needed to determine whether there is also a category of Western SAD with poor insight (7).

IV. SPECTRUM OF ANXIETY/MOOD DISORDERS

DSM-IV characterizes SAD as an anxiety disorder (27). Certainly there are phenomenological and psychobiological overlaps between SAD and other disorders characterized by anxiety and harm avoidance (49). Furthermore, Hudson and Pope put forward the idea of a broad spectrum of affective disorders, noting phenomenological and psychobiological overlaps between a range of mood, anxiety, somatoform, and other psychiatric disorders, one of which would be SAD (63).

A lumping perspective is supported by evidence on comorbidity. The Epidemiological Catchment Area (ECA) study demonstrated psychiatric comorbidity lifetime rates of 69% in individuals with SAD. In 76.8% of subjects it occurred first and in 7.2% of subjects in the same year as another psychiatric disorder (64). The National Comorbidity Survey (NCS) found lifetime rates of psychiatric comorbidity to be 81% in individuals with SAD, again with a trend suggesting that SAD occurred first except in the case of the simple phobias that often preceded SAD (65).

On the other hand, a splitting perspective is supported by differences in symptoms across different anxiety disorders. A patient with panic disorder describes recurrent unexpected panic attacks, including nocturnal panic attacks that can occur in numerous situations (66), whereas individuals with SAD usually experience panic attacks only in social or performance situations, rarely "out of the blue" or nocturnally (21). There are also differences in accompanying somatic complaints, with SAD patients more frequently experiencing blushing, tremors, sweating, and muscle twitching compared to patients with agoraphobia, who commonly suffer from dizziness, palpitations, difficulty breathing, chest pain, tinnitus, blurred vision, and headaches (67). Similarly, anxiety symptoms differ in generalized anxiety disorder and SAD (67–69).

Both splitters and lumpers agree that individuals with generalized SAD are especially vulnerable to the development of both comorbid anxiety disorders and mood disorders, particularly atypical depression (70,71). This is of interest as atypical depression shares interpersonal/rejection sensitivity as a core feature with SAD. Pharmacologically, both SAD and atypical depression have consistently been shown to respond to MAOIs and not tricyclic antidepressants (TCAs) (72,73). Therefore, although it may be useful to differentiate between these disorders for some purposes, the construct of an affective spectrum of disorders may on occasion be helpful in guiding treatment.

A manic episode may be viewed as lying at the extreme end of a spectrum of social inhibition versus disinhibition (63). Increased lifetime rates of bipolar mood disorder (BMD) in individuals with SAD have been reported in both the NCS and ECA studies (64,74), and a 9% lifetime history of bipolar mood disorder (BMD) type II was demonstrated in a group of outpatients with SAD (75). High rates of hypomania were found in SAD subjects responding to either MAOIs or reversible inhibitors of monoamine oxidase type A (RIMAs), with the author raising the possibility of a special subset of SAD patients existing within the bipolar spectrum (76). Conversely, preliminary evidence suggests that gabapentin (which may be useful in bipolar depression) is beneficial in the treatment of generalized SAD (77,78). Further research into the possibility of a continuum of inhibition and disinhibition may be warranted.

V. SPECTRUM OF INCREASED SOCIAL AWARENESS VERSUS SOCIAL DEFICIT

An absence of interest in others may lead to social avoidance in individuals with pervasive developmental disorders (including autism and Asperger's disorder). Several family studies have shown an increased prevalence of SAD in first-degree relatives of autistic patients (79,80), and suggestions have been made that SAD may be the product of a milder version of the same mechanism that leads to the abnormal social interaction seen in autistic patients (49).

Schizoid personality disorder has been described as lying at the extreme of a spectrum of sociability—with no desire for social relationships—whereas APD subjects desire relationships but fear contact and therefore avoid social interactions (15). Individuals with schizoid personality disorder therefore exhibit passive detachment compared to the active avoidance described in APD (12,42).

Conversely, Williams syndrome (a rare genetic syndrome with a specific neuropsychological profile) is characterized by remarkable conversational verbal abilities, hypersociability, and empathy denoting a characteristic behavioral phenotype (81,82). Hypersociability in these patients may be dysfunctional insofar as they are unable to appropriately ascertain the risks of different social interactions.

Thus there is some support for a spectrum that ranges from social deficits (e.g., pervasive developmental disorders and schizoid personality disorder) through to increased social awareness (SAD) to hypersociability (Williams syndrome). As with other putative spectra of social anxiety, further validation is required in order to determine the precise boundaries and underlying neurobiology of this range of symptoms.

VI. MEASURING THE SOCIAL ANXIETY SPECTRUM

The Structured Clinical Interview for Social Anxiety Spectrum (SCI-SHY) is an instrument that addresses the concept of a SAD spectrum, with both self-report and clinician administered versions, each comprising of four domains ("Social Phobic Traits During Childhood and Adolescence," "Interpersonal Sensitivity," "Behavioral Inhibition and Somatic Symptoms," "Specific Anxiety and Phobic Features"). In a small sample the order of administration of these two versions affected the number of symptoms endorsed by patients. Subjects reported more symptoms when the clinician-administrated version was given first, possibly related to patients initially overemphasizing certain novel symptoms described. However, high agreement between scores in both formats was found when the self-report version was administered first. The self-report version of the SCI-SHY is therefore recommended by the authors for use in both clinical and research settings (2).

VII. CONCLUSION

This chapter has covered several approaches to defining the SAD spectrum. Awareness of different dimensions of social anxiety symptoms and conditions may encourage more comprehensive assessment. Given the prevalence of such symptoms, patients with anxiety and mood disorders should be systematically interviewed for SAD, body image/social fear disorders, and deficits in social interaction. Instruments such as the SCI-SHY may also be useful for this purpose. As the psychobiology of SAD advances, it will hopefully be possible to specify the underlying mechanisms that generate these spectra of psychopathology. In the interim, putative dimensions of social anxiety are heuristically useful in the clinical setting insofar as they suggest specific treatment options, since many of the symptoms and conditions that fall on these spectra appear to respond to SSRIs and cognitive behavioral therapy (CBT).

ACKNOWLEDGEMENTS

Dr. Muller and Prof. Stein are supported by the Medical Research Council (MRC) of South Africa.

REFERENCES

1. Cassano GB, Michelini S, Shear MK, Coli E, Maser JD, Frank E. The panic-agoraphobic spectrum: a descriptive approach to the assessment and treatment of subtle symptoms. Am J Psychiatry 1997; 154(6):27–38.
2. Dell'Osso L, Rucci P, Cassano GB, Maser JD, Endicott J, Shear MK, Sarno N, Saettoni M, Grochocinski VJ, Frank E. Measuring social anxiety and obsessive-compulsive spectra: comparison of interviews and self-report instruments. Compr Psychiatry 2002; 42(2):81–87.
3. Stein MB. Phenomenology and epidemiology of social phobia. Int Clin Psychopharmacol 1997; 12(suppl 6):23–26.
4. Chavira DA, Stein MB. The shyness spectrum. CNS Spectrums 1999; 4:20–26.
5. Phillips KA. Body dysmorphic disorder: diagnostic controversies and treatment challenges. Bull Menninger Clin 2000; 64(1):18–35.
6. Stein DJ, Le Roux L, Bouwer C, Van Heerden B. Is olfactory reference syndrome an obsessive-compulsive disorder? Two cases and a discussion. J Neuropsychiatry Clin Neurosci 1998; 10:96–99.
7. Stein DJ, Matsunaga H. Cross-cultural aspects of social anxiety disorder. Psychiatr Clin North Am 2001; 24(4):773–782.
8. Hollander E, Aronowitz BR. Comorbid social anxiety and body dysmorphic disorder: managing the complicated patient. J Clin Psychiatry 1999; 60(suppl 9):27–31.
9. Heimberg RG, Hope DA, Dodge CS, Becker RE. DSM-III-R subtypes of social phobia: comparison to generalized social phobics and public speaking phobics. J Nerv Ment Dis 1990; 178:172–179.
10. Chavira DA, Stein MB, Malcarne VL. Scrutinizing the relationship between shyness and social phobia. Anxiety Disorders 2002; 16:585–598.
11. Zimbardo PG, Pilkonis PA, Norwood RM. The social disease called shyness. Psychol Today 1975; 8:68–72.
12. Schneier FR, Blanco C, Antia SX, Liebowitz MR. The social anxiety spectrum. Psychiatr Clin North Am 2002; 25:757–774.
13. Yerkes RM, Dodson JD. The relation of strength of stimulus to rapidity of habit-formation. J Comp Neurol Psychol 1908; 18(5):459–482.
14. Turner SM, Beidel DC, Townsley RM. Social phobia: relationship to shyness. Behav Res Ther 1990; 28:297–305.
15. Coupland NJ. Social phobia: etiology, neurobiology, and treatment. J Clin Psychiatry 2001; 62(suppl 1):25–35.
16. Biederman J, Hirshfield-Becker D, Rosenbaum J, Faraone S. Temperamental risk factors for anxiety disorders in high risk children. Eur Neuropsychopharmacol 2002; 12(suppl 3):157–158.
17. Kagan J, Snidman N. Early childhood predictors of adult anxiety disorders. Biol Psychiatry 1999; 46:1536–1541.
18. Schwartz CE, Wright CI, Shin LM, Kagan J, Rauch SL. Inhibited and uninhibited infants "grown up": adult amygdala response to novelty. Science 2003; 20;300(5627):1952–1953.

19. Black B, Uhde TW. Psychiatric characteristics of children with selective mutism: a pilot study. J Am Acad Adolesc Psychiatry 1995; 34:847–856.
20. Anstedig KD. Is selective mutism an anxiety disorder? Rethinking its DSM-IV classification. J Anxiety Disord 1999; 13(4):417–434.
21. Yu Moutier C, Stein MB. The history, epidemiology, and differential diagnosis of social anxiety disorder. J Clin Psychiatry 1999; 60(suppl 9):4–8.
22. Dummit ES III, Klein RG, Tancer NK, Asche B, Martin J, Fairbanks JA. Systematic assessment of 50 children with selective mutism. J Am Acad Child Adolesc Psychiatry 1997; 36:653–660.
23. Golwyn DH, Sevlie CP. Phenelzine treatment of selective mutism in four prepubertal children. J Child Adolesc Psychopharmacol 1999; 9:109–113.
24. Stein MB, Walker JR, Forde DR. Setting diagnostic thresholds for social phobia: considerations from a community survey of social anxiety. Am J Psychiatry 1994; 151(3):408–412.
25. Davidson JRT, Hughes DC, George LK, Blazer DG. The boundary of social phobia. Exploring the threshold. Arch Gen Psychiatry 1994; 51:975–983.
26. Stein MB, Torgrud LJ, Walker JR. Social phobia symptoms, subtypes, and severity. Findings from a community survey. Arch Gen Psychiatry 2000; 57: 1046–1052.
27. American Psychiatric Association. Diagnostic and Statistical Manual of Mental Disorders. 4th ed. Washington, DC: American Psychiatric Association; 1994.
28. Kessler RC, Stein MB, Berglund P. Social phobia subtypes in the national comorbidity survey. Am J Psychiatry 1998; 155(5):613–619.
29. Davidson JR. Pharmacotherapy of generalized anxiety disorder. J Clin Psychiatry 2001; 62(suppl 11):46–50.
30. Eng W, Heimberg RG, Coles ME, Schneier FR, Liebowitz MR. An empirical approach to subtype identification in individuals with social phobia. Psychol Med 2000; 30(6):1345–1357.
31. Kendler KS, Neale MC, Kessler RC, Heath AC, Eaves LJ. The genetic epidemiology of phobias in women: the interrelationship of agoraphobia, social phobia, situational phobia and simple phobia. Arch Gen Psychiatry 1992; 49:273–281.
32. Flyer AJ, Mannuzza S, Chapman TF. A direct interview family study of social phobia. Arch Gen Psychiatry 1993; 50:286–293.
33. Stein MB, Chartier MJ, Hazen AL, Kozak MV, Tancer ME, Lander S, Furer P, Chubaty D, Walker JR. A direct-interview family study of generalised social phobia. Am J Psychiatry 1998; 155:90–97.
34. Reiss AL, Freund L. Fragile X syndrome, DSM-III-R, and autism. J Am Acad Child Adolesc Psychiatry 1990; 29:885–891.
35. Pimentel MM. Fragile X syndrome. Int J Mol Med 1999; 3:639–645.
36. Franke P, Leboyer M, Gansicke M, Weiffenbach O, Biancalana V, Cornillet-Lefebre P, Croquette MF, Froster U, Schwab SG, Poustka F, Hautzinger M, Maier W. Genotype-phenotype relationship in female carriers of the permutation and full mutation of the FMRI-I. Psychiatr Res 1998; 80:113–127.

37. American Psychiatric Association. Diagnostic and Statistical Manual of Mental Disorders. 3d ed. Washington, DC: American Psychiatric Association, 1980.

38. McGlashan TH, Grilo CM, Skodol AE, Gunderson JG, Shea MT, Morey LC, Zanarini MC, Stout RL. The collaborative longitudinal personality disorders study: baseline axis I/II and II/II diagnostic co-occurrence. Acta Psychiatr Scand 2000; 102:256–264.

39. Zimmerman M, Coryell WH. Diagnosing personality disorders in the community. A comparison of self-report and interview measures. Arch Gen Psychiatry 1990; 47(6):527–531.

40. Herbert JD, Hope DA, Bellack AS. Validity of the distinction between generalized social phobia and avoidant personality disorder. J Abnorm Psychol 1992; 101:332–339.

41. Holt CS, Heimberg RG, Hope DA. Avoidant personality and the generalized subtype of social phobia. J Abnorm Psychol 1992; 101:318–325.

42. Lydiard RB. Social anxiety disorder and its implications. J Clin Psychiatry 2001; 62(suppl 1):17–24.

43. Dahl AA. The relationship between social phobia and avoidant personality disorder: workshop report 3. Int Clin Psychopharmacol 1996; 11(suppl 3): 109–112.

44. Perugi G, Toni C, Akiskal HS. Anxious-bipolar comorbidity: diagnostic and treatment challenges. Psychiatr Clin North Am 1999; 22:565–583.

45. Liebowitz MR, Schneier F, Campeas R, Hollander E, Hatterer J, Fyer A, Gorman J, Papp L, Davies S, Gully R, Klein DF. Phenelzine vs. atenolol in social phobia. Arch Gen Psychiatry 1992; 49:290–300.

46. Versiani M, Nardi AE, Mundim FD, Alves AB, Liebowitz MR, Amrein R. Pharmacotherapy of social phobia: a controlled study with moclobemide and phenelzine. Br J Psychiatry 1992; 161:353–360.

47. Brown EJ, Heimberg RG, Juster HR. Social phobia subtype and avoidant personality: effect on severity of social phobia, impairment, and outcome of cognitive-behavioural treatment. Behav Ther 1995; 26:467–480.

48. Brawman-Mintzer O, Lydiard RB, Phillips KA, Morton A, Czepowicz V, Emmanuel N, Villareal G, Johnson M, Ballenger JC. Body dysmorphic disorder in patients with anxiety disorders and major depression: a comorbidity study. Am J Psychiatry 1995; 152:1665–1667.

49. Lang AJ, Stein MB. Social phobia: prevalence and diagnostic threshold. J Clin Psychiatry 2001; 62(suppl 1):5–10.

50. Altamura C, Paluello MM, Mundo E, Medda S, Mannu P. Kizu A, Miyoshi N, Yoshida Y, Miyagishi T. Clinical and subclinical body dysmorphic disorder. Eur Arch Clin Neurosci 2001; 251:105–108.

51. Phillips KA, Albertini RS, Siniscalchi JM, Khan A, Robinson M. Effectiveness of pharmacotherapy for body dysmorphic disorder: a chart-review study. J Clin Psychiatry 2001; 62(9):721–727.

52. Phillips KA, Albertini RS, Rasmussen SA. A randomized placebo-controlled trial of fluoxetine in body dysmorphic disorder. Arch Gen Psychiatry 2002; 59(4):381–388.

53. Pryse-Phillips W. An olfactory reference syndrome. Acta Psychiatr Scand 1971; 47:484–509.

54. Matsunaga H, Kiriike N, Matsui T, Iwasaki Y, Stein DJ. Taijin kyofusho: a form of social anxiety disorder that responds to serotonin reuptake inhibitors? Int J Neuropsychopharmacol 2001; 4(3):231–237.

55. Kizu A, Miyoshi N, Yoshida Y, Miyagishi T. A case with fear of emitting body odour resulted in successful treatment with clomipramine. Hokkaido Igaku Zasshi 1994; 69:1477–1480.

56. Clarvit SR, Schneier FR, Liebowitz MR. The offensive subtype of Taijin-kyofu-sho in New York City: the phenomenology and treatment of social anxiety disorder. J Clin Psychiatry 1996; 57:523–527.

57. Kleinknecht RA, Dinnel DL, Kleinknecht EE. Cultural factors in social anxiety: a comparison of social phobia symptoms and taijin kyofusho. J Anxiety Disord 1997; 11(2):157–177.

58. Flament MF, Godart N, Vigan C. The epidemiology and comorbidity of eating disorders. Eur Psychiatry 1998; 13(suppl 4):155s.

59. Godart NT, Flament MF, Lecrubier Y, Jeammet P. Anxiety disorders in anorexia nervosa and bulimia nervosa: co-morbidity and chronology of appearance. Eur Psychiatry 2000; 15:38–45.

60. Stein MB, Heuser IJ, Juncos JL, Uhde TW. Anxiety disorder in patients with Parkinson's disease. Am J Psychiatry 1990; 147:311–317.

61. Oberlander EL, Schneier FR, Liebowitz MR. Physical disability and social phobia. J Clin Psychopharmacol 1994; 14(2):136–143.

62. Lochner C, Vythilingum B, Stein DJ. Olfactory reference syndrome: diagnostic criteria and differential diagnosis. J Postgrad Med 2003; 49(4):328–331.

63. Hudson JI, Mangweth B, Pope HG Jr, De Col C, Hausmann A, Gutweniger S, Laird NM, Biebl W, Tsaung MT. Family study of affective spectrum disorder. Arch Gen Psychiatry 2003; 60(2):170–177.

64. Schneier FR, Johnson J, Hornig CD, Liebowitz MR, Weissman MM. Social phobia: comorbidity and morbidity in an epidemiological sample. Arch Gen Psychiatry 1992; 49:282–291.

65. Magee WJ, Eaton JJ, Wittchen H-U, McGonagle KA, Kessler RC. Agoraphobia, simple phobia and social phobia in the National Comorbidity Survey. Arch Gen Psychiatry 1996; 53:159–168.

66. Stein MB, Chartier M, Walker JR. Sleep in non-depressed patients with panic disorder. Sleep1993; 16(8):724–726.

67. Reich JH, Noyes R, Yates W. Anxiety symptoms distinguishing social phobia from panic and generalized anxiety disorders. J Nerv Ment Dis 1988; 176:510–513.

68. Versiani M, Mundim FD, Nardi AE, Liebowitz MR. Tranylcypromine in social phobia. J Clin Psychopharmacol 1988; 8:279–283.

69. Cameron OG, Thyer BA, Nesse RM, Curtis GC. Symptom profiles of patients with DSM-III-anxiety disorders. Am J Psychiatry 1986; 143:1132–1137.

70. Mannuzza A, Schneier F, Chapman T, Liebowitz M, Klein D, Fyer A. Generalized social phobia: reliability and validity. Arch Gen Psychiatry 1995; 52: 230–237.

71. Wittchen HU, Stein MB, Kessler RC. Social fears and social phobia in a community sample of adolescents and young adults: prevalence, risk factors and comorbidity. Psychol Med 1999; 29:309–323.

72. Thase ME, Trivedi MH, Rush AJ. MAOIs in the contemporary treatment of depression. Neuropsychopharmacology 1995; 12(3):185–219.

73. Simpson HB, Schneier FR, Campeas R, Marshall RD, Fallon BA, Davies S, Klein DF, Liebowitz MR. Imipramine in the treatment of social phobia. J Clin Psychopharmacol 1998; 18:132–135.

74. Kessler RC, Stang P, Wittchen HU, Stein M, Walters EE. Lifetime co-morbidities between social phobia and mood disorders in the US National Comorbidity Survey. Psychol Med 1999; 29:555–567.

75. Perugi G, Frare F, Toni C, Mata B, Akiskal HS. Bipolar II and unipolar comorbidity in 153 outpatients with social phobia. Compr Psychiatry 2001; 42:375–381.

76. Himmelhoch JM. Social anxiety, hypomania and the bipolar spectrum: data, theory and clinical issues. J Affect Disord 1998; 50(2–3):203–213.

77. Wang PW, Santosa C, Schumacher M, Winsberg M, Winsberg ME, Strong C, Ketter TA. Gabapentin augmentation therapy in bipolar depression. Bipolar Disord 2002; 4(5):296–301.

78. Pande AC, Davidson JR, Jefferson JW, Janney CA, Katzelnick DJ, Weisler RH, Greist JH, Sutherland SM. Treatment of social phobia with gabapentin: a placebo-controlled study. J Clin Psychopharmacol 1999; 19:341–348.

79. Smalley SL, McCracken J, Tanguay P. Autism, affective disorders, and social phobia. Am J Med Genet 1995; 60:19–26.

80. Piven J, Palmer P. Psychiatric disorder and the broad autism phenotype: evidence from a family study of multiple-incidence autism families. Am J Psychiatry 1999; 156:557–563.

81. Cassidy SB, Morris CA. Behavioural phenotypes in genetic syndromes: genetic clues to human behaviour. Adv Pediatr 2002; 49:59–86.

82. Galaburda AM, Holinger DP, Bellugi U, Sherman GF. Williams syndrome: neuronal size and neuronal-packing density in primary visual cortex. Arch Neurol 2002; 59(9):1461–1467.

3

Epidemiology of Social Anxiety Disorder

**Carlos Blanco, Carolina Garcia, and
Michael R. Liebowitz**
New York State Psychiatric Institute,
Columbia University
College of Physicians and Surgeons,
New York, New York, U.S.A.

I. INTRODUCTION

Epidemiology is defined as "the study of the distribution of a disease or a psychological condition in human populations and of the factors that influence this distribution" (1). Epidemiological surveys provide information that is essential in addition to the information obtained from clinical samples. First, they provide information about the prevalence, incidence, and rates of help-seeking behavior of the population. Second, representative samples of the general population provide a fuller description of all degrees of severity of a disorder than do clinical samples, which are generally subject to some form of self-selection due to help-seeking bias. Thus, information from epidemiological studies can be used to identify potential vulnerability factors for the development of a disease or disorder. Third, prospective, longitudinal studies of epidemiological samples can be used to investigate the course and clinical consequences of the disorder in the community. This information provides the basis for developing and evaluating preventive and other public health interventions.

Over the last few years, several epidemiological studies in the United States, Europe, and Asian Pacific have provided a deeper picture of social anxiety disorder in relation to its prevalence, incidence, severity, and correlates. Recently, prospective longitudinal studies have started to clarify the natural course of social anxiety disorder and provide insight into risk factors for its development. This chapter reviews the available studies, addressing the prevalence, comorbidity, and natural course of the disorder.

II. PREVALENCE

A. Prevalence in the Community

Although there are significant variations in prevalence findings, the majority of studies conducted in the United States, Europe, and Scandinavia support the view that social anxiety disorder is among the most prevalent of the psychiatric disorders in the general population.

Initial estimates of the prevalence of social anxiety disorder obtained conflicting results. Two large epidemiological studies in the United States have collected data on social anxiety disorder, and their estimates of the prevalence of the disorder have been rather different. The first study, the Epidemiologic Catchment Area (ECA) study, collected data on rates and risk factors for psychiatric disorders based on a probability sample of more than 18,000 adults aged 18 years and over, living in five U.S. communities, using the Diagnostic Interview Schedule (DIS) (2). The ECA assessed only three social fears as part of the Simple Phobia section of the DIS and estimated the lifetime prevalence rate of social anxiety disorder to be approximately 2.4%. Like the results of the ECA, estimates from early studies conducted in the 1980s reported lifetime rates of 1 to 4% (3,4). In contrast, the National Comorbidity Survey (NCS) (5) used a specific social anxiety disorder module based on the criteria of the revised third edition of the *Diagnostic and Statistical Manual of Mental Disorders* (DSM-III-R), as operationalized in the Composite International Diagnostic Interview (CIDI); it found a 1-year prevalence of social anxiety disorder of 13.3% and a lifetime prevalence of 16%.

The estimates from studies conducted in other countries using DSM-III-R and DSM-IV criteria have shown less variability, have been similar to those of the NCS, and have reported lifetime estimates of 7 to 12% and 12-month estimates of 3 to 4% (5–10). It is now generally accepted that the early studies conducted in the 1980s underestimated the true prevalence of social anxiety disorder due to the use of DSM-III criteria and less refined assessment methods and that the estimates from recent studies reflect more accurate estimates. The variability among recent studies is probably due to differences in sampling procedures and cultural variations in the samples of the studies.

For example, samples with a substantial proportion of people more than 50 years old have generally obtained lower prevalence estimates. Although the reasons for this finding are not clear, it is probably due to complete or partial remissions over the years as well as the effect of other comorbid diagnoses, such as major depressive disorder, that might lead to underreporting of social anxiety disorder in older groups.

From the point of view of cross-cultural epidemiology, several studies using the DSM-III criteria for social anxiety disorder in East Asian countries have found significantly lower lifetime prevalence rates than studies conducted in Western countries. A Korean study using the DIS found a lifetime prevalence of 0.5% of DSM-III social anxiety disorder (11), and a Taiwanese study reported lifetime prevalence of 0.6% for DSM-III social anxiety disorder (12). A cross-national study conducted in the United States, Canada, Puerto Rico, and Korea found that the prevalence rates of social anxiety disorder differed by country from 2.6% in the United States to as low as 0.5% in Korea (13). The reasons for these differences are unknown but may involve true differences in prevalence across the countries, cultural inappropriateness of existing instruments to assess social anxiety disorder in non-Western populations, or cultural differences with regard to the emphasis on privacy and willingness to endorse psychiatric symptoms (14).

B. Prevalence in Primary Care

While community surveys provide estimates of the prevalence of a disorder, it is also important from the services point of view to know the prevalence of that disorder in the population of patients seeking medical care, because those patients, if correctly diagnosed, could be readily treated. In many health care systems, most psychiatric care is provided in primary care. Therefore it is important to know the prevalence of social anxiety disorder in primary care. Two studies in Europe (15,16) found that the lifetime prevalence of social anxiety disorder in primary care was 9 to 14%, while the current prevalence was 4.9%, similar to estimates from community surveys. Both studies indicated that the diagnosis of social anxiety disorder was frequently missed and patients not treated, indicating that better detection methods in primary care may help improve the treatment of social anxiety disorder in the population.

III. AGE OF ONSET AND INCIDENCE

Social anxiety disorder generally has its onset in early to late adolescence with estimates of mean age of onset ranging from 10 to 17 years, depending on the type of sample (8,17–21). There is some indication that the prevalence of social anxiety disorder may be increasing in recent cohorts and that this increase may be due exclusively to patients with the generalized form (21). According to this study, the increase is most marked in white, educated, married individuals. There are also some indications that the age of onset of generalized social anxiety disorder is generally lower than that of nongeneralized social anxiety disorder (22,23) and that isolated fears of public speaking seem to occur later than other social fears (21).

IV. DIAGNOSTIC THRESHOLD AND SUBTYPES

Social anxiety is a dimensional phenomenon, and the vast majority of people experience a certain degree of it in one or more social situations. Therefore it is important to establish when the degree of social anxiety is within the normal range and when it should be considered part of a disorder. In an elegant study, Stein et al. (6) assessed changes in the estimated prevalence of social anxiety disorder when different diagnostic (or caseness) thresholds were considered in a community sample of adults from a medium-sized Canadian city. The authors found that 61% of 526 participants believed that they felt much or somewhat more anxious than other people in at least one of the seven social situations surveyed. Speaking to a large audience was the most frequently feared situation (55%), followed by speaking to a small group of familiar people (24.9%), dealing with people in authority (23.3%), attending social gatherings (14.5%), speaking to strangers or meeting new people (13.7%), and eating (7.1%) or writing (5.1%) in front of others. When the threshold for caseness was systematically modified by altering the required level of psychosocial interference or distress or by including or excluding subjects with pure public speaking phobia, the rate of social anxiety disorder varied from 1.9 to 18.7%. Using DSM-III-R criteria, their estimated prevalence was 7.1%—in the neighborhood of the estimates of other population surveys. Similarly, a reanalysis of the NCS (24) found that when the "DSM-IV clinical significance criterion" was required to make a diagnosis, there was a 50% decrease in prevalence of social anxiety (from 7.4 to 3.7%) from the original estimates. A limitation of this study, however, is that there is little consensus among clinicians and researchers on the meaning of the term *clinical significance*.

In addition to the identification of cases, it is important to assess whether all individuals with a diagnosis of social anxiety disorder suffer from the same syndrome or whether they form a heterogeneous group that can be further subdivided. If social anxiety disorder is truly a heterogeneous disorder, refinements in its classification could potentially lead to improved treatment. DSM-IV distinguishes between the generalized and nongeneralized subtypes of social anxiety disorder. Individuals who fear many social situations are classified as suffering from the generalized type, while those suffering only from performance fears or a limited range of social fears are classified as suffering from the nongeneralized subtype. There is no explicit agreement on exactly how many fears constitute the threshold for the generalized subtype, although most clinicians would probably agree that individuals fearing four or more social situations should be classified as suffering from the generalized subtype. Individuals suffering from the generalized subtype tend to be more impaired in psychosocial functioning than those with the nongeneralized subtype. However, this is not an absolute rule, and even individuals with only one fear can be severely impaired.

The nongeneralized subtype seems to be approximately three times more prevalent than the generalized subtype, and there seems to be no evidence suggesting that individuals with the nongeneralized form progress to the generalized form. However, the distinction between those subtypes has not been demonstrated in all studies. Two studies using cluster analyses in clinical samples identified a third subtype intermediate between the generalized and nongeneralized subtypes (25,26), and a third one based on a community sample failed to find a categorical distinction between individuals with the two DSM-IV subtypes. Genetic, neuroimaging, and treatment studies may help clarify the boundaries of each subtype. Some studies (27,28) have found physiological differences between generalized and nongeneralized patients in response to laboratory-simulated performance and social challenges. The results displayed in these studies suggest that nongeneralized patients show a greater increase in heart rate in public speaking settings than generalized patients do in public speaking or social situations. This fits with the utility of beta blockers in the nongeneralized but not the generalized subtype.

V. EARLY DEVELOPMENT, COMORBIDITY, AND NATURAL COURSE

A. Developmental Model

Another potential avenue to improve the treatment of social anxiety disorder is to have a better understanding of its origin and causes. Because social anxiety disorder is characterized by onset in childhood and adolescence and often has a chronic course, it is important to link the course of social anxiety disorder to developmental processes characteristically seen in those who suffer from the disorder.

The evolution of social anxiety disorder has been investigated in the Early Development Stage of Psychopathology Study (EDSP), a 5-year prospective, longitudinal study of 3021 individuals (29). The ESDP found that the majority of cases of social anxiety disorder have emerged by the time an individual has reached the age of 19 years and that, in spite of some variations in severity, few individuals have a stable and spontaneous remission. The developmental study derived from the ESDP suggest that individuals may have a certain predisposition (e.g., genetic factors) that makes them more likely to suffer from social fears and to avoid social interactions. This restrictive behavior, in turn, would interfere with their optimal development and result in disabilities in social and school or professional settings. This suboptimal development could reinforce these social fears and lead to maladaptive behaviors, such as use of alcohol and other drugs, further increasing risk for other comorbid psychiatric disorders. Over time, all these factors would result in decreased quality of life.

B. Comorbidity

Consistent with the developmental model of the EDSP, several cross-sectional studies have shown that comorbidity is common in patients with social anxiety disorder, particularly in those with the generalized subtype (29) (this volume, chapter by Fehm and Wittchen). The disorders most frequently associated with social anxiety disorder are other anxiety disorders, major depression, and substance use disorders, particularly alcohol dependence (9,30–34).

Data from the NCS suggest that individuals with social anxiety disorder are two to three times more likely to develop either major depression or dysthymia than individuals with similar sociodemographic characteristics but no social anxiety disorder (30). Retrospective studies suggest that social anxiety disorder precedes mood disorders in development (35). Moreover, the relationship becomes stronger when considering the number of social fears rather than the type of fear: in subjects with three or more fears, the risk of comorbidity is significantly increased, with an odds ratio of 4.5.

In the EDSP, nondepressed individuals with social anxiety disorder at baseline had an increased likelihood of developing major depressive disorder during the follow-up period compared with individuals without social anxiety disorder. Moreover, individuals with comorbid SAD and depressive disorder at baseline had greater likelihood of depressive disorder persistence or recurrence (OR = 2.3; 95% CI, 1.2 to 4.6) and attempted suicide (OR = 6.1; 95% CI, 1.2 to 32.2). The EDSP survey also studied the probability that individuals with social anxiety disorder have an increase risk for developing substance abuse disorder. The study found that individuals with social anxiety disorder were at greater risk of nicotine and alcohol dependence than were similar individuals without social anxiety disorder (34).

Another issue to consider is the comorbidity between avoidant personality disorder and social anxiety disorder. Criteria for avoidant personality disorder evolved out of the work of Millon, who conceived of persons with avoidant personality disorder as actively avoiding social relationships, in contrast to the passive detachment of schizoid personality disorder. Over the course of revisions in DMS-III-R and DSM-IV, the criteria for avoidant personality have increasingly overlapped with those of social anxiety disorder. Rates of overlap between the two disorders have ranged from 25 to 89% (37–42). Differences in clinical features, including treatment response between groups of patients with these conditions, have tended to be more quantitative than qualitative, which has led some authors to consider whether the conditions might be alternative descriptions of a single population or whether avoidant personality disorder might represent a severe form of social anxiety disorder.

VI. RISK FACTORS

A third avenue to decrease the impact of social anxiety disorder is the identification of characteristics that increase the risk of suffering from this disorder. Identification of high-risk populations may allow the development of specific interventions that may decrease the likelihood of suffering the disorder, or early intervention in cases where symptoms of the disorder are already present.

A number of studies have investigated the role of familial factors in the etiology of social anxiety disorder (this volume, chapter by Stein, Gelernter, and Smoller). Genetic studies found that there is an inherited propensity toward anxiousness rather than a specific heritability of social anxiety (43–47). Another source of familial aggregation of social anxiety disorder is the presence of specific factors in the family environment—such as child-rearing style, restricted exposure to social situations within the family, and parental modeling (this volume, chapter by Bandelow Torrente, and Rüther). Studies regarding both genetic and possible environmental factors have found a higher specificity for the transmission of social anxiety disorder than those focused purely on genetic mechanisms. These factors may shape a general predisposition for anxiety into social anxiety disorder (43).

Behavioral inhibition has also been repeatedly identified as a risk factor for the development of social anxiety disorder (this volume, chapter by Morris). High levels of behavioral inhibition in children are associated with a higher likelihood of developing social anxiety disorder in the future.

In addition to familial and early development factors, some socio-demographic variables have also been shown to constitute risk factors for the development of social anxiety disorder. Probably the most robust finding from epidemiological studies is that women are more likely than men to have social anxiety disorder, although the gender ratio of 3:2 in social anxiety disorder is less pronounced than the gender ratio for other anxiety disorders (5). Furthermore, in clinical settings, the gender ratio is more even. Other factors—such as poor financial situation, low social class, never having been married, unemployment, and poor education—frequently relate to lack of socialization during the early stages of the disorder and have also been suggested as potential risk factors, but there is little information on how to quantify their contribution or explain their interaction with other risk factors.

VII. EPIDEMIOLOGY OF SOCIAL ANXIETY DISORDER IN CHILDREN AND ADOLESCENTS

In contrast with the growing body of data on the epidemiology of social anxiety disorder in adults, much less is known about the epidemiology of social phobia in children. This is not unique to social anxiety disorder but a common fact in the study of anxiety disorders in children. Many of the difficulties conducting research in this area are related to the lack of standardized, widely accepted assessment tools (48). However, it is important to note that even if those tools existed, it would have been difficult to conduct such research prior to the recent explosion of knowledge about social anxiety disorder in adults. Despite those limitations, there has been a recent interest in the epidemiology of social anxiety disorder in children and adolescents.

Studies have estimated the prevalence of social anxiety disorder in children using DSM-III and DSM-III-R at approximately 1% (49,50). Although epidemiological studies have not yet estimated the prevalence of social anxiety disorder in children and adolescents using DSM-IV criteria, it is recognized that social anxiety disorder is one of the most common primary diagnoses in adolescents who present for treatment. Preliminary evidence for this assessment comes from recent studies assessing the lifetime prevalence of social anxiety disorder in adolescents. One study of a sample of 1035 adolescents (ages 12 to 17 years) randomly selected from high schools in Germany found a DSM-IV lifetime prevalence of social anxiety disorder of approximately 16%. The EDSP found a DSM-IV lifetime prevalence of 9.5 and 4.9% in 14- to 24-year-old females and males, respectively. Studies in preadolescents using DSM-IV criteria do not yet exist.

VIII. DISABILITY, QUALITY OF LIFE, AND HEALTH CARE UTILIZATION

Several studies have shown that social anxiety disorder affects the quality of life of the individuals who suffer from it (this volume, chapter by Baldwin and Buis). In an early study, Schneier et al. (51) compared impairment in

32 patients with social anxiety disorder and 14 normal control subjects using the Disability Profile and the Liebowitz Self-Rated Disability Scale. They found that more than half of all patients with social anxiety disorder reported at least moderate impairment at some time in their lives due to social anxiety and avoidance in areas of education, employment, family relationships, marriage/romantic relationships, friendships/social network, and other interests.

Similarly, Wittchen and Beloch (52) compared 65 patients meeting DSM-III-R social anxiety disorder criteria and 65 matched controls who were patients with a history of herpes infection (as a control for chronicity of illness). They used the Short Form of the Medical Outcomes Study (SF-36), a 36-item questionnaire that covers aspects of physical and mental well-being (53). Patients with social anxiety disorder had a significantly lower quality of life, particularly in the domains of mental health, general health, vitality, role limitations, and social function. Patients with comorbid conditions evidenced even greater impairment than those with uncomplicated social anxiety disorder (54,55).

In another study, Wittchen et al. (56) compared 65 patients with uncomplicated social anxiety disorder, 51 with associated comorbidity, 34 with subthreshold social anxiety disorder, and controls in the basis of quality of life, work productivity, and social impairments. They found that current quality of life—particularly in vitality, general health, mental health, role limitations and social functioning—was significantly reduced in all social anxiety disorder groups. On the other hand, patients with comorbidity revealed more severe reductions in quality of life than patients with uncomplicated or subthreshold social anxiety disorder. Overall impairment for the group with subthreshold social anxiety disorder was slightly lower than for the group with uncomplicated social anxiety disorder.

Studies in the United States and in Europe suggest that social anxiety disorder is rarely treated. In the NCS, researchers found that only 13 to 28% of individuals diagnosed with social anxiety disorder ever sought treatment for their condition. Wittchen et al. extended those findings to document that lowest treatment rates were found for pure and comorbid social anxiety disorder, whereas rates for individuals with the generalized subtype were slightly higher.

Moreover, Katzelnick et al. (55) found, in a community cohort of members of a health maintenance organization, that generalized social anxiety disorder is strongly related to decreasing hourly wages and higher health service utilization. The average subject with pure generalized social anxiety disorder is less likely to graduate from college, earns lower wages, and has less likelihood of holding a technical, professional, or managerial job than a healthy person.

IX. CONCLUSION

Over the last few years, epidemiological studies have shown that social anxiety disorder is highly prevalent, generally chronic, and very disabling. There are some indications that it is better understood as a dimensional rather than a categorical construct, and it may include several subtypes. Future research should continue to delineate the role of genetic, environmental (including cultural), and developmental factors in onset and course of social anxiety disorder, as well as its relationship with childhood and other adult anxiety disorders.

ACKNOWLEDGMENTS

Supported in part by grant DA-00482, and a grants from the National Alliance for Schizophrenia and Depression (Dr. Blanco).

REFERENCES

1. Lilienfeld AM. Definitions of epidemiology. Am J Epidemiol 1978; 107:87–90.
2. Schneier FR, Johnson J, Hornig CD, et al. Social phobia: comorbidity in an epidemiologic sample. Arch Gen Psychiatry 1992; 49:282–288.
3. Bland RC, Newman SC, Orn H. Period prevalence of psychiatric disorders in Edmonton. Acta Psychiatr Scand 1988; 77(suppl 338):24–32.
4. Faravelli C, Degl'Innocenti BG, Giardinelli L. Epidemiology of anxiety disorders in Florence. Acta Psychiatr Scand 1989; 79:308–312.
5. Kessler RC, Mc Gonagle KA, Zhao S. Lifetime and 12-month prevalence of DSM-III-R psychiatric disorders in the United States. Results from the National Comorbidity Survey. Arch Gen Psychiatry 1994; 51:8–19.
6. Stein MB, Walker JR, Forde DR. Setting diagnostic thresholds for social phobia: considerations from a community survey of social anxiety. Am J Psychiatry 1994; 151:408–412.
7. Lépine JP, Lellouch J. Diagnosis and epidemiology of agoraphobia and social phobia. Clin Neuropharmacol 1995; 18(suppl 2):15–26.
8. Wittchen HU, Lieb R, Schuster P, et al. When is onset? Investigations into early developmental stages of anxiety and depressive disorders. In: Rapport JL, ed. Childhood Onset of "Adult" Psychopathology, Clinical and Research Advances. Washington, DC: American Psychiatric Press, 1999:259–302.
9. Stein MB, Kean YM. Disability and quality of life in social phobia: Epidemiologia findings. Am J Psychiatry 2000; 157:1606–1613.
10. Faravelli C, Zucchi T, Viviani B, et al. Epidemiology of social phobia: a clinical approach. Eur Psychiatry 2000; 15:17–24.
11. Lee CK, Kwak YS, Yamamoto J, et al. Psychiatric epidemiology in Korea. Part I: gender and age differences in Seoul. J Nerv Ment Dis 1990; 178:242–246.

12. Hwu HG, Yeh EK, Chang LY. Prevalence of psychiatric disorders in Taiwan defined by the Chineses diagnostic interview schedule. Acta Psychiatr Scand 1989; 79:136–147.

13. Weissman MM, Bland RC, Canino GJ, et al. The cross-national epidemiology of social phobia: a preliminary report. Int Clin Psychopharmacol 1996; 11 (suppl 3):9–14.

14. Chapman TF, Manuzza S, Fyer AJ. Epidemiology and family studies of social phobia. In: RG Heimberg, MR Liebowitz, DA Hope, FR Schenier, eds. Social Phobia: Diagnosis, Assessment and Treatment. New York: Guilford Press, 1995:21–40.

15. Bisserbe JC, Weiller E, Boyer P, et al. Social phobia in primary care: level of recognition and drug use. Int Clin Psychopharmacol 1996; 11:25–28.

16. Szádóczky E, Rihmer Z, Papp ZS, et al. The prevalence of affective and anxiety disorders in primary care practice in Hungary. J Affect Disord 1997; 43:239–244.

17. Davidson JRT, Hughes DL, George LK, et al. The epidemiology of social phobia: findings from the Duke Epidemiologic Catchment Area Study. Psychol Med 1993; 23:709–719.

18. Degonda M, Angst J. The Zurich study: XX. Social phobia and agoraphobia. Eur Arch Psychiatr Clin Neurosci 1993; 243:95–102.

19. Faravelli C, Zucchi T, Vivani B, et al. Epidemiology of social phobia: a clinical approach. Eur Psychiatry 2000; 15:17–24.

20. Schneier FR, Johnson J, Hornig CD, et al. Social phobia: comorbidity and morbidity in an epidemiologic sample. Arch Gen Psychiatry 1992; 49:282–288.

21. Heimberg RG, Stein MB, Hirpi E, et al. Trends in the prevalence of social phobia in the United States: a synthetic cohort analysis of changes over four decades. Eur Psychiatry 2000; 15:29–37.

22. Manuzza, S, Schneier FR, Chapman TF, Liebowitz MR, Klein DF, Fyer AJ. Generalized social phobia. Reliability and validity. Arch Gen Psychiatry (1995); 52:230–237.

23. Wittchen HU, Stein MB, Kessler RC. Social fears and social phobia in a community sample of adolescents and young adults: prevalence, risk factors and comorbidity. Psychol Med 1999; 29:309–323.

24. Narrow WE, Rae DS, Robins LN, Regier DA. Revised prevalence estimates of mental disorders in the United States: using a clinical significance criterion to reconcile 2 surveys' estimates. Arch of Gen Psychiatry 2002; 59:115–23.

25. Eng W, Heimberg RG, Coles ME, et al. An empirical approach to subtype identification in individuals with social phobia. Psychol Med 2000; 30:1345–1357.

26. Furmark T, Tillfors M, Stattin H, et al. Social phobia subtypes in the general population revealed by cluster analysis. Psychol Med 2000; 30:1335–1344.

27. Heimberg R, Hope D, Dodge C, Becker R. DSM-III-R Subtypes of social phobia: comparison of generalized social phobics and public speaking phobics. J Nerv Ment Dis 1995; 178:172–179.

28. Levin AP, Saoud JB, Strauman T, Gorman JM, et al. Responses of "generalized" and "discrete" social phobics during public speaking. J Anxiety Disord 1993; 7:207–221.

29. Wittchen HU, Nelson GB, Lachner G. Prevalence of mental disorders and psychosocial impairments in adolescents and young adults. Psychol Med 1998; 28:109–126.

30. Kessler RC, Stang P, Wittchen HU, et al. Lifetime comorbidities between social phobia and mood disorders in the U.S. National Comorbidity Survey. Psychol Med 1999; 29:555–567.

31. Kessler RC, Stan P, Wittchen HU, et al. Lifetime panic-depression comorbidity in the National Comorbidity Survey. Arch Gen Psychiatry 1998; 55:801–808.

32. Lecrubier Y. Comorbidity in social anxiety disorder: impact on disease burden and management. J Clin Psychiatry 1998; 59(suppl 17):33–37.

33. Merikangas K, Angst J, Eaton W, et al. Comorbidity and boundaries of affective disorders with anxiety disorders and substance abuse: results of an international task force. Br J Psychiatry 1996; 168(suppl 30):49–58.

34. Wittchen HU, Stein MB, Kessler R. Social fears and social phobia in a community sample of adolescents and young adults: prevalence, risk factors and comorbidity. Psychol Med 1999; 29:309–232.

35. Kessler RC, Berglund PA, De Wit DJ, et al. Role impairments associated with pure and comorbid generalized anxiety disorder and major depression in two countries. Psychol Med. In press.

36. Stein MB, Fuetsch M, Muller N, Hofler M, Lieb R, Wittchen HU. Social anxiety disorder and the risk of depression. Arch Gen Psychiatry 2001; 58:251–256.

37. Brown EJ, Heimberg RG, Juster HR. Social phobia subtype and avoidant personality disorder: effect on severity of social phobia, impairment, and outcome of cognitive-behavioral treatment. Behav Ther 1995; 26:467–480.

38. Herbert JD, Hope DA, Bellack AS. Validity of the distinction between generalized social phobia and avoidant personality disorder. J Abnorm Psychol 1992; 101:332–339.

39. Holt CS, Heimberg RG, Hope DA. Avoidant personality disorder and the generalized subtype of social phobia. J Abnorm Psychol 1995; 101:318–325.

40. Johnson MR, Lydiard RB. Personality disorders in social phobia. Psychiatr Annu 1995; 25:554–563.

41. Schneier FR, Spitzer RL, Gibbon M, et al. The relationship of social phobia subtypes and avoidant personality disorder. Compr Psychiatry 1991; 32:496–502.

42. Turner SM, Beidel DC, Townsley RM. Social phobia: A comparison of specific and generalized subtypes and avoidant personality disorder. J Abnorm Psychol 1992; 101:326–331.

43. Hudson JL, Rapee RM. The origins of social phobia. Behav Modif 2000; 24:102–129.

44. Kendler DS, Darkowski LM, Prescott CA. Fears and phobias: reliability and heritability. Psychol Med 1999; 29:539–553.

45. Kendler DS, Neale MC, Kessler RC, et al. The genetic epidemiology of phobia in women. The interrelationship of agoraphobia, social phobia, situational phobia, and simple phobia. Arch Gen Psychiatry 1992; 49:273–281.
46. Skre I, Onstad S, Torgerson S, et al. A twin-study of DSM-III-R anxiety disorders. Acta Psychiatr Scand 1993; 88:85–92.
47. Torgerson S. Genetics of neuroses: the effect of sampling variation upon the twin concordance ratio. Br J Psychiatry 1983; 142:126–132.
48. Jablensky A. Epidemiological surveys of mental health of geographically defined populations of Europe. In: Weissman MM, Myers JK, Ross CE, eds. in Community Surveys of Psychiatric Disorders. New Brunswick, NJ: Rutgers University Press, 1986:257–313.
49. Kashani JH, Orvaschel H. A community study of anxiety in children and adolescents. Am J Psychiatry 1990; 147:313–318.
50. McGee R, Fehan M, Williams S, Partridge F, Silva P, Kelly J. DSM-III disorders in a large sample of adolescents. J Am Acad Child Adolesc Psychiatry 1990; 29:611–619.
51. Schneier FR, Heckelman LR, Garfinkel R, Campeas R, et al. Functional impairment in social phobia. J Clin Psychiatry 1994; 55(suppl 8):322–331.
52. Wittchen HU, Belloch E. The impact of social phobia and quality of life. Int Clin Psychopharmacol 1996; 11(suppl 3):15–23.
53. Ware JE, Gandek B, Group IP. The SF-36 Health Survey: development and use in mental health research and the IQOLA project. Int J Mental Health 1994; 23(suppl 2):49–73.
54. Wittchen HU, Stein MB, Kessler RC. Social fears and social phobia in a community sample of adolescents and young adults: prevalence, risk factors and comorbidity. Psychol Med 1999; 29:309–323.
55. Katzelnick DJ, Kobak KA, DeLeire T, et al. Impact of generalized anxiety disorder in managed care. Am J Psychiatry 2001; 158(suppl 12):1999–2007.
56. Wittchen M, Sonntag H, Mueller N, Liebowitz M. Disability and quality of life in pure and comorbid social phobia: findings from a controlled study. Eur Psychiatry 2000; 15:46–58.

4

Comorbidity in Social Anxiety Disorder

Lydia Fehm and Hans-Ulrich Wittchen
Dresden University of Technology
Dresden, Germany

I. INTRODUCTION

Is comorbidity an artifact of our current way of conceptualizing and defining mental disorders, or does it provide useful information in terms of etiology, pathogenesis, and therapeutic or preventive issues? This remains a core question despite the fact that many researchers have addressed it in the past two decades from various perspectives. The main obstacle for a better understanding of comorbidity is the fact that researchers still define and evaluate comorbidity with a considerable degree of variability in terms, for example, of the scope of disorders considered, consideration of temporal relationships among each other, and the level of detail with regard to both predictors and critical outcomes (e.g., disability, treatment response). As a result, the literature sometimes has a confusing mix of partly contradictory findings. It seems fair to state that this situation applies not only to mood and anxiety disorders in general but also to social anxiety disorder (SAD) in particular. This chapter begins with a brief discussion of critical conceptual issues and then reviews several facets of comorbidity in social anxiety disorder, emphasizing potential etiological and clinical implications.

A. Critical Issues in Dealing with Comorbidity

"Comorbidity is defined as the presence of more than one disorder in a person in a defined period of time" (1). This more general definition of comorbidity has been found to apply equally well in epidemiological, basic, and clinical contexts. It also highlights the critical aspects that need consideration in interpreting comorbidity findings:

1. *Unit of analysis*: As indicated by the word *morbus*, the term *comorbidity* should be restricted to generally accepted and clearly defined "disorders," such as those defined by the *International Classification of Diseases*, 10th ed. (ICD-10) or by the *Diagnostic and Statistical Manual of Mental Disorders*, 4th ed. (DSM-IV). Unfortunately some authors have also used this term to study syndromal overlap—for example, by including subthreshold manifestations of disorders. This approach can lead to conceptual problems and result in findings that are difficult to interpret and to compare.

2. *Scope of disorders*: Without defining clearly what range of disorders is studied, the interpretation of findings is difficult. Despite the fact that DSM-IV, for example, operationalizes about 500 disorders, most studies have examined only a restricted range of disorders. Some studies examined the association of SAD with only one or two disorders (i.e., major depression and alcohol dependence), others have used a much wider scope (all specific anxiety disorders, all mood, or substance use disorders), and a few even go beyond this range by covering somatoform, eating, psychotic and general medical disorders. As a result of this choice, some will come to the conclusion that only 20 to 30% of SAD cases are comorbid and those with a much broader definition will find 70 to 80% comorbidity rates. Further, studies also frequently fail to indicate whether the DSM-IV differential diagnostic rules (hierarchies) are considered, which also have a remarkable effect on resulting comorbidity figures.

3. *Time frame and temporal resolution*: Much of the confusion in this field comes from the quite variable time period of risk: clinicians are used to consider primarily the cross-sectional picture, with time frames of 2 to 4 weeks, and sometimes even 6 months. In epidemiological and etiological research, however the co-occurrence of disorders is usually regarded for 1 year or even the whole lifespan (lifetime comorbidity). It is evident that the choice of time frame will dramatically influence rates of comorbidity (the longer the time span, the higher the rates). This issue is also confounded with another critical aspect rarely specifically addressed—namely, the age of the study group. Let us assume that the longer SAD persists, the higher the probability for major depression. This might imply that in adolescents there is only a moderate comorbidity with depression but that in adults comorbidity

rates are considerably increased. Yet it should be noted that even this pattern could be complicated—for example, if one assumes that SAD is getting milder or even remits spontaneously in late life, the association might get weaker again. Further, it must be emphasized that comorbidity findings also vary as a function of the level of detail regarding the temporal resolution. Prospective-longitudinal studies, usually interested in the sequencing of disorders, frequently use quite detailed descriptors for onset, offset, and duration (sequential comorbidity). In contrast to cross-sectional findings, such longitudinal methods have been shown to considerably increase the probability of a subject reporting comorbid conditions.

4. *Assessment and other methodological issues*: In addition, numerous other more technical factors play a role, such as: How are the units in question determined (e.g., by loosely structured clinical diagnoses or by standardized diagnostic instruments)? How was the study population sampled (e.g., representative community versus patients in specialized treatment settings)? How was the comorbidity rate calculated (e.g., simple percentage versus odds ratios)? How were possible confounding factors dealt with?

Each of these critical factors significantly influences the resulting comorbidity rates. Since most studies differ from each other in one or more of these aspects, it is confusing yet understandable that comorbidity findings for SAD and for most other disorders are quite variable.

Beyond the already complex determination of the size and the breadth of comorbidity in SAD, a more challenging issue is the exploration of pathogenesis. Over the past decade, for example, several longitudinal epidemiological studies have revealed that people with primary hypertension at early stages in life not only have an increased cross-sectional risk for other somatic disorders but also show a complex cascade of increased risks for developing diabetes, nephropathy, cardiovascular disease, and other arteriosclerotic conditions. The demonstration of these temporal relationships among disorders has resulted in searches for the mechanism involved and resulted in improved strategies of long-term care and management. Similar considerations apply to psychiatric disorders in general and SAD in particular. The core questions in this perspective are as follows: 1) Is disorder A (for example, SAD) an explicit cause of disorder B (depression), so that B would be a direct consequence of disorder A? 2) Is A an indirect cause of disorder B—for example, by lowering the threshold for the onset of B? 3) Are A and B caused by a third common factor—e.g., a genetic vulnerability? Whereas the former perspective has been associated with the "splitter" model, the latter is frequently described as being the "lumper's" perspective (2).

Clearly such an endeavor is much more challenging in terms of design, assessment, and statistical analyses, and it should also be noted that the three patterns are not exclusive but may also overlap or interact. Furthermore, different causal patterns may play a role during the course of the disorder (e.g., onset versus fluctuations in symptomatology).

With these critical methodological considerations in mind, we begin by presenting cross-sectional results assessing lifetime comorbidity retrospectively. Then, several stimulating studies using longitudinal designs are discussed, aiming at a determination of temporal patterns of comorbidity. Finally, we discuss the implications of comorbidity for the course of SAD as well as for treatment outcome.

II. SAD COMORBIDITY IN CROSS-SECTIONAL DESIGNS

Overall, comorbidity seems to be the rule rather than the exception—which is true not only for SAD but also for the majority of other psychiatric disorders. For SAD, epidemiological studies in the community yield lifetime comorbidity rates with any other mental disorder between 69 (3) and 81% (4). Similar rates were also reported in a study among primary care attenders (81%) (5). Data collected in clinical samples can be expected to reveal even higher rates, because patients in clinical treatment can be too severely impaired, demoralized, and sensitized to report all their symptoms. In particular SAD sufferers in clinical settings should reveal higher rates for depression, as it has been reported that these patients are more likely to seek treatment or to receive professional attention when being demoralized and meeting criteria for depressive disorders (3,6).

Three groups of disorders were particularly frequently studied and proved to be strongly associated with SAD: other anxiety disorders, mood disorders, and substance problems/disorders. Yet it should be noted that these studies mostly did not pay attention to other disorders. For example, associations with sleep disorders, somatoform disorders, and so on were rarely studied.

A. Other Anxiety Disorders

Epidemiological community studies find fairly consistently that up to 50% of persons with SAD report at least one other anxiety disorder: 57% (4) and 50% (7). Lower rates emerge when only cross-sectional patterns (e.g., other current disorders) are regarded: 9.1% in the ECA[*] (8) and 19.2% in a French primary care study[†] (9).

---

[*]ECA: Epidemiologic Catchment Area study; 4 U.S. regions, $N = 13,537$; adults.
[†]Region of Paris, France; $N = 2096$ of whom 405 were interviewed; adults.

On the level of single disorders, high comorbidity rates are reported for specific phobia [ranging from 37.6% in the NCS[*] (4) to a high of 60.8% in the ECA (10)] as well as for agoraphobia [ranging from 8.8% in the EDSP[†] (7), to 45% in the ECA (10)] and panic disorder [ranging from 4.7% in the ECA (3), to 26.9% in the "Zürich Study" (11,12)]. Somewhat lower rates are reported for generalized anxiety disorder (2 to 27%) (4,7,10); obsessive compulsive disorder (2 to 19%) (3,7,10); and posttraumatic stress disorder (5 to 16%) (4,7,10).

Thus there is considerable agreement from various cross-sectional community studies that among subjects with SAD, the vast majority also suffer from at least one other anxiety disorder. In two studies, differences of SAD generalized versus nongeneralized subtype were also explored. The generalized subtype is characterized not only by higher degrees of impairment and higher help-seeking rates (13) but also by stronger comorbidity (14).

B. Mood Disorders

Among subjects with SAD in the community, roughly 41% are estimated to also suffer from mood disorders (OR = 3.74; 95% CI = 3.14 to 4.45) (4). It is noteworthy that all affective disorders showed strong and significant associations with SAD [depression, odds ratios ranging from 2.69 (7) to 6.8 (10); dysthymia, 2.7 (6) to 5.03 (7); bipolar disorders, 4.60 (4) to 6.8 (10)].

When only the percentages of comorbidity are regarded, a different but (due to the neglect of differing base rates) incorrect picture would emerge: e.g., 16.6% of all respondents having lifetime comorbid major depression and 12.5% comorbid dysthymia but only 4.7% bipolar disorder (3).

It is noteworthy that this association is seen not only in adult samples such as the NCS (major depression OR = 3.65, dysthymia OR = 3.15, mania OR = 4.60; (4)) but also in adolescents and young adults up to age to 24 (EDSP: major depression OR = 2.69, dysthymia OR = 5.03, (7)). Thus, social anxiety disorder is closely associated with mood disorders (6, 15–17). The generalized subtype of SAD reveals generally higher associations, whereas pure speaking phobias and other discrete SADs have a considerably lower risk for comorbidity with depressive disorders (13,14).

C. Alcohol and Substance Abuse

Alcohol and substance use problems constitute a third group of disorders frequently dealt with in epidemiological studies. Most studies have examined

---

[*]NCS: National Comorbidity Survey, United States; $N = 8098$; age 15 to 54.
[†]EDSP: Early Developmental Stages of Psychopathology; $N = 3021$; age: 14 to 24.

the association with alcohol use and alcohol disorders; however, more recently smoking and nicotine dependence have been addressed as well (18). In a case-control design we demonstrated that adult cases with SAD drink and smoke significantly more than subjects without SAD as well as subjects in the control group with recurrent herpes infections (19). In community studies SAD subjects were found to be significantly more likely to also meet criteria for either alcohol abuse or dependence [e.g., abuse: OR = 2.2; 95% CI = 1.64 to 2.96, (3); dependence: OR = 2.17; 95% CI = 1.78 to 2.64; (4)]. This could not be confirmed for a younger sample in the EDSP [alcohol abuse/dependence: OR = 1.14, 95% CI = 0.76 to 1.72; (7)]. It is noteworthy that no consistently elevated risk for illegal substance disorders was found: significant association for drug abuse, OR = 2.85; 95% CI = 2.04 to 4.00 (3), and drug dependence, OR = 2.56; 95% CI = 1.93 to 3.40 (4), were found in some studies, but other studies yielded different results—e.g., drug abuse, OR = 1.24, 95% CI = 0.85 to 1.81 (4), and OR = 1.67, 95% CI = 0.89 to 3.13 (7).

Clinical samples have revealed even higher associations between social anxiety disorder and alcohol dependence, estimating that about 25% of patients with social anxiety disorder also meet criteria for (lifetime) alcohol dependence (20). In contrast to anxiety and mood disorders, the generalized and nongeneralized subtype seem not to differ with regard to the degree of comorbidity with substance problems (13,14).

D. Eating Disorders

Eating disorders deserve special interest from an etiopathogenic and differential diagnostic perspective (symptoms of eating disorders are diagnostic exclusionary criteria for SAD in DSM-IV), yet this association has rarely been dealt with in community studies. In a representative sample of over 3000 adolescents and young adults, only slightly higher rates of eating disorders among SAD sufferers were found (OR = 1.99; 95% CI = 0.93 to 4.27) (7). A similar association was found in the "Zürich Study" for binge eating (OR = 2.8) (12). However, it is noteworthy that for clinical samples with eating disorders, various reports have pointed to high rates of SAD: 55% patients with anorexia nervosa, 45 to 59% bulimics, and 36.4% obese binge eaters were found to have SAD (21,22). It remains open to question whether this considerable difference between epidemiological and clinical study findings is due to selection biases, methodological differences, or special characteristics in treatment of eating disorders.

E. Body Dysmorphic Disorder

Only recently attention was drawn to the relation of social anxiety disorder to body dysmorphic disorder (BDD) (see, for example, Refs. 23 and 24).

BDD can be a debilitating and chronic disorder characterized by an imagined defect in appearance (25,26). Although community surveys are unavailable, clinical studies indicate a strong association of BDD and SAD: it is estimated that among BDD patients, between 10 and 23% (24,27,28) also meet criteria for SAD. It is noteworthy that one of the studies presented evidence for similarities of SAD and BDD on the level of information processing (29). There are also indications that SAD precedes BDD in most to all cases examined [80% (30)/100% (28)].

F. General Medical Disorders

Only a fragmentary picture exists for the relation of SAD and general medical disorders. This is remarkable, since the SAD exclusionary criteria include conditions like Parkinson's disease, stuttering, and other potentially socially embarrassing somatic conditions as potential diagnostic exclusionary criteria. Community findings, however, have revealed that among all SAD subjects, only very few have general medical conditions that would apply for this exclusion rule (7).

Beyond these findings, the ECA study (10) revealed elevated risks of participants with social anxiety disorder for peptic ulcer disease (OR: 2.0; 95% CI: 1.1 to 3.6) and neurological disorders (OR: 3.0; 95% CI: 1.1 to 13.8). However, no significant association emerged for the other eleven chronic medical conditions considered in the study. A similar picture emerges within a more recent study in Germany with a representative adult sample in the community (Fehm and Jacobi, unpublished data; for details of this study, see Ref. 31). Table 1 reveals significant associations between SAD and ulcers, endocrine disorders, and musculoskeletal diseases. Whereas neurological disorders as a group showed no significant association with SAD, Parkinson's disease alone was significantly more prevalent in SAD (not taking into account the DSM-IV exclusionary rule). It must be noted that with the exception of Parkinson's disease, these associations may not be specific pathological patterns for SAD but rather may reflect a strong association of psychiatric and medical problems, which can also be found in other conditions.

One study analyzed the relationship between SAD and essential tremor in detail, examining SAD both preceding and following the onset of essential tremor (32). In this study, 21.6% of essential tremor cases had a lifetime diagnosis of SAD, and its onset occurred about as often before the onset of essential tremor as after it. Much higher rates of SAD were found among patients with spasmodic torticollis, characterized by intermittent or sustained deviations of the head and neck. Up to 41.3% of the patients with spasmodic torticollis also met criteria for current SAD (33). The vast

TABLE 1 Comorbidity of Social Anxiety Disorder and Selected Somatic Disorders in a Representative Adult Sample (12-month Prevalence Rate; $N = 4170$)

Somatic disorder	Prevalence (%)		
	no SAD	SAD	OR
Hypertension	13.1	11.0	.91
Cardiac diseases—e.g., angina pectoris	2.95	1.24	.46
Cerebrovascular diseases—e.g., stroke	0.8	1.1	1.66
Chronic-obstructive pulmonary diseases—e.g., asthma	7.5	12.8	1.81
Ulcers, gastritis	7.5	15.7	2.24[a]
Endocrine disorders—e.g., thyroid gland disease	11.3	23.1	2.05[a]
Metabolic syndromes—e.g., high cholesterol	14.5	20.7	1.93
Neurological diseases—e.g., migraine	10.7	17.2	1.50
Parkinson's disease alone	.07	.78	14.31[a]
Musculoskeletal diseases—e.g., different forms of arthritis	26.3	33.9	1.81[a]
Allergies—e.g., hay fever, neurodermatitis	23.8	28.5	1.12
Any somatic disorder	69.91	77.96	1.56

Key: SAD, social anxiety disorder; OR, odds ratio.
[a] $p < 0.05$.

majority (80%) reported the onset of SAD after the onset of spasmodic torticollis.

IV. TEMPORAL PATTERNS OF COMORBIDITY

From a lifelong perspective, two simple theoretical assumptions can be made to explain the considerable degree of comorbidity observed with SAD and other disorders (Fig. 1):

1. Preexisting disorders may promote the development of SAD as well as its onset and presentation. This hypothesis has, however, found almost no consistent support from longitudinal studies to date. Since the first onset of SAD is almost invariably during childhood or early adulthood at the latest (7,34) and no consistent childhood psychopathological disorder has been found to precede SAD, it is unlikely that this assumption is valid.
2. SAD is much more likely to enhance the risk of a wide variety of other disorders, and there is also evidence that comorbid disorders beginning after the onset of SAD may influence the course of SAD

as well as presentation, associated degree of disability, and help-seeking behavior.

3. As a third more complex variant, the concurrence of the two disorders with or without a common etiological basis has to be considered. Three candidates are currently being explored in prospective family investigations: familial transmission, family climate, and behavioral inhibition as a temperamental precursor (35). But also the style of child rearing, restricted exposure to social situations within the family, as well as parental modeling have been discussed as possible source of familial aggregation of SAD (36).

On the basis of both retrospective cross-sectional data as well as prospective longitudinal data, there is little doubt that SAD is mostly a primary disorder within the temporal course. This is true for anxiety disorders (3,4,37) with the exception of specific phobias developing more often before the onset of SAD than after it (38) as well as for depressive disorders (3,5,6,17,39,40) and substance abuse disorders (34,41) but less so for bipolar disorders (Fig. 2).

Most studies providing insight into temporal patterns rely on retrospective data, which may be subject to recall biases. Only longitudinal studies allow controlling for those possible sources of error.

One of those studies compared cases of SAD without current or previous depression at baseline to persons with no mental disorders and found a significantly higher risk (OR: 3.5; 95% CI: 2.0 to 6.0) for patients with SAD to develop a depressive episode during the follow-up period of about 4 years (42). Further strong indications were found for SAD as being a risk factor for a more malignant course in terms of number of and duration of

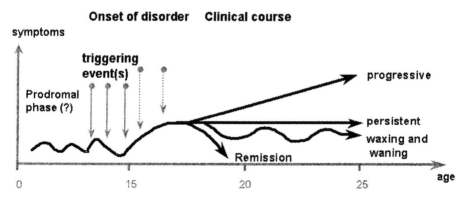

FIGURE 1 Developmental model for onset and course in social anxiety disorder.

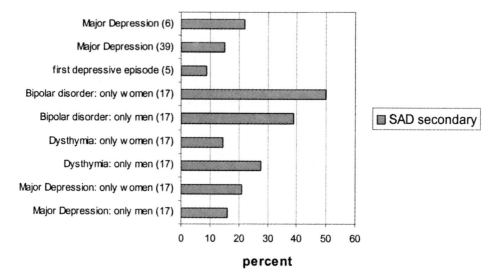

FIGURE 2 Temporal relations of social anxiety disorder and affective disorders.

episodes as well as suicidality (42). Persons with SAD and depressive disorder at baseline were at a significantly higher risk for experiencing new depressive episodes or higher persistence of present episodes (OR: 2.3; CI 95%: 1.2 to 4.6). The role of SAD as a risk factor for alcohol abuse is inconsistent: one prospective study examining the temporal pattern of SAD and alcoholism found no significantly higher risk for individuals with SAD to abuse alcohol or develop dependence on it. However, another study revealed that even subthreshold SAD is associated with an increased risk of developing a drinking problem (OR: 2.41) as well as alcohol abuse/dependence (OR: 2.30) (8). This may point to alcohol as a means of coping with social situations that are routinely avoided by individuals with full-blown SAD. The possible risk role of SAD recently received further support in a prospective longitudinal study among adolescents and young adults, where SAD was identified as a significant baseline predictor of regular as well as hazardous use of alcohol as well as of the persistence of already existing alcohol dependence over a 4- to 5-year follow-up period (43).

V. IMPLICATIONS OF COMORBIDITY/ PROGNOSTIC ISSUES

Comorbidity has been shown to have multiple implications: disability and quality of life have been shown to be significantly reduced in pure SAD subjects in community samples; further, both measures are considerably worse when comorbid conditions are present. Particularly strong moderators of the degree of disability are depressive disorders (Ref. 44, pp. 148 and 149). There are also indications that the natural (untreated) course of SAD in community samples is worse in comorbid as compared to pure (uncomplicated) SAD (10,45), although it should be noted that prospective follow-up studies investigating treated patients could not affirm these relationships (46,47).

Consistent with these indications that comorbid SAD is associated with increased levels of suffering, affected subjects are more likely to seek treatment and/or to be in treatment than those with uncomplicated SAD (6,48). In fact, it has been assumed that people with SAD receive treatment only when this is complicated by depression, whereas the influence of the subtype (generalized versus nongeneralized) seems to have an even higher impact, with the generalized subtype being associated with higher treatment rates (7).

The role of comorbidity for treatment response, in turn, has not been extensively researched. The level of pretreatment depression was identified as a predictor of treatment outcome (49), as treatment groups with either comorbid anxiety or depressive disorders had higher posttreatment scores in impairment (50). Individuals with comorbid conditions were more impaired before treatment, but treatment responses did not differ accordingly.

VI. CONCLUSION

Clearly, after two decades of research, it is become apparent that comorbidity is not simply an artifact of our currently deficient classificatory models and assessment modes. Although still conceived as a nuisance in clinical practice, this overview has shown that comorbidity in SAD provides valuable clues for a better understanding of the pathogenesis of SAD and the clinical and public health implications of this disorder. Despite the fact that the core questions of common underlying vulnerabilities across diagnostic boundaries is still unresolved, current diagnostic models provide a reliable way to diagnose the disorder and to communicate the diagnosis effectively to patients and their significant others. This alone enhances the earlier recognition of a "silent" disorder such as SAD by health care practitioners and thus enhances the chance for the provision of early treatment. Based on the evidence presented above, this seems to be of utmost importance in SAD as a disorder that not only occurs early in the person's life, affecting social roles and performance dramatically, but more importantly raises considerably the risk for secondary disorders. We have highlighted that in particular the incidence of depression and substance abuse disorders is not only strongly increased but, further, that these conditions more frequently run a malignant course. These findings strongly suggest the need to determine whether earlier and more effective interventions by psychological and drug therapies will be able to significantly reduce the complex pattern of secondary comorbidity associated with SAD.

REFERENCES

1. Wittchen H-U. What is comorbidity—fact or artefact? Br J Psychiatry 1996;168(suppl 30):7–8.
2. Wittchen HU, Kessler RC, Pfister H, Lieb R. Why do people with anxiety disorders become depressed? A prospective-longitudinal community study. Acta Psychiatr Scand 2000;102:14–23.
3. Schneier FR, Johnson J, Hornig CD, Liebowitz MR, Weissman MM. Social phobia. Comorbidity and morbidity in an epidemiologic sample. Arch Gen Psychiatry 1992;49:282–288.
4. Magee WJ, Eaton WW, Wittchen HU, McGonagle KA, Kessler RC. Agoraphobia, simple phobia, and social phobia in the national comorbidity survey. Arch Gen Psychiatry 1996;53:159–168.
5. Weiller E, Bisserbe J-C, Boyer P, Lépine JP, Lecrubier Y. Social phobia in general health care: an unrecognised undertreated disabling disorder. Br J Psychiatry 1996;168:169–174.
6. Kessler RC, Stang P, Wittchen H-U, Stein M, Walters EE. Lifetime co-morbidities between social phobia and mood disorders in the US National Comorbidity Survey. Psychol Med 1999;29:555–567.
7. Wittchen H-U, Stein MB, Kessler RC. Social fears and social phobia in a community sample of adolescents and young adults: prevalence, risk factors and co-morbidity. Psychol Med 1999;29:309–323.
8. Crum RM, Pratt LA. Risk of heavy drinking and alcohol use disorders in social phobia: a prospective analysis. Am J Psychiatry 2001;158:1693–1700.
9. Lecrubier Y. Comorbidity in social anxiety disorder: impact on disease burden and management. Clin Psychiatry 1998;59:33–37.
10. Davidson JRT, Hughes DL, George LK, Blazer DG. The epidemiology of social phobia: findings from the Duke Epidemiological Catchment Area Study. Psychol Med 1993;23:709–718.
11. Degonda M, Angst J. The Zürich Study XX. Social phobia and agoraphobia. Eur Arch Psychiatr Clin Neurosci 1993;243:95–102.
12. Angst J. Comorbidity of anxiety, phobia, compulsion and depression. Int Clin Psychopharmacol 1993;8:21–25.
13. Kessler RC, Stein MB, Berglund P. Social phobia subtypes in the National Comorbidity Survey. Am J Psychiatry 1998;155(5):613–619.
14. Stein MB, Chavira DA. Subtypes of social phobia and comorbidity with depression and other anxiety disorders. J Affect Disord 1998;50:11–16.
15. Rihmer Z, Szadoczky E, Furedi J, Kiss K, Papp Z. Anxiety disorders co-morbidity in bipolar I, bipolar II and unipolar major depression: results from a population-based study in Hungary. J Affect Disord 2001;67(1–3):175–179.

16. Zimmerman M, Chelminski I, McDermut W. Major depressive disorder and axis I diagnostic comorbidity. J Clini Psychiatry 2002;63(3):187–193.

17. de Graaf R, Bijl RV, Spijker J, Beekmann ATF, Vollebergh WAM. Temporal sequencing of lifetime mood disorders in relation to comorbid anxiety and substance use disorders. Findings from the Netherlands Mental Health Survey and Incidence Study. Soc Psychiatry Psychiatr Epidemiol 2003;38:1–11.

18. Sonntag H, Wittchen HU, Höfler M, Kessler RC, Stein MB. Are social fears and DSM-IV social anxiety disorder associated with smoking and nicotine dependence in adolescents and young adults? Eur Psychiatry 2000;15: 67–74.

19. Wittchen H-U, Fuetsch M, Sonntag H, Müller N, Liebowitz M. Disability and quality of life in pure and comorbid social phobia. Findings from a controlled study. Eur Psychiatry 2000;15(1):46–58.

20. Lépine J-P, Pélissolo A. Social phobia and alcoholism: a complex relationship. J Affect Disord 1998;50:S23–S28.

21. Godart NT, Flament MF, Lecrubier Y, Jeammet P. Anxiety disorders in anorexia nervosa and bulimia nervosa: co-morbidity and chronology of appearance. Eur Psychiatry 2000;15:38–45.

22. Schwalberg MD, Barlow DH, Alger SA, Howard LJ. Comparison of bulimics, obese binge eaters, social phobics, and individuals with panic disorder on comorbidity across DSM-III-R anxiety disorders. J Abnorm Psychol 1992;101(4): 675–681.

23. Schneier FR, Blanco C, Antia SX, Liebowitz MR. The social anxiety spectrum. Psychiatr Clin North Am 2002;25(4):757–774.

24. Stangier U, Hungerbühler R, Meyer A, Wolter M. Diagnostische Erfassung der Körperdysmorphen Störung [Assessment of body dysmorphic disorder: a pilot study]. Nervenarzt 2000;71:876–884.

25. Phillips KA. Body dysmorphic disorder: the distress of imagined ugliness. Am J Psychiatry 1991;148:1138–1149.

26. Phillips KA. Body dysmorphic disorder: diagnosis and treatment of imagined ugliness. J Clin Psychiatry 1996;57:61–65.

27. Brawman-Mintzer O, Lydiard RB, Phillips KA, Morton A, Czepowicz V, Emmanuel N, Villareal G, Johnson M, Ballenger CJ. Body dysmorphic disorder in patients with anxiety disorders and major depression: a comorbidity study. Am J Psychiatry 1995;152(11):1665–1667.

28. Wilhelm S, Otto MW, Zucker BG, Pollack MH. Prevalence of body dysmorphic disorder in patients with anxiety disorders. J Anxiety Disord 1997; 11(5):499–502.

29. Buhlmann U, McNally RJ, Wilhelm S, Florin I. Selective processing of emotional information in body dysmorphic disorder. J Anxiety Disord 2002;16(3): 289–298.

30. Phillips KA, McElroy SL, Keck PE, Pope HG, Hudson JI. Body dysmorphic disorder: 30 cases of imagined ugliness. Am J Psychiatry 1993;150:302–308.

31. Jacobi F, Wittchen HU, Hölting C, Sommer S, Lieb R, Höfler M, Pfister H. Estimating the prevalence of mental and somatic disorders in the community:

aims and methods of the German National Health Interview and Examination Survey. Int J Methods Psychiatr Res 2002;11(1):1–18.

32. Schneier FR, Barnes LF, Albert SM, Louis ED. Characteristics of social phobia among persons with essential tremor. J Clin Psychiatry 2001;62(5):367–372.

33. Gündel H, Wolf A, Xidara V, Busch R, Ceballos-Baumann AO. Social Phobia in spasmodic torticollis. J Neurol Neurosurg Psychiatry 2001;71:499–504.

34. Wittchen H-U, Fehm L. Epidemiology and natural course of social fears and social phobia. Acta Psychiatr Scand 2003;108(suppl 417):4–18.

35. Lieb R, Wittchen H-U, Höfler M, Fuetsch M, Stein MB, Merikangas KR. Parental psychopathology, parenting styles, and the risk of social phobia in offspring: a prospective longitudinal community study. Arch Gen Psychiatry 2000; 57(9):859–866.

36. Hudson JL, Rapee RM. The origins of social phobia. Behav Modif 2000;24(1):102–129.

37. Faravelli C, Zucchi T, Viviani B, Salmoria R, Perone A, Paionni A, Scarpato B, Vigliaturo D, Rosi S, D'adamo D, Bartolozzi D, Cecchi C, Abrardi L. Epidemiology of social phobia: a clinical approach. Eur Psychiatry 2000;15:17–24.

38. Merikangas KR, Angst J. Comorbidity and social phobia: evidence from clinical, epidemiologic, and genetic studies. Eur Arch Psychiatry Clin Neurosci 1995;244:297–303.

39. Schatzberg AF, Samson JA, Rothschild AJ, Bond TC, Regier DA. McLean Hospital Depression Research Facility: early-onset phobic disorders and adult-onset major depression. Br J Psychiatry 1998;173 (suppl 34):29–34.

40. Van Amerigen M, Mancini C, Styan G, Donison D. Relationships of social phobia with other psychiatric illness. J Affect Disord 1991;21:93–99.

41. Merikangas KR, Angst J, Eaton W, Canino G, Rubio-Stipec M, Wacker H, Wittchen HU, Andrade L, Essau C, Whitaker A, Kraemer H, Robins LN, Kupfer DJ. Comorbidity and boundaries of affective disorders with anxiety disorders and substance misuse: results of an international task force. Br J Psychiatry 1996;168 (suppl 30):58–67.

42. Stein MB, Fuetsch M, Müller N, Höfler M, Lieb R, Wittchen HU. Social anxiety disorder and the risk of depression: a prospective community study of adolescents and young adults. Arch Gen Psychiatry 2001;58:251–256.

43. Zimmermann P, Wittchen HU, Höfler M, Pfister H, Kessler RC, Lieb R. Primary anxiety disorders and the development of subsequent alcohol use disorders: a four-year community study of adolescents and young adults. Psychol Med 2003;33:1211–1222.

44. Müller N. Die soziale Angststörung bei Jugendlichen und jungen Erwachsenen: Erscheinungsformen, Verlauf und Konsequenzen. Münster: Waxmann, 2002.

45. DeWit DJ, Ogborne A, Offord DR, MacDonald K. Antecedents of the risk of recovery from DSM-III-R social phobia. Psychol Med 1999;29:569–582.

46. Reich J, Goldenberg I, Goisman RM, Vasile RG, Keller M. A prospective follow-along study of the course of social phobia: II. Testing for basic predictors of course. J Nerv Ment Dis 1994;182(5):297–301.

47. Last CG, Perrin S, Hersen M, Kazdin AE. A prospective study of childhood anxiety disorders. J Am Acad Child Adolesc Psychiatry 1996;35(11):1502–1510.

48. Lecrubier Y, Wittchen HU, Faravelli C, Bobes J, Patel A, Knapp M. A European perspective on social anxiety disorder. Eur Psychiatry 2000;15:5–16.

49. Chambless DJ, Tran GQ, Glass CR. Predictors of response to cognitive-behavioural group therapy for social phobia. J Anxiety Disord 1997;11:221–240.

50. Erwin BA, Heimberg RG, Juster H, Mindlin M. Comorbid anxiety and mood disorders among persons with social anxiety disorder. Behav Res Ther 2002;40:19–35.

5

Burden of Social Anxiety Disorder

David S. Baldwin and Christel Buis
University of Southampton,
Southampton, United Kingdom

I. INTRODUCTION

Social anxiety disorder (social phobia) is one of the most common mental disorders. Recent epidemiological studies have reported a lifetime prevalence for social anxiety disorder of around 13 to 14% (1,2). Being so common and having a typical onset in midadolescence (3) and a lengthy course (4), social anxiety disorder is responsible for considerable and prolonged individual suffering. It is also associated with marked impairment in social and occupational function, reduction in quality of life, increased risk of alcohol and drug abuse, and an increased risk of attempted suicide. The condition is therefore also associated with a substantial economic burden.

II. SOCIAL AND OCCUPATIONAL FUNCTIONING

The typical onset of symptoms by midadolescence interferes with academic progress, entry into employment, and ability to form and maintain interpersonal relationships. In an early case-control study using the Disability Profile and Liebowitz Self-Rated Disability Scale to assess lifetime and cross-sectional functional impairment, patients with social anxiety disorder ($n = 32$) were more impaired across a range of measures than matched

65

healthy controls. More than half of the patients reported significant impairment in a number of domains including education, employment, and family and romantic relationships (5).

The social and occupational impairment associated with social anxiety disorder was examined through data collected in primary health care centers in France in parallel with the World Health Organization Study on Psychological Problems in General Health Care (2). More than 50% of the patients ($n = 38$) who fulfilled criteria for social anxiety disorder had either moderate or severe disability in areas relating to daily routine and performance. On average, patients with social anxiety disorder reported 5.4 disability days in

TABLE 1 Disability in Social Anxiety Disorder with or Without Comorbid Depression—Results from the French Primary Care Study

	Social anxiety disorder		
Variable	Without depression $N = 16$	With depression $N = 22$	Healthy controls $N = 152$
Social disability schedule Percent of patients with moderate or severe disability			
Adjustment to daily routine	33.3	75.0[b]	22.5
Performance	53.3[b]	62.5[b]	19.1
Contact with others	40.0[b]	37.5[b]	10.7
Other daily activities	26.7	72.7[b]	20.4
Disability days (mean in past month)	1.4	9.6[b]	1.9
Alcohol abuse or dependence	25.0	31.8	-
Risk of suicide			
History of suicidal thoughts	50.0[a]	77.3[a]	14.5
History of suicide attempts	6.3	45.5[c]	5.3
Overall health (percent fair or poor)	43.8[a]	77.3[a,c]	12.7

Sources: Refs. 2 and 6.
[a] $p < 0.05$ versus controls.
[b] $p < 0.01$ versus controls.
[c] $p < 0.05$ versus subjects with social anxiety disorder without depression.

TABLE 2 Disability and Quality of Life in Social Anxiety Disorder—Results from the Canadian Community Resident Study

Variable	Odds ratio[a]	95% CI	Wald X^2 (df $= 1$)	p value
Dysfunction in main activity	8.48	4.57–15.71	46.06	<0.001
Dysfunction in other activities	7.94	4.70–13.42	60.03	<0.001
Troubled relationships	1.87	0.87–3.99	2.61	0.11
Inability to perform usual activities at least 1 day in last month	8.77	3.99–19.29	29.12	0.001
Failed a grade at school	1.77	1.38–2.28	20.14	<0.001
Leaving school early	1.77	1.39–2.26	21.36	<0.001
Dissatisfaction				
Main activity	1.82	1.21–2.75	8.13	<0.005
Family life	2.76	1.71–4.46	17.32	<0.001
Friends	5.95	2.50–14.15	16.24	<0.001
Leisure	2.41	1.65–3.52	20.67	<0.001
Income	1.90	1.47–2.45	24.15	<0.001
Poor score on Quality of Well-Being Scale	3.03	2.01–4.56	28.24	<0.001

[a]Odds ratios were derived from multiple logistic regression analyses with simultaneous entry of predictors (e.g., age, gender, etc.) and are adjusted for all other predictors in the model.

the previous month, significantly greater than the 2.3 disability days reported by the control group ($n = 152$).

In this study, the presence of comorbid depression was associated with greater functional disability in patients with social phobia. More than 70% of patients with comorbid social phobia had moderate or severe disability, compared to 30% of patients with social phobia uncomplicated by depression. Similarly, comorbid social phobia was associated with 9.6 disability days in the preceding month, compared to 1.4 disability days in patients without depression (6).

Further evidence for the substantial functional impairment associated with social anxiety disorder comes from the results of a more recent epidemiological study involving over 8000 residents aged 15 to 64 years in Ontario, Canada (7). Using the Composite Diagnostic Interview to assign DSM-III-R (*Diagnostic and Statistical Manual of Mental Disorders*, third revised edition) diagnoses, people with social phobia were impaired on a broad spectrum of measures. When compared to controls, those with generalized social phobia showed significantly more impairment in daily activities and dysfunction in interpersonal relationships. Social phobia was also associated with a significantly greater likelihood of failing to make a grade at school and of dropping out of school before graduation, these associations again being most marked in those with generalized social phobia (7).

III. QUALITY OF LIFE

The effects of social anxiety disorder on self-rated quality of life have not been studied extensively. The prospective epidemiological study of depressive, neurotic, and psychosomatic syndromes (the well-known "Zürich Study") in a community sample of young adults (8) found that quality of life in subjects with DSM-III–defined social anxiety disorder was poor compared to the general population. The domains of quality of life that were most affected were work, relationships (partners and friends), and retrospective perceptions of childhood (9).

A case-control study compared quality of life in 65 patients with DSM-III-R social anxiety disorder without comorbidity and 65 matched controls (patients with chronic herpes infection as a control for chronicity). Using a 36-item questionnaire developed for the Medical Outcomes Study (the SF-36) (10), subjects with social anxiety showed significantly lower scores on the domains of mental health, general health, vitality, role limitations, and social function (11).

The impact of social anxiety disorder on quality of life varies from that seen with other anxiety disorders. In a comparative study in patients with panic disorder, obsessive compulsive disorder, or social anxiety disorder, there was no difference in overall score on the Illness Intrusiveness Rating Scale, which assesses the perception of interference across 13 functional domains. However, patients with social anxiety disorder reported significantly more impairment in certain domains, including social relationships, self-expression, and self-improvement (12).

In the Canadian epidemiological study described earlier, people with social phobia were significantly more likely than controls to rate themselves as "low functioning" on the Quality of Well-Being Scale (13) and to report significantly greater dissatisfaction with work, family life, friends, leisure activities, and income. This effect was seen with or without lifetime comorbid depression (7).

IV. RISK OF SUBSTANCE MISUSE

The results of several epidemiological studies indicate that social anxiety disorder is associated with increased rates of alcohol abuse and dependence (14) (see also this volume, Fehm and Wittchen). In the Epidemiologic

Catchment Area study, the lifetime prevalences for alcohol and drug abuse in social phobia were 18.8 and 13.0%, respectively (15). Similar findings were seen in the National Comorbidity Survey, in which the lifetime prevalences for alcohol and drug abuse were 10.9 and 5.3%, respectively, the lifetime prevalence for alcohol and drug dependence being 23.9% and 14.8% (1).

Typically, social anxiety symptoms precede the development of substance misuse. In the Epidemiologic Catchment Area study, social anxiety disorder preceded alcohol abuse in 85% and drug abuse in 77% of community-based residents with comorbid conditions (15). These observations are supported by the findings of the National Comorbidity Survey, in which alcohol abuse or dependence occurred first in 6.4% of subjects and drug abuse or dependence in only 3.8%, in those with comorbid conditions (1). Further support is provided by the findings of the Zürich study, in which the typical pattern of onset was social anxiety disorder followed by depression and the later development of alcoholism in patients with the comorbid condition (16).

The findings of the French primary care study suggest that the association between social phobia and substance misuse, seen in community surveys, is not dependent upon the presence of comorbid depression. The prevalence of either harmful use or dependence on alcohol was 25.0% in those without depression and 31.8% in those with depression, but this difference was not significant (6).

Secondary analysis of data from the United Kingdom Psychiatric Morbidity Surveys indicates that social phobia was associated with a nonsignificant trend toward higher levels of alcohol dependence than in the general population. However, drug dependence and problems were significantly more frequent in the group with social phobia than in the population without mental health problems. This association was most marked in patients without comorbid depression (17).

Social anxiety disorder is also associated with an increased risk of cigarette smoking. The findings of the Early Developmental Stages of Psychopathology study, a prospective epidemiological survey of over 3000 subjects aged between 14 and 24 years (18), indicate that the prevalences of smoking in subjects with or without social anxiety disorder were 31.9 and 17.8%, respectively (19).

V.   RISK OF SUICIDE

When compared to the general population, patients with social anxiety disorder are at increased risk of attempted suicide. Traditionally this increase is regarded as being particularly remarkable in those patients with comorbid depression (15,20). However, a recent study of members of a United States Health Maintenance Organization found that 21.9% of subjects with generalized social anxiety disorder without comorbidity had attempted suicide (21).

The results of the French primary care study emphasize the role of comorbid depression in raising the risk of attempted suicide in social phobia. When compared to controls, suicidal thoughts were significantly more common in patients with social anxiety disorder with or without comorbid depression. However, a history of suicide attempts was significantly increased only over the rate in control, in those patients with comorbid depression (6).

VI. UTILIZATION OF HEALTH SERVICES

Despite the high level of associated impairment, patients with social anxiety disorder may be less likely than people with other anxiety disorders to seek help for their mental health problems. For example, the Duke Epidemiologic Catchment Area Survey found that 32.6% of the respondent subjects had consulted their doctor with psychological complaints, but only 3% had sought help for the symptoms of social anxiety disorder (22).

These early findings were confirmed in larger and more recent epidemiological studies. For example, in the National Comorbidity Survey, when people with social anxiety disorder were compared to people with agoraphobia, fewer had sought professional help (19 versus 41%), and fewer had used medication (6.2 versus 21.6%) (1).

Furthermore, analysis of data from the United Kingdom Psychiatric Morbidity Surveys indicated that people with social anxiety disorder used overall health services significantly less frequently than the population without mental health problems. However, consultations with general practitioners were significantly more frequent in the group with social phobia (27%) than in controls (27%) (17).

VII. ECONOMIC CONSEQUENCES

There have been few investigations of the economic burden associated with social anxiety disorder. Taken together, anxiety disorders account for around one-third of all costs associated with psychiatric illness (23). Much of this cost is attributable to reduced or lost work productivity—that is, it represents indirect costs rather than the direct costs arising from use of health and social services.

Epidemiological studies and analyses of Health Maintenance Organization data indicate that people with social phobia are more likely to be unemployed or absent from work and to have reduced productivity compared to the general population. (21,24). For example, in a primary care study (11), patients with social anxiety disorder showed a reduction in work productivity of around 12% compared to controls. In addition, 11% of patients were unemployed, compared to 3% of controls; furthermore, 8% of patients reported taking time off work because of their condition, amounting to an average of 12 hours in the previous week, and 23% reported a substantial impairment in working performance due to their symptoms (11).

The secondary analysis of data from the United Kingdom Psychiatric Morbidity Surveys indicates that social anxiety disorder is associated with a substantial economic burden. When compared to those without psychiatric morbidity ($n = 8501$), subjects with probable social anxiety disorder ($n = 63$), identified by an algorithm based on responses during the Clinical Interview Schedule–Revised (25), showed a substantial economic deficit. They were less likely to be in the highest socioeconomic groups and had lower employment rates and household incomes compared to those with no psychiatric morbidity (17). Using 1997–1998 prices, the annual costs of health services, lost employment, and benefits were notably greater in subjects with social phobia compared to the population without mental health problems. Social phobia was associated with significantly greater costs arising from consultations with general practitioners and with significantly greater costs arising from social security benefits (17).

TABLE 3 Economic Burden of Social Phobia

	Social phobia only $N = 36$		Comorbid social phobia $N = 27$		No mental health problems $N = 8185$	
Variable	Mean	SD	Mean	SD	Mean	SD
Physician visits	96.10	216.41	164.58	234.44	66.12	196.78
Inpatient	11.59	86.64	216.87	684.54	345.55	2465.5
Outpatient	110.40	121.00	157.16	146.59	110.42	173.93
Home visits	27.63	191.50	183.21	456.46	34.49	173.26
Counseling	177.13	680.77	30.03	98.84	89.98	770.30
Total health care costs	451.84	821.25	751.85	927.77	379.09	969.69
Cost of days off work	538.49	634.65	320.92	677.17	594.76	2245.2
Social security benefits	1106.22	1506.32	1816.52	2422.45	794.16	1519.04

Annual costs of health services, lost employment and benefits (£ at 1997/1998 prices).
Results from the United Kingdom Psychiatric Morbidity Survey.

VIII. IMPACT OF TREATMENT UPON DISABILITY AND WORK PRODUCTIVITY

Although social anxiety disorder is associated with considerable and persistent impairment, the results of randomized controlled trials indicate that effective relief of symptoms can result in a substantial reduction in disability. Most treatment studies (see later chapters) include measures of symptom-rated disability, and it is gratifying to see that disability can be reduced, sometimes even after short-term treatment in patients with long-lasting symptoms.

For example, the results of an international, multicenter, randomized, placebo-controlled, parallel-group, flexible-dose study (26) ($n = 290$) indicate that paroxetine was efficacious in reducing symptom-rated disability, as rated by the three-item Sheehan Disability Scale (27). There were significant advantages for paroxetine over placebo on the work item after 4 weeks of double-blind treatment, the family life item after 6 weeks, and the social life item at 12 weeks in patients with a mean duration of social anxiety disorder of over 15 years. Similar findings have been seen in other placebo-controlled studies with paroxetine.

These findings are supported by the results of an analysis of pooled data ($n = 1736$) from five multicenter, randomized, double-blind, placebo-controlled, parallel-group, flexible-dose 12-week treatment studies with extended-release venlafaxine (two of which also involved paroxetine as a comparator) (28). There were significant advantages for both venlafaxine and paroxetine over placebo on all three items of the Sheehan Disability Scale; furthermore the proportion of patients left with only mild disability at study endpoint was significantly higher with the two active treatments than with placebo.

IX. CONCLUSIONS

Social anxiety disorder is typically associated with a long-lasting, substantial, and pervasive impairment of social and occupational function, reduced quality of life, increased risk of substance misuse and dependence, elevated risk of attempted suicide, and a considerable economic burden. Short-term treatment studies indicate that effective relief of symptoms is associated with a reduction in symptom-related disability. Given the concern about cost containment in health service provision, studies of the cost-effectiveness of acute and continuation treatment in patients in primary care settings are needed.

REFERENCES

1. Magee WJ, Eaton WW, Wittchen HU, McGonagle KA, Kessler RC. Agoraphobia, simple phobia, and social phobia in the National Comorbidity Survey. Arch Gen Psychiatry 1996; 53: 159–168.

2. Weiller E, Bisserbe JC, Boyer P, Lépine JP, Lecrubier Y. Social phobia in general health care: an unrecognised, undertreated disabling condition. Br J Psychiatry 1996; 168: 169–174.

3. Beidel DC. Social anxiety disorder: etiology and early clinical presentation. J Clin Psychiatry 1998 (suppl 17): 27–31.

4. Reich J, Goldenberg I, Vasile R, Goisman R, Keller M. A prospective follow-up study of the course of social phobia. Psychiatry Res 1994; 54: 249–268.

5. Schneier FR, Heckelman LR, Garfinkel R, Campras R. Functional impairment in social phobia. J Clin Psychiatry 1994; 55: 322–331.

6. Lecrubier Y, Weiller E. Comorbidities in social phobia. Int Clin Psychopharmacol 1997; 12: 517–521.

7. Stein MB, Kean YM. Disability and quality of life in social phobia: epidemiological findings. Am J Psychiatry 2000; 157: 1606–1613.

8. Angst J, Dobler-Mikola MA, Binder J. The Zurich Study: a prospective epidemiological study of depressive, neurotic and psychosomatic syndromes. I. Problem, methodology. Eur Arch Psychiatr Neurol Sci 1984; 234: 13–20.

9. Bech P, Angst J. Quality of life in anxiety and social phobia. Int Clin Psychopharmacol 1996; 11 (suppl 3): 97–100.

10. Ware JE, Gandek B. The SF-36 health survey: development and use in mental health research and the IQOLA Project. Int J Mental Health 1994; 23: 49–73.

11. Wittchen HU, Beloch E. The impact of social phobia on quality of life. Int Clin Psychopharmacol 1996; 11 (suppl 3): 15–24.

12. Antony MM, Roth D, Swinson RP, Huta V, Devins GM. Illness intrusiveness in individuals with panic disorder, obsessive-compulsive disorder, or social phobia. J Nerv Ment Dis 1998; 186: 311–315.

13. McDowell I, Newell C. Measuring Health: A Guide to Rating Scales and Questionnaires. New York: Oxford University Press, 1987.

14. Lépine JP, Pélissolo A. Social phobia and alcoholism: a complex relationship. J Affect Disord 1998; 50 (suppl): S23–S28.

15. Schneier FR, Spitzer RL, Gibbon M, Fyer AJ, Liebowitz MR, Weissman MM. Social phobia. Comorbidity in an epidemiological sample. Arch Gen Psychiatry 1992; 49:282–288.

16. Angst J, Vollrath M, Merikangas KR, Ernst C. Comorbidity of anxiety and depression in the Zurich cohort study of young adults. In: Maser J, Cloninger CR (eds). Comorbidity of mood and anxiety disorders. Washington, DC: American Psychiatric Press, 1990.

17. Patel A, Knapp M, Henderson J, Baldwin DS. The economic consequences of social phobia. J Affect Disord 2002; 68: 221–233.

18. Wittchen HU, Stein M, Kessler RC. Social fears and social phobia in a community sample of adolescents and young adults: prevalence, risk factors and comorbidity. Psychol Med 1999; 29: 309–323.

19. Nelson CB, Wittchen HU. Smoking and nicotine dependence. Results from a sample of 14- to 24-years old in Germany. Eur Addict Res 1998; 4: 42–49.

20. Lépine JP, Lellouch J. Diagnosis and epidemiology of agoraphobia and social phobia. Clin Neuropharmacol 1995; 18 (suppl 2): S15–S26.

21. Katzelnick DJ, Kobak KA, DeLire T, et al. Impact of generalised social anxiety disorder in managed care. Am J Psychiatry 2001; 158: 1999–2007.
22. Davidson JRT, Hughes DL, George LK, et al. The epidemiology of social phobia: findings from the Duke Epidemiological Catchment Area study. Psychol Med 1993; 23: 709–718.
23. DuPont RL, Rice DP, Miller LS, Shiraki SS, Rowland CR, Harwood HJ. Economic costs of anxiety disorders. Anxiety 1996; 2: 167–172.
24. Wittchen HU, Sonntag H, Mueller N, Liebowitz M. Disability and quality of life in pure and comorbid social phobia: findings from a controlled study. Eur Psychiatry 2000; 15: 46–58.
25. Lewis G, Pelosi AJ. Manual of the Revised Clinical Interview Schedule (CIS-R). London: Institute of Psychiatry, 1990.
26. Baldwin DS, Bobes J, Stein DJ, Scharwachter I, Faure M, on behalf of the Paroxetine Study Group. Paroxetine in social phobia/social anxiety disorder. Br J Psychiatry 1999; 175: 120–126.
27. Sheehan D. The Anxiety Disease. New York: Scribner, 1983.
28. Baldwin DS, DeMartinis, Mallick R. Patient-reported functioning in social anxiety disorder and improvement with treatment: a comparison of venlafaxine XR, paroxetine and placebo. Eur Neuropsychopharmacol. In press.

6

Diagnosis of Social Anxiety Disorder in Children

Tracy L. Morris
West Virginia University,
Morgantown, West Virginia, U.S.A.

As a symptom state, nearly all humans have personal experience with the feeling of social anxiety. For most individuals, the feeling state is transitory, or limited to relatively circumscribed developmental periods. For others, social anxiety is a chronic condition resulting in significant functional impairment. Social anxiety disorder is defined in the fourth edition of the Diagnostic and Statistical Manual of Mental Disorders (DSM-IV) as a "marked and persistent fear of one or more social or performance situations in which the person is exposed to unfamiliar people or to possible scrutiny by others" (1). In order to qualify for a diagnosis of social anxiety disorder, children must demonstrate capacity for age-appropriate social relationships. Pervasive developmental disorder must be considered as an alternative diagnosis for children who demonstrate deficits in social relatedness even with family members and others with whom they have extended contact. Further, diagnosis of social anxiety disorder requires that the child experience anxiety-related symptoms in the presence of other children, not merely in interaction with adult authority figures. Reticence only in the presence of adults, while potentially disconcerting, falls within the normative scope of shyness and is not necessarily grounds for intervention.

As childhood shyness is a relatively common phenomenon, which for many children subsides as they age, how do clinicians distinguish between normative and pathological social anxiety? This question is generally answered with reference to the extent of functional impairment in social relationships and/or academic performance as well as the level of distress experienced by the child. Escape from, and avoidance of, social situations are particularly salient features of social anxiety disorder. However, as children often do not have the freedom to avoid many social situations (e.g., school), responses such as clinging to parental figures, freezing, or tantruming may be observed when children are unable to avoid feared stimuli. Self-deprecatory cognitions and fear of negative evaluation are common among children with social anxiety disorder—even when faced with objective evidence to the contrary. Intense physiological responses—including heart palpitations, trembling, sweating, and blushing—are also common in anticipation of, throughout, and/or following social performance situations. Fear that others will notice these physiological reactions further exacerbates the child's social concerns.

Social anxiety disorder typically begins in early childhood, with a mean age of onset of 11 years reported for the generalized form (2). Due to the pervasive deleterious effects of social anxiety on children's social and academic functioning, early detection and diagnosis are crucial in order that proper intervention may be delivered. Early intervention can serve to avert a lifetime of dysfunction and distress. Unfortunately, relatively few children meeting criteria for social anxiety disorder are identified and referred to appropriate treatment providers. This is due in part to limits in children's understanding of their own emotional states, and ability to communicate them, limited ability of parents and teachers to detect mild to moderate levels of anxiety in children, and the often expressed hope of parents that their children will simply "grow out of it."

Accurate assessment of social anxiety disorder requires an appreciation of child development. In order to determine whether a given behavior is age-appropriate, one must have an understanding of the behaviors and skills that children should demonstrate across various ages. Unfortunately, many clinicians have not received adequate training in "normal" child development and thus have limited ability to ascertain whether certain behaviors are indeed "abnormal." Normative information regarding social, cognitive, emotional, and physical development is necessary to place behaviors in a proper context.

I. STRANGER ANXIETY AND BEHAVIORAL INHIBITION

Stranger anxiety tends to arise among infants around 8 months of age and peaks between 12 to 18 months. For most infants this is expressed as an initial wariness of unfamiliar persons followed by a gradual warming and willingness to interact with the stranger over a period of a few minutes. For other infants and toddlers, this stranger anxiety is exemplified by extreme distress, crying, and protestation that fails to subside. Young children who demonstrate extreme wariness and withdrawal in the face of novelty have been termed behaviorally inhibited (3). These behaviorally inhibited children refrain from exploration, prefer to remain in close proximity to their mothers, rarely initiate verbal interaction, and smile at significantly lower rates than do other children. Approximately 15% of children are classified as behaviorally inhibited. Comprehensive assessment of behavioral inhibition generally involves structured observation of the child's responses to familiar and unfamiliar settings, objects, and people (including same-age peers and adults). Children who behave in an inhibited manner across multiple contexts—and with both adults and peers—tend to be those who will manifest the highest levels of anxiety over time (4).

Not surprisingly, behavioral inhibition has been suggested as an early precursor to social anxiety disorder. Behavioral inhibition is prevalent among children of parents with anxiety disorders (5–7) and with social anxiety disorder in particular (8). Likewise, cross-sectional and prospective investigations of toddlers and preschoolers have found that inhibited children are at elevated risk for social anxiety disorder (9–11).

II. ASSESSMENT OF SOCIAL ANXIETY IN CHILDREN

Comprehensive evaluation and diagnosis of social anxiety disorder in children requires examination of behavioral, cognitive, and physiological responses across multiple social contexts. Diagnostic assessment tools include clinical interviews, child self-report measures, parent- and teacher-completed questionnaires, behavioral observation, and peer reports. The hazards of relying on only a single source of information cannot be overstated. Nonetheless, the diagnostician's task is not merely to obtain a substantial quantity of assessment data but also to integrate and gauge the potential relevance of data from multiple sources.

A. Clinical Interviews

Semistructured diagnostic interviews offer several advantages, including broad assessment of a wide range of symptoms potentially experienced by children within configurations demonstrated to have adequate or better psychometric properties. This is of significant advantage over unstructured intake interviews, which may be subject to the personal biases or limitations in knowledge of classification on the part of the interviewer. More detailed and targeted information may be acquired through branching question sequences (12,13). The downside of semistructured interviews includes the long time required to become proficient in administration and the relatively lengthy time to administer and score the interviews in comparison with that of questionnaire measures. However, the accuracy and thoroughness of diagnostic information would seem to take precedence over mere time-related concerns. More often than not, sufficient time taken to complete a thorough evaluation will more than pay off in terms of accuracy of differential diagnosis and identification of proper target behaviors for intervention.

The most widely used and highly regarded interviews for the assessment of childhood psychopathology include the Schedule for Affective Disorders and Schizophrenia for School-Aged Children (14), the Diagnostic Interview Schedule for Children (15), and the Diagnostic Interview for Children and Adolescents–Revised (16). Although these interviews generally have demonstrated acceptable psychometric properties, particularly for disruptive behavior disorders, they have demonstrated weaknesses with respect to anxiety disorders (17).

In an attempt to improve on this state of affairs, Silverman and Albano (18) developed the Anxiety Disorders Interview Schedule for DSM-IV–Child and Parent Versions (ADIS-IV-C/P) (18). The ADIS-IV-C/P was designed specifically to diagnose childhood anxiety disorders and to differentiate anxiety from other affective and disruptive behavior disorders. Parent and child interviews are administered separately and then integrated to derive diagnoses. Since its release, the ADIS-IV-C/P has become the interview of choice for child anxiety researchers.

Although intended for children of ages 6 to 18, the ADIS-IV-C/P has been administered to children as young as 4 years of age (19). Excellent psychometric properties have been reported (20). The interview has been used in most of the published treatment trials for childhood anxiety and has been shown to be sensitive to treatment effects (21–24).

B. Clinician Ratings

Clinician ratings provide for quick and expedient assessment of symptom level and overall functioning. The Hamilton Anxiety Rating Scale (25), though developed for adults, has been validated for use with adolescents (26). The Pediatric Anxiety Rating Scale (27) is a 50-item checklist that assesses symptoms of social anxiety, separation anxiety, generalized anxiety, and specific phobias. Data are gathered during separate or joint interviews with parents and children and then rated by the clinician on seven dimensions (e.g., frequency, avoidance, severity of distress). Adequate psychometric properties have been demonstrated.

The Liebowitz Social Anxiety Scale for Children and Adolescents (LSAS-CA) (28) is a 24-item clinician-rated measure that is based on the adult Liebowitz Social Anxiety Scale (29). The LSAS-CA comprises two scales assessing social interactions and performance situations. Separate ratings are provided for anxiety level and avoidance. Initial psychometric reports support the reliability and sensitivity of the measure (30,31).

C. Child Self-Report

Child self-report measures should be considered a standard part of any assessment protocol, given the largely subjective nature of anxiety. Global self-report measures provide a general index of overall anxiety, whereas syndrome-specific measures assess symptoms within more circumscribed contexts and are more closely related to individual anxiety disorder diagnoses. The Revised Children's Manifest Anxiety Scale (RCMAS) (32), State-Trait Anxiety Inventory for Children (STAI-C) (33), and Fear Survey Scale for Children–Revised (FSSC-R) (34) represent the first-generation of global self-report measures of childhood anxiety. While serving a worthy purpose at the time they were initially released, these measures have been criticized as being mere downward extensions of adult self-reports. Further, these measures do not reflect the current diagnostic system and generally have failed to adequately discriminate among different forms of psychopathology (35,36).

The next generations of self-report measures have been designed to better address issues of discriminative validity and treatment sensitivity. The Multidimensional Anxiety Scale for Children (MASC) (37) is a 45-item scale that yields a Total Anxiety Disorder Index and four main factor scores: Social Anxiety, Physical Symptoms, Harm/Avoidance, and Separation/Panic. The MASC has demonstrated strong psychometric properties and is becoming one of the most accepted measures of child anxiety (38–40). The Spence Children's Anxiety Scale (SCAS) (41,42) consists of 45 items, assessing Social Anxiety, Generalized Anxiety, Separation Anxiety, Panic/Agoraphobia Obsessions/Compulsions, Fear of Physical Injury, as well as Social Desirability. The SCAS has demonstrated good internal consistency and test–retest reliability. The Screen for Child Anxiety Related Emotional Disorders–Revised (SCARED-R) (43,44) is a 66-item self-report instrument with subscales encompassing Social Anxiety, Generalized Anxiety, Separation Anxiety, Panic, OCD, PTSD, and three types of Specific Phobias (blood-injection-injury, animal, environmental phobias). The SCARED-R has demonstrated strong psychometric properties and sensitivity to treatment effects (45).

Two self-report measures have been designed specifically to assess social anxiety in children. The Social Anxiety Scale for Children–Revised (SASC-R)

(46) includes 22 items assessing a range of subjective experiences and behavioral consequences associated with social anxiety. The SASC-R is comprised of three factors: Fear of Negative Evaluation (FNE), Social Avoidance and Distress with new or unfamiliar peers (SAD-New) and generalized social avoidance and distress (SAD-G). The SASC-R and its parallel version for adolescents (SASC-A) have demonstrated excellent psychometric properties. The Social Phobia and Anxiety Inventory for Children (SPAI-C) (47,48) was designed specifically to assess the DSM construct of social anxiety disorder and comprises 26 items assessing a range of social fears experienced by children and adolescents (8 to 14 years) in multiple social settings (e.g., home and school). Several items require the child to indicate level of fear or distress experienced in three different contexts: familiar peers, unfamiliar peers, and adults. The SPAI-C has demonstrated excellent psychometric properties. The measure has not only successfully discriminated children with social anxiety disorder from normal controls but also, more significantly, has been shown to discriminate children with social anxiety disorder from children with other anxiety disorders. Moderate associations have been found between the SPAI-C and SASC-R, indicating that the two measures assess similar but not identical constructs (49,50).

D. Parent Report

The Child Behavior Checklist (CBCL) (51) is the most widely used global parent-report measure of childhood psychopathology. Separate versions are available for children of ages 2 to 3 years and for those of ages 4 to 16. The CBCL comprises over 100 items assessing social and academic functioning and a range of problem behaviors. Scores are derived for two broad-band scales (Internalizing and Externalizing) and nine content areas (e.g., Anxious/Depressed; Social Problems; Withdrawn). The CBCL has high short- and long-term retest reliability, good predictive validity, and moderate ability to discriminate referred and nonreferred children (51,52).

Although to date there have been no published measures designed specifically as parent reports of social anxiety in children, child self-report measures have been adapted to allow comparison across informants. For example, Beidel and colleagues (53) have reported a modest correlation between child and parent versions of the Social Phobia and Anxiety Inventory for Children. Further examination of the psychometric properties of the parent-report version of the SPAI-C is in progress.

E. Parent-Child Agreement

A challenging dilemma for diagnosticians is how to evaluate and integrate information obtained from multiple informants. Clinicians and researchers must take care not to assume that parents are the "gold standard" for all information about their children. Child, parent, teacher, and peer reports may all play a significant role in diagnostic assessment. Each informant may provide uniquely relevant information (54). When reports differ, possible bases for cross-informant disagreement should be examined. Potential reasons why discrepant information may be obtained across reporters include: 1) bias or error on the part of one or more of the respondents; 2) actual variability in the child's behavior across the situations observed by the informants; 3) limited access to the child's private events (cognitions, affect, and physiological responses); 4) denial of the problem; or 5) intentional false reporting in service of an ulterior motive such as qualification for treatment or financial services (55).

Correlations across child, parent, and teacher reports have generally been found to be small to moderate (56). Cross-informant agreement is generally higher between child and teacher reports than between child and parent reports. Child and parent reports typically tend to be more highly correlated for younger children than for older children (57). However, accuracy of assessment for very young children can be extremely difficult, as self-reports are of limited value with children below reading age and many parents may not be aware that certain behaviors are abnormal or developmentally inappropriate. For example, 40% of parents whose 3-year-olds displayed clinically significant behavioral or emotional problems failed to identify these as significant concerns (58). Concordance across child, parent, and teacher reports has been shown to decrease in adolescence, as children begin to spend proportionally more private time with peers (59). Differential patterns of agreement have also been found for child gender, with parent reports (from mothers and fathers) more highly correlated with child self reports for boys than for girls.

With respect to type of symptoms under consideration, parent-child agreement is typically higher for externalizing than for internalizing symptoms (60,61). This is not surprising given the more readily observable nature of disruptive behavior in contrast to the more subjective components of anxiety and affective disorders. Along these lines, parents have been found to report higher frequencies and intensities of externalizing symptoms, while children tend to report higher levels of internalizing symptoms (61–64). Lowered sensitivity to and detection of internalizing symptoms in children on the part of adults contributes in part to the fact that children with anxiety and depression are less likely to receive treatment than are children with disruptive behavior disorders (65,66).

Parental psychopathology has been suggested as a potential factor related to discrepancies in parent-child agreement. Maternal anxiety and depression have been implicated in potential reporting biases (67,68). Mothers who are depressed and anxious have been found to report higher levels of internalizing and externalizing symptoms for their children (69) than do mothers who are not anxious or depressed. Perhaps these mothers are merely more sensitive to actual internalizing symptoms in their children, but this pattern has typically been labeled as overreporting. In a study of children of parents with social anxiety disorder (19), number of anxiety symptoms endorsed for the parent significantly correlated with the number of anxiety disorders for the child. Some authors have suggested that parents with social anxiety may be more likely to perceive social inhibition in their children as a projection of their own social concerns (8,68). Further research is necessary to determine whether parent perceptions of anxiety in their children are indeed biased overreports or sensitive reflections from parents who are intimately acquainted with the subtleties of anxiety. At any rate, thorough evaluation will incorporate assessment of the family system. Intervention efforts will differ depending on whether parents are affected by their own anxiety. Parents with anxiety disorders may model dependency, reinforce anxious behaviors (e.g., school refusal), and/or discourage their children's attempts at separation. Parental anxiety may have to be addressed prior to—or at least concurrently with—treatment for the child's social anxiety disorder in order that the parent may more fully engage in social exposure assignments as part of standard cognitive-behavioral intervention.

F. Behavioral Observation

Any comprehensive assessment of social anxiety will include observation of the child. In an ideal world, observation would take place across several settings in the naturalistic environment—notably those in which anxiety is most often elicited (e.g., at school, in the classroom, and on the playground during recess). Granted, it can be difficult for many clinicians to leave the office to conduct extensive observation. With forethought and planning, analogous situations may be arranged within the clinic to provide the proper setting events in which relevant skills and anxious behaviors may be displayed. For instance, children may be asked to read aloud or deliver an impromptu speech in the presence of the clinician and other staff or to initiate conversation with other children and adults in the waiting room. Behavioral assessment tasks have been of considerable utility not only as diagnostic assessment tools but also as measures of treatment outcome in clinical trials of cognitive-behavioral therapy for social anxiety disorder (21).

G. Peer Reports

School is the primary social setting for children over 5 years of age. While teacher reports serve as the gold standard for assessment of academic functioning, peer reports have no substitute in terms of ascertaining the child's level of integration in the social group. Assessments of children's peer relations may be of particular value in evaluating generalization of treatment effects. Peer status is typically obtained through sociometric nomination methods in which each child in a classroom names three children with whom he or she most likes to play and three with whom he or she least likes to play. Peer status is then classified based on the extent to which the child is liked or disliked by his or her peers (70). Alternatively, sociometric rating procedures may be employed in which children rate each of their classmates on various dimensions using Likert-type scales. In the Revised Class Play procedure (71), children are asked to assign classmates to roles in an imaginary play. For example, children may be asked which classmate is the most shy, most fearful, most outgoing, and so on. In addition to peer reports, direct observation of children's interactions with classmates can provide key information regarding social behavior, interaction style, skills, and deficits that may be identified as targets for intervention. It is important to keep in mind that many children who are socially anxious with peers are able to interact quite skillfully with adults; thus, important behaviors may be missed in the absence of peer observation. Among children, athletic ability, trendy attire, skill with video games, and use of current slang are important social variables that must be considered in evaluation of age-appropriate behavior, whether or not adults wish this to be the case.

H. Recommended Assessment Protocol

Clearly, one will not always be in a position to collect as extensive an assessment battery as one might prefer. If social anxiety disorder is suspected (based on the initial referral question or uncovered during broad-band screening), a reasonable diagnostic protocol would include administration of the Social Phobia and Anxiety Inventory for Children (child self-report) and the Anxiety Disorders Interview Schedule (child and parent interviews). Additionally, it is recommended that children self-monitor anxiety-provoking situations and use of coping responses via a daily diary (21,72). Diary sheets may be sent home with the child and returned at the time of the next appointment. Self-monitoring should continue throughout treatment to assist in target selection. The assessment protocol should be repeated following the treatment course in order to document outcome.

III. COMORBIDITY AND DIFFERENTIAL DIAGNOSIS

Social anxiety disorder is highly comorbid (this volume, chapter by Baldwin and Buis). The most frequently associated conditions include school refusal, other anxiety disorders, and depression. Children who meet criteria for multiple anxiety disorders tend to manifest earlier age of onset, extended chronicity, and higher intensity of anxiety symptoms than do children who meet criteria for only a single anxiety disorder.

A. School Refusal

School refusal may be related to one of several different functions: a child may fear separation from a parent (as with separation anxiety disorder) or ridicule by peers (as with social anxiety), or may avoid school subsequent to academic difficulties (as a consequence of a learning disability or attention deficit hyperactivity disorder), or as part of a general pattern of noncompliance (as with oppositional defiant disorder). It is imperative that clinicians conduct a thorough functional analysis of school refusal behavior to select appropriate targets and methods for intervention. In a study of children with anxiety-related school refusal, 30% met criteria for social anxiety disorder (73). Socially anxious children are likely to withdraw from social encounters in the school setting and may soon experience perceived or actual lack of reinforcement or even punishment from the social environment. Social isolation from peers may impair the development of age-appropriate social skills and further exacerbate the potential for social anxiety.

B. Separation Anxiety Disorder

The hallmark feature of separation anxiety disorder is excessive concern over separation from parental attachment figures. Although the child may have considerable difficulty articulating the reasons behind his or her separation fears, targeted interviewing generally will reveal that the child anticipates coming to harm and/or fears harm to the parental figure(s) if they are separated. While on the surface similar behaviors may be manifest in the two conditions (e.g., clinging, school refusal), social anxiety is not a dependency on the caretaker but rather a fear of approaching social interaction in which scrutiny by others is possible. In contrast to children with separation anxiety disorder, those with social anxiety will not express significant fear or distress when left at home with babysitters or during overnight stays with close friends or relatives. These disorders may co-occur; in such cases, separate avenues of treatment must be engaged. As effective treatment of social anxiety inevitably will involve social encounters apart from parents, it may be best to address the separation anxiety first.

C. Generalized Anxiety Disorder

The diagnosis of generalized anxiety disorder requires that the child experience numerous cognitive and physiological symptoms across multiple areas.

These fears and anxieties must not merely be associated with social concerns; otherwise a diagnosis of social anxiety disorder would be more appropriate. Generalized anxiety disorder is highly comorbid with social anxiety disorder in adults, with rates ranging from 15 to 50% across samples. Beidel and Turner have reported 16% comorbidity within their samples of children with social anxiety disorder (74).

D. Depression

Comorbidity rates of 8 to 10% have been reported for social anxiety and depression in child samples (21,75). Children who are depressed may resist attending social events, but they do so for different reasons than children who are socially anxious. Children who are depressed will report that they are tired or do not have sufficient energy to participate (and at high levels of depression will indeed appear to be fatigued). Unfortunately, children with social anxiety disorder are at elevated risk for the development of depression subsequent to decreased social engagement and reinforcement, as well as maladaptive cognitions of worthlessness.

E. Attention-Deficit Hyperactivity Disorder (ADHD)

Restless, fidgety, and noncompliant behavior in classroom settings may be interpreted by teachers and other adults as a result of anxiety, but more often there are seen as indications of ADHD. Inability to concentrate in academic contexts may be related to either condition; as such, full psychological assessment (including achievement testing) and functional analysis is necessary. Further, anxiety and ADHD may co-occur, with estimates upward of 20% having been reported (76). Social anxiety may be a legitimate outcome for children with ADHD, who may be ridiculed or disliked by their peers for engaging in disruptive, impulsive, or aggressive behavior or failure to perform academically. Realization of lowered peer status among children with ADHD is increasingly likely as they age and develop a better understanding of themselves and others. Early intervention for attentional and academic problems will serve to reduce the likelihood that these children will develop a dislike for school and distress in social settings. In cases where children legitimately meet criteria for ADHD and an anxiety or mood disorder, the disruptive behavior disorder tends to overshadow the identification and treatment of anxiety and depression (56). Clinicians should be cautioned not to overlook the possibility of co-occurring anxiety when children are referred for evaluation of ADHD.

IV. CONCLUDING COMMENTS

Social anxiety is an early-onset, chronic disorder. Most adults with social anxiety disorder report that they have felt shy and uncomfortable in social situations most of their lives. The onset of social anxiety disorder in childhood places the individual at considerable risk for the later development of depression and substance abuse. It is essential that pediatricians, family physicians, and mental health professionals develop an awareness of social anxiety disorder and implement adequate screening procedures so that children may be referred for appropriate intervention. Accurate detection and diagnosis of social anxiety disorder will go a long way toward improving the quality of life for countless children and adolescents.

REFERENCES

1. American Psychiatric Association. Diagnostic and Statistical Manual of Mental Disorders. 4th ed. Washington, DC: APA, 1994.
2. Manuzza A, Schneier F, Chapman T, Leibowitz M, Klein D, Fyer A. Generalized social phobia: Reliability and validity. Arch Gen Psychiatry 1995; 52:230–237.
3. Kagan J, Reznick JS, Snidman N, Gibbons J, Johnson MO. Childhood derivatives of inhibition and lack of inhibition to the unfamiliar. Child Dev, 1988; 59:1580–1589.
4. Rubin K, Hastings P, Stewart S, Henderson H, Chen X. The consistency and concomitants of inhibition: Some of the children, all of the time. Child Dev 1997; 68:467–483.
5. Battaglia M, Bajo S, Strambi LF, Brambilla F, Castronovo C, Vanni G, Bellodi L. Physiological and behavioral responses to minor stressors in offspring of patients with panic disorder. J Psychiatr Res 1997; 31:365–376.
6. Manassis K, Bradley S, Goldberg S, Hood J, Swinson R. Behavioural inhibition, attachment and anxiety in children of mothers with anxiety disorders. Can J Psychiatry 1995; 40:87–92.
7. Rosenbaum JF, Biederman J, Hirshfeld-Becker DR, Kagan J, Snidman N, Friedman D, Nineberg A, Gallery DJ, Faraone SV. A controlled study of behavioral inhibition in children of parents with panic disorder and depression. Am J Psychiatry 2000; 157:2002–2010.
8. Cooper P, Eke M. Childhood shyness and maternal social phobia: a community study. Br J Psychiatry 1999; 174:439–443.
9. Biederman J, Hirshfeld-Becker DR, Rosenbaum JF, Herot C, Friedman D, Snidman N, Kagan J, Faraone SV. Further evidence of association between behavioral inhibition and social anxiety in children. Am J Psychiatry 2001; 158:1673–1679.
10. Hirshfeld DR, Rosenbaum JF, Biederman J, Bolduc EA, Faraone SV, Snidman N, Reznick JS, Kagan J. Stable behavioral inhibition and its

association with anxiety disorder. J Am Acad Child Adolesc Psychiatry 1992; 31:103–111.

11. Schwartz C, Snidman N, Kagan J. Adolescent social anxiety as an outcome of inhibited temperament in childhood. J Am Acad Child Adolesc Psychiatry 1999; 38:1008–1015.

12. McClellan JM, Werry JS. Research on psychiatric diagnostic interviews for children and adolescents: introduction. J Am Acad Child Adolesc Psychiatry 2000; 39:19–27.

13. Silverman WK. Structured diagnostic interviews. In: Ollendick TH, King NJ, eds. International Handbook of Phobic and Anxiety Disorders in Children and Adolescents: Issues in Clinical Child Psychology. New York: Plenum, 1994: 293–315.

14. Ambrosini P. Historical development and present status of the Schedule for Affective Disorders and Schizophrenia for School-Age Children (K-SADS). J Am Acad Child Adolesc Psychiatry 2000; 39:49–58.

15. Shaffer D, Fisher P, Lucas CP, Dulcan MK, Schwab-Stone ME. NIMH Diagnostic Interview Schedule for Children Version IV (NIMH DISC-IV): description, differences from previous versions, and reliability of some common diagnoses. J Am Acad Child Adolesc Psychiatry 2000; 39:28–39.

16. Reich W, Welner Z. Diagnostic Inventory for Children and Adolescents–Revised: parent version. Toronto: Multi-Health Systems, 1988.

17. Shaffer D, Fisher P, Dulcan MK, Davies M, et al. The NIMH Diagnostic Interview Schedule for Children Version 2.3 (DISC-2.3): description, acceptability, prevalence rates, and performance in the MECA study. J Am Acad Child Adolesc Psychiatry 1996; 35:865–877.

18. Silverman WK, Albano AM. The Anxiety Disorders Interview Schedule for Children for DSM-IV (Child and Parent Versions). San Antonio, TX: Psychological Corporation, 1996.

19. Mancini C, Van Ameringen M, Szatmari P, Fugere C, Boyle M. A high-risk pilot study of the children of adults with social phobia. J Am Acad Child Adolesc Psychiatry 1996; 35:1511–1517.

20. Silverman WK, Saavedra LM, Pina AA. Test-retest reliability of anxiety symptoms and diagnoses with the Anxiety Disorders Interview Schedule for DSM-IV: child and parent versions. J Am Acad Child Adolesc Psychiatry 2001; 40:937–944.

21. Beidel DC, Turner SM, Morris TL. Behavioral treatment of childhood social phobia. J Consult Clin Psychology 2000; 68:1072–1080.

22. Hayward C, Varady S, Albano AM, Thienemann M, Henderson L, Schatzberg AF. Cognitive-behavioral group therapy for social phobia in female adolescents: results of a pilot study. J Am Acad Child Adolesc Psychiatry 2000; 39:721–734.

23. Kendall P, Flannery-Schroeder E, Panichelli-Mindel S, Southam-Gerow M, Henin A, Warman M. Therapy for youths with anxiety disorders: a second randomized trial. J Consult Clin Psychol 1997; 65:366–380.

24. Spence SH, Donovan C, Brechman-Toussaint M. The treatment of childhood social phobia: the effectiveness of a social skills training-based,

cognitive-behavioral intervention, with and without parental involvement. J Child Psychol Psychiatry 2000; 41:713–726.

25. Hamilton M. The assessment of anxiety states by rating. Br J Med Psychol 1959; 32:50–55.

26. Clark D, Donovan J. Reliability and validity of the Hamilton Anxiety Scale in an adolescent sample. J Am Acad Child Adolesc Psychiatry 1994; 33:354–360.

27. Research Units on Pediatric Psychopharmacology Anxiety Study Group. The Pediatric Anxiety Rating Scale (PARS): development and psychometric properties. J Am Acad Child Adolesc Psychiatry 2002; 41:1061–1069.

28. Masia CL, Hofmann SG, Klein RG, Liebowitz MR. The Liebowitz Social Anxiety Scale for Children and Adolescents (LSAS-CA). Available from Carrie L. Masia, Ph.D., NYU Child Study Center, 215 Lexington Avenue, New York, 10016.

29. Liebowitz MR. Social phobia. Mod Probl Psychopharmacol 1987; 22:141–173.

30. Storch EA, Masia CL, Pincus D, Klein R, Liebowitz M. Initial psychometric properties of the Liebowitz Social Anxiety Scale for Children and adolescents. Poster presented at the annual meeting of the Anxiety Disorders of America Association, Atlanta, GA.

31. Masia CL, Klein RG, Storch EA, Corda B. School-based behavioral treatment for social anxiety disorder in adolescents: results of a pilot study. J Am Acad Child Adolesc Psychiatry 2001; 40:780–786.

32. Reynolds CR, Richmond BO. Factor structure and construct validity of "What I Think and Feel." The Revised Children's Manifest Anxiety Scale. J Personality Assess 1978; 43:281–283.

33. Spielberger CD. Manual for the State-Trait Anxiety Inventory (Form V). Palo Alto, CA: Consulting Psychologists Press, 1983.

34. Ollendick TH. Reliability and validity of the revised fear survey schedule for children (FSSC-R). Behav Res Ther 1983; 21:685–692.

35. Perrin S, Last CG. Do childhood anxiety measures measure anxiety? J Abnorm Child Psychol 1992; 20:567–578.

36. Stark D, Kaslow NJ, Laurent J. The assessment of depression in children: are we assessing depression or the broad-band construct of negative affectivity? J Emot Behav Disord 1993; 1:149–159.

37. March J. Manual for the Multidimensional Anxiety Scale for Children (MASC). Toronto: Multihealth Systems, 1998.

38. Greenhill LL, Pine D, March J, Birmaher B, Riddle M. Assessment measures in anxiety disorders research. Psychopharmacol Bull 1998; 34:155–164.

39. Langley AK, Bergman L, Piacentini JC. Assessment of childhood anxiety. Int Rev Psychiatry 2002; 14:102–113.

40. The Multidimensional Anxiety Scale for Children (MASC): factor structure, reliability, and validity. Toronto: Multi-Health Systems, 1998.

41. Spence SH. Structure of anxiety symptoms among children: a confirmatory factor-analytic study. J Abnorm Psychol 1997; 106:280–297.

42. Spence SH. A measure of anxiety symptoms among children. Behav Res Ther 1998; 36:545–566.

43. Birmaher B, Khetarpal S, Brent D, Cully M, Balach L, Kaufman J, McKenzie Neer S. The Screen for Child Anxiety Related Emotional Disorders (SCARED): scale construction and psychometric characteristics. J Am Acad Child Adolesc Psychiatry 1997; 36:545–553.

44. Muris P, Merckelbach H, Schmidt H, Mayer B. The revised version of the Screen for Child Anxiety Related Emotional Disorders (SCARED-R): factor structure in normal children. Personality Ind Diff 1999; 26:99–112.

45. Muris P, Mayer B, Bartelds E, Tierney S, Bogie N. The revised version of the Screen for Child Anxiety Related Emotional Disorders (SCARED-R): Treatment sensitivity in an early intervention trial for childhood anxiety disorders. Br J Clin Psychol 2001; 40:323–336.

46. La Greca AM, Stone WL. Social anxiety scale for children-revised: factor structure and concurrent validity. J Clin Child Psychol 1993; 22:17–27.

47. Beidel DC, Turner SM, Morris TL. A new inventory to assess child social phobia: the Social Phobia and Anxiety Inventory for Children. Psychol Assess 1995; 7:73–79.

48. Beidel DC, Turner SM, Morris TL. Social Phobia and Anxiety Inventory for Children. North Tonawanda, NY: Multi-Health Systems, 1998.

49. Epkins C. A comparison of two self-report measures of children's social anxiety in clinical and community samples. J Clin Child Adolesc Psychol 2002; 31: 69–79.

50. Morris TL, Masia CL. Psychometric evaluation of the social phobia and anxiety inventory for children: concurrent validity and normative data. J Clin Child Psychol 1998; 27:459–468.

51. Achenbach TM. Manual for the Child Behavior Checklist/2-3 and 1992 Profile. Burlington, VT: University of Vermont Department of Psychiatry, 1992.

52. Koot HM, Van Den Oord EJCG, Verhulst FC, Boomsma DI. Behavioral and emotional problems in young preschoolers: cross-cultural testing of the validity of the Child Behavior Checklist/2-3. J Abnorm Child Psychol 1997; 25:183–196.

53. Beidel DC, Turner SM, Hamlin K, Morris TL. The Social Phobia and Anxiety Inventory for Children (SPAI-C): external and discriminative validity. Behav Ther 2000; 31:75–87.

54. Bird H, Gould M, Staghezza B. Aggregating data from multiple informants in child psychiatry epidemiological research. J Am Acad Child Adolesc Psychiatry 1992; 35:1440–1448.

55. Mash EJ, Dozois DJA. Child psychopathology: a developmental-systems perspective. In: Mash EJ, Barkley RA, eds. Child Psychopathology. New York: Guilford, 1996:3–60.

56. Mesman J, Koot HM. Child-reported depression and anxiety in preadolescence: I. Associations with parent- and teacher-reported problems. J Am Acad Child Adolesc Psychiatry 2000; 39:1371–1378.

57. Krain AL, Kendall PC. The role of parental emotional distress in parent report of child anxiety. J Clin Child Psychol 2000; 29:328–335.

58. Stallard P. The behaviour of 3-year-old children: prevalence and parental perception of problem behavior: a research note. J Child Psychol Psychiatry 1993; 34:413–421.

59. Jensen PS, Rubio-Stipec M, Canino G, Bird HR, Dulcan MK, Schwab-Stone ME, Lahey BB. Parent and child contributions to diagnosis of mental disorder: are both informants always necessary? J Am Academy of Child and Adolescent Psychiatry 1999; 38:1569–1579.

60. Edelbrock C, Costello AJ, Dulcan MK, Conover NC, Kala R. Parent-child agreement on child psychiatric symptoms assessed via structured interview. J Child Psychol Psychiatry 1986; 32:666–673.

61. Manassis K, Tannock R, Mendlowitz S, Laslo D, Maselis M. Distinguishing anxiety disorders psychometrically. J Am Acad Child Adolesc Psychiatry 1997; 36:1645–1646.

62. Cantwell DP, Lewinsohn PM, Rohde P, Seeley JR. Correspondence between adolescent report and parent report of psychiatric diagnostic data. Journal of the American Academy of Child and Adolescent Psychiatry 1997; 36:610–619.

63. Crawford AM, Manassis K. Familial predictors of treatment outcome in childhood anxiety disorders. J Am Acad Child Adolesc Psychiatry 2001; 40:1182–1189.

64. Herjanic B, Reich W. Development of a structured psychiatric interview for children: agreement between child and parents on individual symptoms. J Abnorm Child Psychol 1997; 25:21–31.

65. Cohen P, Kasen S, Brooks JS, Struening EL. Diagnostic predictors of treatment patterns in a cohort of adolescents. J Am Acad Child Adolesc Psychiatry 1991; 30:989–993.

66. Wu P, Hoven CW, Bird HR, et al. Depressive and disruptive disorders and mental health service utilization in children and adolescents. J Am Acad Child Adolesc Psychiatry 1999; 39:1081–1090.

67. Fergusson DM, Lynskey MT, Horwood LJ. The effect of maternal depression on maternal ratings of child behavior. J Abnorm Child Psychol 1993; 21:245–269.

68. Richters JE. Depressed mothers as informants about their children: a critical review of the evidence for distortion. Psychol Bull 1992; 112:485–499.

69. Chilcoat HD, Breslau N. Does psychiatric history bias mothers' reports? An application of a new analytic approach. J Am Acad Child Adolesc Psychiatry 1997; 36:971–979.

70. Coie JD, Dodge KA, Coppotelli H. Dimensions and types of social status: a cross-age perspective. Dev Psychol 1982; 18:557–570.

71. Matsen AS, Morrison P, Pelligrini DS. A revised class play method of peer assessment. Dev Psychol 1985; 21:523–533.

72. Beidel DC, Neal AM, Lederer AS. The feasibility and validity of a daily diary for the assessment of anxiety in children. Behav Ther 1991; 22:505–517.

73. Last CG, Strauss CC. School refusal in anxiety disordered children and adolescents. J Am Acad Child Adolesc Psychiatry 1990; 29:31–35.

74. Beidel DC, Turner SM. Shy Children, Phobic Adults: The Nature and Treatment of Social Phobia. Washington DC: American Psychological Association, 1998.
75. Strauss CC, Last CG. Social and simple phobias in children. J Anxiety Disord 1993; 1:141–152.
76. Last CG, Strauss CC, Francis G. Comorbidity among childhood anxiety disorders. J Nerve Ment Dis 1987; 175:726–730.

7

Assessing Social Anxiety Disorder with Rating Scales: Practical Utility for the Clinician

**Joshua D. Lipsitz and
Michael R. Liebowitz**

New York State Psychiatric Institute, Columbia University
College of Physicians and Surgeons,
New York, New York, U.S.A.

In the past few decades, numerous rating scales have been developed for the assessment of social anxiety disorder. Several recent reviews provide scholarly consideration of the psychometric properties of these instruments (1–7). Rather than restate specifics as to their reliability and validity, this chapter emphasizes social anxiety rating scales from the standpoint of their clinical relevance. In other words, it considers which scales are most useful for the needs of specific clinical situations. As such, this review is limited to commonly used instruments that have demonstrated adequate reliability, validity, and sensitivity to treatment based on empirical studies. The scales considered in this chapter are presented in Table 1. For a more comprehensive review of available scales for assessing social anxiety disorder, the reader is referred to reviews cited above.

TABLE 1 Features of Commonly Used Rating Scales for Social Anxiety Disorder

	Description	Scores (subscales)	Cutoffs	Advantages	Drawbacks
Clinician-Rated Scales:					

Liebowitz Social Anxiety Scale: (Liebowitz, 1987)	24 items
	Fear + avoidance (0–3)
		Total score
		1. Performance
		2. Social/interaction
		  1. Fear
		  2. Avoidance
			Range: 0–144
			Cutoffs:
			≥30 = for SAD
			≥60 = for generalized SAD
				Easy to administer
				Widely used
				Subscale scores for Performance vs. social interaction and fear vs. avoidance
					No specific coverage of physical symptoms

Brief Social Phobia Scale (Davidson et al., 1991)	11 items (0–4)	Total score 1. Fear 2. Avoidance 3. Physical symptoms	Range: 0–72 Cutoff: ≥20 = SAD	Brief. Covers fear, avoidance, and physical symptoms	Limited item coverage
ADIS Clinician Severity Scale (Dinardo et al., 1994)	Fear and avoidance 13 social situations 14 physical and cognitive symptoms	None	Range: 0–8 Cutoff: ≥4 = SAD	Yields DSM-IV diagnosis	No overall score Limited psychometric data
Self-Rated Scales:					
Social Phobia Scale (Mattick and Clark, 1989)	20 items (0–4) Anxiety related to being observed by others	Total score	Range: 0–80 Cutoff: ≥24 = for SAD	Brief, simple format For assessing performance fears	Limited to performance fears No specific assessment of avoidance

Measure	Items	Score	Range/Cutoff	Strengths	Weaknesses
Social Interaction Anxiety Scale (Mattick and Clark, 1989)	20 items (19-item version in Mattick and Clark, 1989) (0–4)	Total score	Range: 0–80 Cutoff: ≥34 = for SAD ≥42 = for GSAD	Brief, simple format for assessing interactional fears	Limited to interactional situations No specific assessment of avoidance
Social Phobia and Anxiety Inventory (Turner et al., 1989)	45 items (0–6) Cognitive/physical avoidance symptoms of SAD	Social phobia scale (32 items) Agoraphobia scale (13 items) Total score = social phobia (minus) agoraphobia score	Total/difference Score 0–192 Cutoffs: ≥80 = SAD ≥60 = lower threshold for screening	Usable for individuals age 14 and over Thorough coverage of SAD symptoms Useful if patient has panic symptoms	Lengthy and somewhat complex to fill out and score
The Social Phobia Inventory (Connor et al., 2000)	17 items (0–4) Derived from BSPS	Total score 1. Fear 2. Avoidance 3. Physical symptoms	Range: 0–68 Cutoff: 19 = SAD	Brief, simple format Subscales for fear, avoidance, and physical symptoms	Limited item coverage
Fear Questionaire-Social Phobia Scale (Marks and Mathews, 1979)	5 items (0–8)	Total social phobia score	Range: 0–40	Brief. Assesses impairment/distress	No direct assessment of fear or anxiety in the situation

I. DIAGNOSTIC THRESHOLD

A rating scale may help to answer the question "Does this individual have social anxiety disorder?" Although a final diagnostic decision should be based on a thorough diagnostic interview rather than a rating scale, the appropriate diagnostic threshold for social anxiety is often difficult to discern (8). "When is it social anxiety disorder and when is it just shyness within the normal range?" To answer this question, the clinician may benefit from guidance provided by results of a standardized scale. Such quantitative results put an individual's symptoms in context and allow direct comparison with groups of individuals whose symptoms meet criteria for social anxiety disorder. Such information may be especially useful in a screening situation (e.g., in a medical setting or school setting) in which the individual is not seeking treatment for social anxiety disorder. Establishing a threshold for diagnosis may also be a challenge as the patient's symptoms improve (e.g., with treatment) and the clinician needs to decide if the patient has indeed "recovered" from the disorder.

Rating scales determine overall severity based on the pervasiveness of social fears (e.g., the number of situations which are feared or avoided) as well as the intensity of the fear and avoidance in each situation. As such, rating scales are most directly informative about generalized social anxiety disorder. In clinical samples, individuals seeking treatment for a specific social anxiety syndrome (e.g., fear of public speaking) usually have increased anxiety in a variety of social situations (9) and their scores will be elevated on social anxiety scales. However, an individual with a truly circumscribed social anxiety disorder (i.e., intense anxiety in one situation but low levels of anxiety in nearly all other situations) may obtain a low overall score on social anxiety scales and may even score low on pertinent subscales (e.g., performance), which generate this score based on a variety of other situations. Scales are available for assessment of specific social fears (e.g., Personal Report of Confidence as a Speaker) (10); these are considered in, for example, Clark et al. (1).

Other clinical questions that may be answered by a rating scale:

1. *How severe is this patient's social anxiety disorder?* Rating scales quantify symptoms and place each individual along a range of severity relative to others with the same diagnosis. A single clinician may have experience with a limited number of patients with social anxiety disorder and may have difficulty identifying where a patient's symptoms lie along a range of severity. A score on a rating scale will help put each patient's symptoms in perspective. Is this among the most severe cases of social anxiety disorder, among the milder cases, or somewhere in between? Such information may be useful in assessing the need for treatment, setting realistic goals for treatment, and in selecting appropriate treatment strategies.

2. *What is the full clinical picture of this patient's social anxiety disorder?* Although it may be possible to assess the full range of social anxiety disorder symptoms based on an unstructured clinical interview, rating scales help provide systematic coverage of an array of commonly feared situations. Often, patients focus on anxiety in a specific situation or a few situations. The rating scale forces the clinician to "cover the bases" by evaluating an array of possible symptoms. This will provide systematic assessment of a range of symptoms that may not be reported spontaneously.

3. *Have the patient's social anxiety disorder symptoms changed over time?* This question is most often asked to determine a patient's response to treatment. A patient's own perception of progress or lack thereof may fail to capture the full breadth of illness. Research suggests, for example, that patients with social anxiety disorder will selectively attend to negative aspects of social situations (e.g., Ref. 11) and may also recall negative features selectively (12). This may make it difficult for the individual with social anxiety disorder to accurately gauge his or her own progress. Alternatively, a patient may focus only on that situation which is most salient at the time. Rating scales allow the patient and clinician to attend to a range of situations in order to measure overall change.

II. IMPORTANT FEATURES OF RATING SCALES

1. *Item content.* From a clinician's standpoint, the most important feature of a given scale is the content or "coverage" of the scale. What types of symptoms are asked about? How specific are questions about symptoms? All social anxiety disorder scales include a sample of commonly feared social situations. However, some scales include a few general items (e.g., "social gatherings") and others include specific situations (e.g., parties, casual gatherings etc.). As shown in Table 2, there is considerable overlap in the social situations assessed by various available scales. The table includes only those items that are covered by (i.e., common to) two or more of the scales listed. Some scales include a few additional items and some include several additional items, which are not covered by other scales.

2. *Components of the disorder assessed.* In addition to the sample of social situations selected, scales differ with regard to the components of social anxiety disorder that are assessed. Table 2 lists five components of social anxiety disorder: fear, avoidance, endurance with dread (anxiety while in the situation), physical symptoms, and impairment or distress. With the exception of physical symptoms, all of these components are included in the fourth edition of the *Diagnostic and Statistical Manual of Mental Disorders* (DSM-IV) diagnostic criteria for social anxiety disorder. As shown, only

TABLE 2 Overlapping Social Situations and Components of Anxiety Among Rating Scales

	LSAS[a]	BSPS[b]	ADIS[c]	SIAS[d]	SPS[e]	SPAI[f]	SPIN[g]	FQ[h]
Public speaking/ performing	✓	✓	✓		✓	✓	✓	✓
Eating in public	✓	✓	✓		✓	✓		✓
Drinking in public	✓	✓			✓	✓		✓
Public bathrooms	✓	✓	✓		✓			
Participating/ speaking up in a small group	✓		✓		✓			
Working while being observed	✓	✓					✓	
Writing while being observed	✓		✓		✓	✓		
Entering room with others seated	✓				✓			
Center of attention	✓				✓	✓	✓	✓
Conscious of own voice					✓	✓		
Dating/trying to pick up someone	✓	✓	✓	✓				
Parties/social gatherings	✓	✓	✓	✓		✓	✓	
Initiating a conversation			✓			✓		
Maintaining a conversation			✓	✓				
Being ignored				✓		✓		
Discussing intimate feelings				✓		✓		
Being embarrassed/ humiliated		✓		✓		✓	✓	
Being criticized		✓				✓	✓	✓
Talking to authority figures	✓	✓	✓	✓		✓	✓	
Talking to strangers	✓	✓	✓			✓	✓	
Disagreeing with someone	✓			✓		✓		
Being assertive	✓		✓			✓		
Making eye contact	✓			✓				

TABLE 2 (Cont.)

	LSAS[a]	BSPS[b]	ADIS[c]	SIAS[d]	SPS[e]	SPAI[f]	SPIN[g]	FQ[h]
Fear	✓	✓	✓	✓	✓	✓	✓	
Avoidance	✓	✓	✓			✓	✓	✓
Endurance with dread	✓	✓	✓	✓	✓	✓	✓	
Physical symptoms		✓	✓			✓	✓	
Impairment/distress			✓					✓

[a]Liebowitz Social Anxiety Scale.
[b]Anxiety Disorders Interview Schedule.
[c]The Social Phobia Scale.
[d]Social Phobia Inventory.
[e]The Brief Social Phobia Scale.
[f]The Social Interaction Anxiety Scale.
[g]The Social Phobia and Anxiety Inventory.
[h]Fear Questionnaire.

two scales directly assess impairment or distress and some scales assess only fear and not avoidance.

3. *Method of administration.* How is this scale administered? Some scales are rated by the clinician, based on information from the individual being assessed as well as other sources of information (e.g., clinical observation, information from other informants). These are referred to as clinician-rated scales. Another type of rating scale is filled out by the individual with little or no assistance from a clinician. These are self-rated scales. Because the type of information ascertained by each may differ, a thorough assessment would include both clinician ratings and self ratings.

4. *Length of the scale.* One of the most important practical questions in selecting a scale is its length. How many items are included? Longer scales usually provide the most comprehensive coverage. Such scales may provide a wealth of material to the clinician above and beyond a global score of severity. On the other hand, the more items, the longer it will take to administer. Thus, the importance of a longer versus shorter scale may depend on the needs of the situation and the type of patient who is being evaluated.

5. *Type of scores generated by the scale.* Does the scale generate an overall global score of severity? Are there additional subscale scores or factor scores that will provide additional information about specific types of symptoms (e.g., fear versus avoidance, physical symptoms).

6. *Time frame.* Scales may vary with regard to the time frame being assessed. A scale may assess symptoms for the current day, or for the past week, 2 weeks, or month. Because social anxiety depends on exposure to

situations, which do not all occur on a daily basis, an interval of less than a week may provide too limited a view. On the other hand, an interval of more than a week may render the scale insensitive to change over time.

III. CLINICIAN-RATED SCALES

A. Clinician Judgment

A key feature of the clinician-rated scales is that they require the clinician to make some judgment about symptoms. In some clinician-rated scales, such as the Liebowitz Social Anxiety Scale (13), the respondent may first choose among levels of severity much as would be done in a self-rated scale. However, clinicians will use additional information and their own clinical judgment to determine the final rating. On a basic level, the clinician can ensure that the individual understands the meaning of questions and can help clarify vague wordings of queries and response choices. On a more sophisticated level, the clinician considers information reported in the context of the patient's history, observable behavior, and other sources of information, such as relative informants. If a patient denies anxiety in one or more situations but becomes visibly uncomfortable talking to the evaluator, the evaluator may adjust a rating based on this observation. Alternatively, the evaluator may gently challenge the patient about this discrepancy to determine whether this is an exception or if the patient may be minimizing the problem.

B. Use of Clinician-Rated Scales During an Initial Evaluation

A clinician-rated scale can be included as part of an intake evaluation or initial consultation. Many patients with social anxiety disorder are unaware of the full extent of their symptoms and may also minimize the pervasiveness of their difficulties unless situations are asked about directly. It is best to get general information about the individual's life (e.g., marital status, occupation, living situation) and some history of symptoms before asking for specifics about symptoms. This allows the clinician to put specific symptoms in context. Avoidance of dating, for example, will have different implications for someone who is in a steady relationship as compared to someone who is unattached. Difficulty with public speaking may be more or less of a problem for someone depending on actual job responsibilities.

C. Use for Repeated Evaluations

For the patient in treatment, a clinician-rated scale may be repeated at intervals to measure change in symptoms over time. In choosing how often to administer the scale, the clinician should balance the requirement of information with the additional demands this places on the clinician and patient. Although weekly ratings are ideal to track progress over time, this may not be necessary in clinical practice, and the optimal interval may be 1 month to 6 weeks. A more frequent schedule of administration may be employed if the patient's symptoms are not improving as expected and adjustments or augmentation of treatment are needed.

IV. THE LIEBOWITZ SOCIAL ANXIETY SCALE

The Liebowitz Social Anxiety Scale (LSAS) (14) (Liebowitz, unpublished) is the most widely used clinician rated scale for assessment of social anxiety disorder. It covers 24 situations, 13 of which involve social interactions (social), and 11, which involve being observed in social situations (performance). Each situation is rated independently for fear: 0 (none), 1 (mild), 2 (moderate), 3 (severe); and for avoidance: 0 (never, 0%), 1 (occasionally, 1 to 33%), 2 (often, >33 to $<67\%$), 3 (usually, >67 to 100%). Items are rated for severity in the past week. The patient is handed a sheet with response choices to help them select their response.

Although items of the LSAS were initially selected in an informal process, based in clinical knowledge of patients with social anxiety disorder, the scale has generally stood up well under psychometric scrutiny, showing good internal consistency, and convergent and discriminant validity (15–17). The LSAS has proven sensitive to treatment effects for both pharmacological (14,18) and cognitive behavior therapy treatments (19). The LSAS has been a primary outcome measure in numerous multi-center trials. Important features of the LSAS, such as rating fear and avoidance independently, have since been adopted by a number of social anxiety disorder rating scales.

A. Fear versus Avoidance

An important feature of the LSAS, since adopted by many other social anxiety scales, is the attempt to assess fear vs. avoidance of social situations. It should be noted that "fear" in the LSAS emphasizes how anxious the person feels when in the situation (i.e., "endurance with dread" in DSM-IV) and not just how much the person fears going into the situation (anticipatory anxiety). Individuals with social anxiety disorder may differ across the dimensions of fear and avoidance. A patient may have severe fear and anxiety in the situation, but force himself or herself to confront it. Conversely, an individual may avoid a situation completely but deny more than mild anxiety or fear when in the situation.

The relative severity of fear versus avoidance may be influenced by internal factors such as personality factors but may also be a function of the demands of different situations. Individuals may opt out of situations that are not essential but may keep confronting feared situations if this is, for example, a requirement of their job. In the course of treatment for social anxiety disorder, changes in level of fear may be more prominent than changes in level of avoidance (20). However, in most clinical samples, social anxiety and avoidance seem to decrease in parallel.

B.   Performance versus Interactional Situations

The second division in the LSAS is between social/interactional situations and performance situations. For the most part, performance items involve situations that individuals can do comfortably when alone but have trouble completing in front of others, such as giving a speech. Social items involve situations that are inherently interpersonal—for example, being the center of attention (Liebowitz, unpublished). These two factors have not held up well based on confirmatory factor analysis (21). Safren and colleagues propose instead a four-factor model of social situations in the LSAS, which includes social interaction, public speaking, observation by others, and eating and drinking in public. However, this four-factor model is complex, especially if further subdivided by fear versus avoidance, and the clinical utility of these four subdivisions is yet to be established.

C.   Rating Based on Hypothetical Exposure

Because patients do not have the opportunity to expose themselves to all possible social situations, they may have difficulty describing their level of fear and avoidance of some situations in real terms. To the question "How much have you avoided parties in the past week?" the patient may answer "I don't know. I haven't been invited to any parties in the past week." In such situations, the LSAS asks the individual to describe level of fear based on hypothetical opportunities. Thus, if patients had no opportunity to encounter a party in the past week, the clinician would ask them to describe how fearful they would have been and how much they would have avoided the situations if the opportunity had presented itself. This enables the clinician to make a complete rating at each assessment session. Since individuals with social anxiety disorder may underestimate their ability to perform in a situation however, such hypothetical ratings may be subject to bias. The validity of ratings based on hypothetical exposure versus those based on actual experience requires further research.

D. Ranges and Thresholds

Scores on the LSAS overall can range from 0 to 144. Scores of 30 or above usually indicate that social anxiety disorder is present. Scores of 60 or above indicate generalized social anxiety disorder. In clinical samples or patients seeking treatment for generalized social anxiety disorder, average scores range from 80 to 95 and scores above 100 are not uncommon. A score between 30 and 60 may indicate that generalized social anxiety disorder is subthreshold or partially remitted. On the other hand, it may indicate that social anxiety disorder is clinically significant but limited to a few social situations. An individual with a severe circumscribed social anxiety disorder (such as fear of performing, taking tests, using public bathrooms) and little anxiety in other situations may score fairly low on the LSAS.

E. Identifying Patients with Generalized Social Anxiety Disorder (GSAD)

In addition to the cutoffs recommended below, 10 items of the LSAS have been found to discriminate between individuals with GSAD and those without GSAD (22). These include talking to authority figures, going to a party, talking with someone you don't know well, meeting a stranger, entering a room when others are seated, disagreeing with someone, looking someone in the eye, trying to pick up someone, hosting a party, and resisting a high pressure salesperson.

F. Comment

Like any clinician-administered scale, the utility of the LSAS presumes clinical competence on the part of the rater administering the scale and consistency in how the ratings are applied across occasions. Although no specialized training is needed, the rater should be familiar, through clinical experience and training, with the range of severity of fear and avoidance in social anxiety disorder. Up until now, the LSAS has been employed without the benefit of explicit administration and scoring guidelines. However, a detailed manual has recently become available (Liebowitz, unpublished).

G. Self-Report and Computer-Assisted Administration

The LSAS has been used successfully as a self-report instrument (23–26). The self-report version has been found to have similar psychometric properties to the clinician rated LSAS (24,26). Turk (7) suggests that self-administration of the LSAS may be useful only if the items are accompanied by specific instructions which define clearly what is meant by "fear" and "avoidance" and also clarify that ratings are based on hypothetical fear and avoidance when there was no occasion to confront the situation in the past week.

Kobak and colleagues report on successful computer administration of the LSAS (27). This computer administration, which was tested in a randomized medication trial of social anxiety disorder, was similar to the paper and pencil self-report except that response options were presented and scored by computer. Results generally support the reliability, validity, and equivalence of the two scales (clinician-rated LSAS and computer-administered LSAS).

The clinician-administered LSAS bases ratings primarily on the individual's reports rather than direct clinical observation. As such it may not require the degree of clinician input that is required in other clinician rated instruments such as the Hamilton Depression Scale (28) or the Positive and Negative Symptoms Scale (29). The initial success of self-report and computer administration suggests that for many patients with social anxiety disorder, the added contribution of clinical judgment may not be essential to evaluation of social anxiety disorder severity. Because these non-clinician formats are still relatively new and the LSAS has not been used this way in a large controlled study, further research is needed.

V. BRIEF SOCIAL PHOBIA SCALE (BSPS)

The Brief Social Phobia Scale (BSPS) is an 11-item scale that rates social anxiety and avoidance in 7 commonly feared social situations and 4 types of physical symptoms upon exposure to feared situations (30). Each of the 7 social situation items is rated on a 5-point scale for fear (0 to 4; none, mild, moderate, severe, extreme) and avoidance (0 to 4; never, rare, sometimes, frequent, always). The four physiologic symptoms are rated on a single 5-point scale (0 to 4; none, mild, moderate, severe, extreme). Psychometric properties based on the overall scale score and the fear and avoidance subscales are good (30,31). Furthermore, the BSPS has been shown to be sensitive to change with pharmacological treatment (32). However, the physiologic symptoms subscale has not demonstrated good internal consistency (30).

A. Features

Similar to the LSAS, the BSPS rates fear and avoidance independently. However, for the sake of brevity, the BSPS includes categories that are more general (e.g., "doing something while being watched") as compared to the more specific situations listed in the LSAS. Interestingly, the BSPS includes two items, which focus on specific negative outcomes in a social situation (being embarrassed and being criticized) rather than fear of the situation per se. In this manner, the BSPS provides a direct prompt and rating of social evaluative concerns, which are common for patients with social anxiety disorder.

The BSPS rates items based on the past week, although the user has the flexibility to assess other time frames. Items in the BSPS should be asked sequentially. The score sheet with 11 items and the anchor points can be handed to the patient. Similar to the LSAS, the BSPS provides the flexibility to rate items based on "thoughts about the situation" if these situations were not encountered in the previous week (30).

B. Comment

The main advantage of the BSPS is its brevity and its ability to collect direct information about physiologic symptoms. Although the items of the physiological symptoms subscale may not represent a unitary dimension, it may still be useful for the clinician to systematically record common physical symptoms that occur and to rate how severe these may be. Because it may take less time to administer than the LSAS, the BSPS may be especially useful in situations in which time pressure is a major concern.

VI. ADIS-IV SOCIAL PHOBIA CLINICIAN SEVERITY SCALE (CSR)

Although not a formal rating scale, another clinician rating system we find useful comes from the social anxiety disorder module of the Anxiety Disorders Interview Schedule (ADIS) (33). The ADIS includes a Clinician Severity Scale (CSR), which first provides two general introductory questions and then asks the clinician to rate degree of fear and avoidance in 13 commonly feared social situations. The CSR also provides an optional "other" item in which the clinician may list other social situations that the patient may fear and avoid. Ratings range from 0 (absent) to 8 (very severe fear or always avoids). The clinician also rates (on the same scale of 0 to 8) the presence/severity of 14 physical and cognitive symptoms. The CSR correlates highly with self-report measures of social anxiety and avoidance (34). In our own studies, interrater reliability was high (0.81) for CSR assessed by two independent assessors.

A. Comment

An advantage of the CSR over other rating scales is that it covers all diagnostic criteria (including, for instance, impairment and distress) for a DSM-IV diagnosis of social anxiety disorder. Thus a clinician can systematically ascertain a diagnosis and also rate specific symptoms using a single instrument. Disadvantages are that the CSR does not yield an overall severity score and psychometric data are still limited.

VII. SELF-REPORT SCALES

Self-rated scales are completed by the individual being evaluated with limited or no help from a clinician. The biggest advantage of self-rated instruments is their minimal time burden on clinical staff. Patients can be handed rating forms while sitting in a waiting room waiting to see their doctor (assuming that these can be filled out with some level of privacy). This process can be repeated weekly in the office or as a homework assignment with little added time for the clinician. For screening purposes, a class of hundreds of students can fill out self-rated forms with limited need for staff time, other than to check the forms for completion, enter data, and tabulate scores. Another advantage of self-rated forms is that they avoid the problem of unreliability across clinical raters. Most treatment studies now involve several sites and multiple clinical raters at each site. If raters differ in how they rate symptoms on the same scale, error variance will increase. This will make it more difficult to detect treatment differences.

VIII. THE SOCIAL INTERACTION ANXIETY SCALE (SIAS)

The SIAS is a 20-item self-rated scale, which rates social anxiety in a variety of social-interaction situations. Mattick and Clarke (35) developed the SIAS and the Social Phobia Scale (below) based on analyses of items taken from preexisting scales as well as additional items derived from clinical interviews. Those items that pertained to ongoing interaction with people in dyads or small groups were assigned to the SIAS. Items relevant to anxiety about being observed by others formed the Social Phobia Scale. These categories correspond roughly to the social and performance subscales of the LSAS. All SIAS items are rated on a five-point scale: 0 (not at all), 1 (slightly), 2 (moderately), 3 (very), 4 (extremely). Each item of the SIAS is a statement about how the respondent feels in a specific social situation. All but three items are negative statements. The remaining three positive statements are reverse scored (e.g., I find it easy to think of things to talk about).

The SIAS has good internal consistency and test-retest reliability (36). It correlates closely with the LSAS social (interactional) subscale. The SIAS discriminates between patients with and without social anxiety disorder and between patients with generalized and with nongeneralized social anxiety disorder (37). In addition, the SIAS has been shown to be sensitive to change in social anxiety symptoms in patients treated for this disorder (3).

A. Features

As shown in Table 2, the SIAS is less focused on observable behavior (i.e., avoidance) than some other social anxiety scales. It addresses several aspects of fear and anxiety by using a variety of words in different situations. Eight items describe feeling "tense," "nervous," "uncomfortable," or "unsure" in specific social situations. Seven items use the general word "difficult/difficulty" (or "easy" in reverse scored items) to capture the trouble caused by social anxiety in that situation.

The SIAS rates social anxiety without attempting to extract components such as fear or avoidance. Thus, an items such as, "I have difficulty talking to attractive persons of the opposite sex" might be rated positively due to 1) actual avoidance of these situations, 2) subjective feelings of discomfort, 3) impaired performance in this situation, or 4) more than one of the above. Remaining items capture negative "worry" or negative beliefs about outcomes in social situations. Based on these wordings, it is not surprising that the SIAS correlates highly with a measure of worry and that this scale score is also elevated in individuals with generalized anxiety disorder (38).

B. Comment

The SIAS is a simple, user-friendly scale for assessing social/interactional fears. It is commonly used in tandem with the Social Phobia Scale (below). Beyond a few specific cognitive symptoms, ratings of reactions to each situation are global (e.g., "tension," or "unease") rather than specific ratings of reactions such as physical symptoms. Rating a single dimension of fear on each item enhances the simplicity of this scale. As noted earlier, fear and avoidance are highly correlated in clinical samples. However, the clinician interested in specific information about baseline avoidance and behavioral change will not obtain such information from the SIAS.

IX. SOCIAL PHOBIA SCALE (SPS)

The Social Phobia Scale (SPS) (36) is a 20-item measure of social anxiety related to being observed by others. As described above, items taken from a larger pool of items were analyzed and those that pertained to anxiety about being observed formed the SPS. As with the SIAS, each SPS item is rated on a five-point scale 0 (not at all), 1 (slightly), 2 (moderately), 3 (very), 4 (extremely) (0 to 4; not at all, slightly, moderately, very, extremely). The SPS is often administered together with the SIAS, with each scale intended to provide information about a different aspect of social anxiety disorder.

The SPS has good internal consistency and test–retest reliability (36). Factor analysis indicates that the SPS may actually be best represented by two factors, anxiety about being observed by others and fear that others will notice anxiety symptoms (39). The SPS correlates highly with the performance subscale of the LSAS and discriminates individuals with social anxiety disorder from individuals without this disorder. Consistent with the content coverage, which is salient for both circumscribed and generalized SAD, the SPS does not discriminate patients with generalized social anxiety disorder from those with non-generalized social anxiety disorder (38).

A. Features

The SPS rates 20 individual statements on a scale ranging from 0 (not at all characteristic or true of me) to 4 (extremely characteristic or true of me). All items are negative statements and higher scores on each item contribute to the total score. Much like the SIAS, the SPS focuses on thoughts and feelings of anxiety rather than avoidance of situations per se. Several items describe fears or worries about specific outcomes or symptoms the patients may experience in a given social situation (e.g., "I worry about shaking or trembling when I'm being watched by other people"). Other items describe feelings in less precise terms such as feeling "tense," self conscious," or "anxious" when confronted with certain social situations.

B. Comment

The SPS is an easy to use self-rated scale for assessing performance related anxiety in social situations. It might be administered alone when performance fears are most problematic and the patient is not troubled by interactional fears. For most patients with generalized social anxiety disorder, the SPS is best administered together with the SIAS. As with the SIAS, the absence of specific information about avoidance behavior may be a limitation for the clinician who is focused on specific information about this dimension.

X. SOCIAL PHOBIA AND ANXIETY INVENTORY (SPAI)

The Social Phobia and Anxiety Inventory (SPAI) (9,40) is a 45-item self-report scale for assessing social anxiety disorder. However, many "items" contain multiple questions so the scale actually requires 109 individual ratings. Each item is rated on a seven-point scale: 0 (never), 1 (very infrequent), 2 (infrequent), 3 (sometimes), 4 (frequent), 5 (very frequent), 6 (always). The SPAI was designed to provide comprehensive coverage of several component symptoms of social anxiety disorder (cognitive, physical, behavioral/avoidance) based on DSM-III criteria for social phobia. In addition, the SPAI contains an agoraphobia subscale to assess, and then factor out avoidance that is due to agoraphobia rather than social anxiety. As shown in Table 2, The SPAI covers all salient dimensions of social anxiety disorder, except for impairment and distress.

The SPAI has good internal consistency for the overall scale and subscales and good two-week test-retest reliability (40). It has been demonstrated to be sensitive to change with both behavior therapy (41) and pharmacotherapy (e.g., Ref. 42) treatments. Findings of one study suggest that there may be justification for the author's inclusion of a separate agoraphobia scale. Peters (43) found that compared to the SIAS and SPS, the SPAI did a better job of discriminating patients with social anxiety disorder from those who were diagnosed with panic disorder.

A. Features

The SPAI is unique in that it includes two scales, a social phobia scale and an agoraphobia scale. The social phobia scale includes 32 items which consist of both interactional and performance situations. Seventeen of these 32 items ask for ratings of anxiety in specific situations for four different human variations: 1) with strangers, 2) with authority figures, 3) with members of the opposite sex, and 4) with people in general. The remaining items include questions focusing on physical and cognitive symptoms of social anxiety. The agoraphobia scale includes 13 items, which cover fear and avoidance linked to fear of panic attacks and related symptoms.

The SPAI attempts to isolate symptoms of social anxiety as distinct from anxiety symptoms that are part of agoraphobia. The authors propose that a difference score (social phobia score minus the agoraphobia score) should be used, as it is the truest measure of severity of social anxiety disorder. However, many studies find high rates of comorbidity between social anxiety disorder and panic disorder (44) and panic symptoms may play an important role in social anxiety pathology (45). Thus the wisdom of subtracting agoraphobia symptoms from the overall measure of severity has been questioned. Some recommend using the SPAI social phobia subscale alone rather than deriving the SPAI difference score (46).

B. Comment

The SPAI is the most ambitious of the commonly used rating scales for social anxiety. It is very thorough in its coverage of several social phobia situations and human variations on these situations (e.g., with stranger? with authority figure? and so on). It also includes extensive detail about specific anxious thoughts and physical symptoms. This type of information may be helpful in providing a profile of relative strengths and weakness. However, the SPAI takes longer to administer than other self-report measures (longer than the

SIAS and SPS combined) and its multilayered construction may be too complex for some respondents. The seven-point ratings may provide some additional nuance, but subtle differences in rating levels may be challenging to rate (e.g., it may be difficult to decide between 3, "infrequent," and 4, "sometimes"). The scoring system of the SPAI is also somewhat complex and may seem cumbersome for the clinician who is not actively involved in quantitative research.

XI. SOCIAL PHOBIA INVENTORY (SPIN)

The Social Phobia Inventory (SPIN) (47) is a relative newcomer among social anxiety disorder scales. Modeled after the clinician-rated BSPS (30), the authors sought to cover the multiple dimensions of fear, avoidance and physical symptoms, but to avoid the length and complexity if the SPAI. The SPIN includes 17 items, each rated on a five-point scale: 0 (not at all), 1 (a little bit), 2 (somewhat), 3 (very much), 4 (extremely). Initial data suggest that the SPIN has good internal consistency, test-retest reliability, and validity as well as sensitivity to treatment effects (47).

A. Features

The SPIN includes the four physical symptoms items from the BSPS. The remaining seven social-situation items of the BSPS were each divided into separate items for both fear and avoidance, except for speeches, which is rated for avoidance only. In this manner the SPIN avoids the scoring complexity of the BSPS, which requires the clinician to rate each item on two dimensions. The SPIN correlates highly with the BSPS.

B. MINI SPIN

Seeking to further streamline the process of screening for social anxiety disorder, Connor and colleagues (48) selected the three SPIN items, which best discriminated between patients diagnosed as having GSAD and those who did not have this diagnosis. The three items are:

1. Fear of embarrassment causes me to avoid doing things and speaking to people.
2. I avoid activities in which I am the center of attention.
3. Being embarrassed or looking stupid are among my worst fears.

Although the SPIN with the highest rate of endorsement overall was "Avoids speeches," this item failed to discriminate between individuals with and without generalized social anxiety disorder so it was not included. Using a cutoff of 6, this trio of items provided impressive sensitivity (89%) and specificity (90%) in identifying GSAD cases in a large managed care population (48).

C. Comment

The SPIN may have promise as an alternative self rated scale, although further research is needed. Results with the MINI SPIN are intriguing. Although the MINI SPIN does not provide much in the way of descriptive information, results suggest that the MINI SPIN may have utility as a brief screening device in settings in which time is very limited. One might also consider that the clinician should be especially attentive to the three MINI SPIN questions in conducting a clinical interview. The discriminative sensitivity of the first and last items in particular reinforces the importance of assessing the focus of fear as both of these items focus on feelings of embarrassment.

XII. FEAR QUESTIONNAIRE SOCIAL PHOBIA SUBSCALE (FQ-SOCIAL)

Finally, another very brief assessment scale bears mention. Developed by Marks and Matthews (49), the Fear Questionnaire includes 15 items, 5 of which comprise the social phobia subscale (FQ-Social). Each item of the fear questionnaire is rated on a nine-point scale ranging from 0 (would not avoid it) to 8 (always avoid it). The FQ-Social predates the acceptance of the formal diagnostic category of social phobia/social anxiety disorder. It has demonstrated adequate reliability (49) and correlates with more recently developed clinician rated and self rated scales (24,36). The FQ-Social has also been shown to be sensitive to treatment with cognitive behavior therapy (e.g., Ref. 50).

A. Comment

The FQ-Social is unique among self-rated scales in that it assesses impairment/distress directly. Since impairment and distress are pivotal criteria of the diagnosis of social anxiety disorder, it is interesting that more recent scales have not incorporated questions to assess these criteria.

XIII. CONCLUSION

Several rating scales are available for assessing social anxiety disorder. Many of these are relatively brief and simple to administer and could be easily incorporated into an initial evaluation or treatment session. Individual scales vary with regard to mode of administration, item coverage, and dimensions of social anxiety assessed. However, all rating scales are similar in rating level of anxiety in a sample of commonly feared social situations. Studies comparing rating scales to one another find that scales are significantly intercorrelated (e.g., Ref. 3). The choice of which scale or scales to use with a given patient at a given time will depend on the clinical question being addressed, the time demands of the situation, and the style and focus of the clinician.

Although not developed for this purpose, rating scales may also serve a therapeutic function for individuals with social anxiety disorder. The structured inquiry about cognitive, physical, and behavioral symptoms may aid with psychoeducation about the components of this disorder. The systematic and direct inquiry about a range of social situations may help the patient overcome minimizing. Discussion of the empirical evidence of progress based on change in scores over time may assist in cognitive restructuring. In our own research clinic, some patients volunteer that they were surprised and relieved to find that situations that they had always thought were uniquely problematic for them were actually included in a routine checklist. Other patients have expressed satisfaction and a renewed perspective after they answer "no" to a few scale items. In this way, they discover that a number of social situations that are apparently problematic for others are not really a problem for them.

ACKNOWLEDGMENT

The authors gratefully acknowledge the assistance of Lani Sherman in the preparation of this chapter.

REFERENCES

1. Clark DB, Feske U, Macia CL, et al. Systematic assessment of social phobia in clinical practice. Depress Anxiety 1997; 6:47–61.
2. Cox BJ, Swinsin RP. Assessment and measurement. In: Stein MB ed. Social Phobia: Clinical and Research Perspectives. Washington, DC: American Psychiatric Press, 1995:261–291.
3. Ries BJ, Mcneil DW, Boone ML, Turk CL, Carter LE. Assessment of contemporary social phobia verbal report instruments. Behav Res Ther 1998; 36:983–984.
4. Hart TA, Jack MS, Turk CS, Heimberg RG. Issues for the measurement of social anxiety disorder (social phobia). In: Westenberg HGM, Denboer JA, eds. Focus on Psychiatry: Social Anxiety Disorder. Amsterdam: Syn-Thesis, 1999: 133–155.
5. McNeil DW, Ries BJ, Turk CL. Behavioral Assessment: Self-report, physiology, and overt behavior. In: Heimberg RG, Liebowitz MR, Hope DA, Schneier FR

eds. Social Phobia: Diagnosis, Assessment, and Treatment. New York: Guilford Press, 1995:202–231.

6. Tharwani HM, Davidson JRT. Symptomatic and functional assessment of social anxiety disorder in adults. Psychiatr Clin North Am 2001; 24(4):643–659.

7. Turk C. Assessment of social phobia. In: Heimberg RG, Becker RE, eds. Cognitive-Behavioral Group Therapy for Social Phobia: Basic Mechanisms and Clinical Strategies. New York: Guilford Press, 2002:107–126.

8. Stein MB, Walker JR, Forde DR. Setting diagnostic thresholds for social phobia: considerations from a community study of social anxiety. Am J Psychiatry 1994; 152:408–412.

9. Turner SM, Beidel DC, Dancu CV, et al. An empirically derived inventory to measure social fears and anxiety: the Social Phobia and Anxiety Inventory. Psychol Assess 1989; 1:35–40.

10. Paul G. Insight versus Desensitization in Psychotherapy: An Experiment in Anxiety Reduction. Palo Alto, CA: Stanford University Press, 1966.

11. Hope DA, Rapee RM, Heimber RG, Dombeck M. Representations of the self in social phobia: vulnerability to social threat. Cogn Ther Res 1990; 19:399–417.

12. Coles ME, Heimberg RG. Memory biases in the anxiety disorders: current status. Clin Psychol Rev 2002; 22:587–627.

13. Liebowitz MR. Social phobia. Mod Probl Psychopharmacol 1987; 22:141–173.

14. Liebowitz MR, Schneier FR, Campeas R, et al. Phenalzine vs atenolol in social phobia: a placebo controlled comparison. Arch Gen Psychiatry 1992; 49:290–300.

15. Brown EJ, Heimberg RJ, Juster HR. Social Phobia Subtype and avoidant personality disorder: Effects on severity of social phobia, impairment, and outcome of cognitive-behavioral treatment. Behav Ther 1995; 26:467–487.

16. Heimberg RG, Horner KJ, Juster HR, et al. Psychometric properties of Liebowitz Social Phobia Scale. Psychol Med 1999; 29:199–212.

17. Holt CS, Heimberg RG, Hope DA, Liebowitz MR. Situational domains of social phobia. J Anxiety Disord 1992; 6:63–77.

18. Stein MB, Liebowitz MR, Lydiard RB, et al. Paroxetine treatment of generalized social phobia: A randomized controlled trial. JAMA 1998;280:713.

19. Heimberg RG, Liebowitz MR, Hope DA, et al. Cognitive-behavioral group therapy vs phenelzine therapy for social phobia: 12-week outcome. Arch Gen Psychiatry 1998; 55:1133–1141.

20. Slaap BR, van Vliet IM, Westenberg HG, Den Boer JA. Responders and non-responders to drug treatment in social phobia: differences at baseline and prediction of response. J Affect Disord 1996; 39(1):13–19.

21. Safren SA, Heimberg RG, Horner KJ, Juster HR, Schneier FR, Liebowitz MR. Factor structure of social fears: the Liebowitz Social Anxiety Scale. J Anxiety Disord 1999; 13:253–270.

22. Johnson MR, Emmanuel N, Ware M, Mintzer O, Book S, Jones C, Crawford M, Kapp R, Morton A, Ballenger J, Lydiard RB. Differentiating generalized from specific phobia by responses on the Liebowitz Social Anxiety Scale. Poster presented at the 16th annual convention of the Anxiety Disorders Association of America, Orlando, FL, 1996.

23. Cox BJ, Swinson RP, Direnfeld DM. A comparison of social phobia outcome measures in cognitive-behavioral group therapy. Behav Modif 1998; 22:285–297.

24. Fresco DM, Coles ME, Heimberg RG, Liebowitz MR, Hami S, Stein MB, Goetz D. The Liebowitz Social Anxiety Scale: A comparison of the psychometric properties of the self-report and the clinician administered formats. Psychol Med 2001; 31:1025–1035.

25. Mancini C, van Ameringen M, Oakman JM. Assessing the clinical utility of a self-report version of the Liebowitz Social Anxiety Scale. Paper presented at the 19th National Conference of the Anxiety Disorders Association of America, San Diego, CA, March 1999.

26. Oakman J, van Ameringen M, Mancini C, Farvolden, P. A confirmatory factor analysis of a self-report version of the Liebowitz Social Anxiety Scale. J Clin Psychol 2003; 59(1):149–161.

27. Kobak KA, Schaettle SC, Greist JH, Jefferson JW, Katzelnick DJ, Dottl SL. Computer-administered rating scale for socal anxiety in a clinical drug trial. Depress Anxiety 1998; 7:97–104.

28. Hamilton M. A rating scale for depression. J Neurol Neurosurg Psychiatry 1960; 23:56–62.

29. Kay SR, Fiszbein A, Opler LA. The positive and negative syndrome scale (PANSS) for schizophrenia. Schizophr Bull 1987; 13(2):261–276.

30. Davidson JRT, Potts NLS, Richichi EA, et al. The Brief Social Phobia Scale. J Clin Psychiatry 1991; 52:48–51.

31. Davidson JRT, Miner CM, DeVeaugh-Geiss J, et al. The Brief Social Phobia Scale: a psychometric evaluation. Psychol Med 1997; 27:161–166.

32. Davidson JRT, Potts N, Richichi E, et al. The treatment of social phobia with clonazepam and placebo. J Clin Psychopharmacol 1993; 13:423–428.

33. DiNardo PA, Brown TA, Barlow DH. Anxiety Interview Schedule for DSM-IV (ADIS IV). Albany, NY: Greywind Publications, 1994.

34. Hope DA, Laguna LB, Heimberg RG, Barlow DH. The relationship between ADIS clinician's severity rating and self-report measures among social phobics. Depress Anxiety 1997; 4:120–125.

35. Mattick RP, Peters L, Clark JC. Exposure and cognitive restructuring for social phobia: a controlled study. Behav Ther 1989; 20:3–23.

36. Mattick RP, Clarke JC. Development and validation of measures of social phobia scrutiny fear and social interaction anxiety. Behav Res Ther 1998; 36: 455–470.

37. Heimberg RG, Mueller G, Holt CS, Hope DA, Liebowitz MR. Assessment of anxiety in social interaction and being observed by others: the Social Interaction Anxiety Scale and the Social Phobia Scale. Behav Ther 1992; 23:53–73.

38. Brown EJ, Turovsky J, Heiberg RG, Juster HR, Brown TA, Barlow DH. Validation of the Social Interaction Anxiety Scale and the Social Phobia Scale across the anxiety disorders. Psychol Assess 1997; 9:21–27.

39. Safren SA, Turk CL, Heimberg RG. Factor structure of the Social Interaction Anxiety Scale and the Social Phobia Scale. Behav Res Ther 1998; 36:443–453.

40. Turner SM. Beidel DC, Dancu CV, et al. Social Phobia and Anxiety Inventory Manual. North Tonawanda, NY: Multihealth Systems, 1996.

41. Beidel DC, Turner SM, Cooley MR. Assessing reliable and clinically significant change in social phobia: validity of the Social Phobia and Anxiety Inventory. Behav Res Ther 1993; 31:331–337.

42. Van Ameringen MA, Lane RM, Walker JR, et al. Sertraline treatment of generalized social phobia: a 20-week, double-blind, placebo-controlled study. Am J Psychiatry 2001; 158:275–281.

43. Peters L. Discriminant validity of the Social Phobia and Anxiety Inventory (SPAI), the Social Phobia Scale (SPS) and the Social Interaction Anxiety Scale (SIAS). Behav Res Ther 2000; 38:943–950.

44. Sanderson WC, Dinardo PA, Rapee RM, et al. Syndrome comorbidity in patients diagnosed with DSM-III-R anxiety disorder. J Abnorm Psychol 1990; 99:308–312.

45. Jack MS, Heimberg RG, Mennin DS. Situational panic attacks: impact on social phobia with and without panic disorder. Depress Anxiety 1999; 10: 112–118.

46. Herbert JD, Bellack AS, Hope DA. Concurrent validity of the Social Phobia and Anxiety Inventory. J Psychopathol Behav Assess 1991; 13:357–368.

47. Connor KM, Davidson JRT, Churchill LE, et al. Psychometric properties of the Social Phobia Inventory. Br J Psychiatry 2000; 176:379–386.

48. Connor KM, Kobak KA, Churchill LE, Katzelnick D, Davidson JRT. MINI-SPIN: a brief assessment for generalized social anxiety disorder. Depress Anxiety 2001; 14:137–140.

49. Marks IM, Mathews AM. Brief standard self-rating for phobic patients. Behav Res Ther 1979; 17:263–267.

50. Heimberg RG, Dodge CS, Hope DA, Kennedy CR, Zollo LJ. Cognitive behavioral group treatment for social phobia: Comparison with a credible placebo control. Cog Ther Res 1990; 14:1–23.

8

Cross-Cultural Aspects of Social Anxiety Disorder

Soraya Seedat
University of Stellenbosch,
Cape Town, South Africa

Toshihiko Nagata
Osaka City University Medical School,
Osaka, Japan

I. INTRODUCTION

Although it is acknowledged that culture can impact on the physiological, behavioral, and cognitive manifestations of social anxiety disorder (SAD) (1), there are relatively few cross-cultural studies in existence. A question that arises in cross-cultural research on SAD is how to measure, in a standardized way, the different components of social anxiety in different cultural groups and how to determine to what extent these emotions and behaviors are attributable to cultural affiliation when two populations differ on language, customs, attitudes, beliefs, and social structure. Certainly, studies on SAD in culturally different samples within a country are more numerous than cross-national or multinational studies, probably because samples within a country are more easily accessed than samples across countries (2). Additionally, convenience samples (e.g., college students) are often selected for cross-cultural research on shyness and SAD on the premise that similar samples drawn from western cultures are not different with respect to the anxious and phobic responses they display. This contention is illustrated by the widespread use of similar assessment instruments and treatment modalities for SAD across cultures (2). Conversely, it has been argued that results from one sample are not simply generalizable to other samples drawn from similar cultural settings. This view is supported by findings of a recent study on cross-cultural differences in social anxiety among students sampled from three western countries (the United States, the Netherlands, and Turkey). Comparison of the levels of social anxiety across the three groups revealed that American students had higher levels of social anxiety than did Dutch and Turkish students. American students also demonstrated fewer social skills than the other two groups, who did not differ in this regard (2). This chapter considers the impact of culture on the prevalence, clinical presentation, and treatment of SAD.

II. PREVALENCE OF SAD: TRANSCULTURAL VARIATIONS

Another question that arises in cross-cultural research concerns is "What have prevalence studies taught us about the patterns of SAD across countries?" As shown in Table 1, several epidemiological studies have documented cross-cultural differences in lifetime rates of SAD. Earlier studies, based on criteria of the *Diagnostic and Statistical Manual of Mental Disorders*, third edition (DSM-III), documented lower lifetime rates (0.4 to 0.6%) in East Asian countries, such as Taiwan and Korea, compared with western countries (e.g., Germany, United States, France, and New Zealand), where rates about four times as high were recorded (2.5 to 4.0%) (3). Higher rates of SAD were also documented in females across all countries. However, differences were observed in the symptom profile and age of onset of SAD. For example, Korean respondents were less likely to endorse fears of speaking in front of a group but were more likely to report fears of speaking to strangers than were respondents in the United States, Canada, or Puerto Rico. Compared with other countries, the age of onset in Korea was approximately 10 years after age of onset in the United States.

Arguably, lifetime rates in Asian countries may not reflect true low prevalence but may reflect differences in methodology, social habits, and population response rates (4). The fact that diagnostic criteria used in epidemiological studies were developed in western settings and may, therefore, not take into account culture-specific symptoms of social anxiety needs to be considered, as this can lead to underrecognition or misidentification of the problem. Furthermore, findings may illustrate differences in the thresholds

TABLE 1 Lifetime Prevalence of DSM-III Social Anxiety Disorder

Region	Country (city)	Prevalence			Onset		
		Male	Female	Overall	Male	Female	Overall
East Asian	Korea (Seoul and rural regions)	0.1	1.0	0.5	23.2(11.5)	24.8(12.1)	24.3(12.1)
	Taiwan (Taipei)	0.2	1.0	0.6	—	—	—
	(Small town)	0.6	0.5	0.5	—	—	—
	(Rural village)	0.4	0.5	0.4	—	—	—
Caribbean	Puerto Rico	0.8	1.1	1.0	20.6(11.5)	19.4(9.9)	19.8(10.3)
North American	USA (5 US sites)	2.1	3.1	2.6	15.9(9.8)	15.8(8.2)	15.8(8.6)
	Canada (Edmonton)	1.3	2.1	1.7	16.9(10.7)	13.3(7.6)	14.6(8.7)
European	France (Paris)	2.1	5.4	(4.1)	—	—	—
	Switzerland (Zürich)	3.1	4.4	3.8	—	—	—
	Italy (Florence)	—	—	1.0	—	—	—
	Germany (Munich)	—	—	2.5	—	—	—
	Iceland	2.5	4.5	3.5	—	—	—
Oceania	New Zealand (Christchurch)	4.3	3.5	3.0	—	—	—

Sources: Korea, USA, Canada and Puerto Rico (6), Taiwan (55), France (56), Switzerland (57), Italy (58), Germany (59), Iceland (60), and New Zealand (61).

for social anxiety–related experiences in different cultural groupings (5). It is interesting to note that more recent epidemiological studies have documented higher lifetime rates of SAD and more comparable rates across countries. This may be attributed in part to changes in the diagnostic criteria between DSM-III and DSM-IV to include a more heterogenous group (i.e., individuals who fear a diverse range social and performance situations). For example, a cohort analysis of trends in social phobia in the United States over the past four decades found an increased prevalence over time, particularly of the generalized subtype (6). Further, very similar lifetime rates were found in four large community studies conducted in Italy (6.6%) (7), France (7.3%) (8), Germany (7.3%) (9), and the United States (7.2%) (12).

Findings relating to ethnic differences have not been entirely consistent. In the aforementioned cohort analysis by Heimberg et al. (6), higher rates were documented in the United States in Caucasian and in educated and married persons; however, in epidemiological data from the National Comorbidity Survey (11), comparable rates of social anxiety were recorded among Caucasians, African Americans, and Hispanics. Okazaki (12) found in a college sample of Asian and Caucasian American students that Asian Americans scored significantly higher than Caucasian Americans on measures of social anxiety and depression (12). Higher levels of avoidance and distress in social situations were also reported by Asian Americans who were less acculturated (greater acculturation reflecting greater adoption of mainstream beliefs and practices and entry into primary group relations). In the aforementioned sample, self-construal variables predicted social anxiety and not depression: variables denoting emphasis on the self as part of a group (interdependent self-construals) were better predictors of social anxiety than variables denoting emphasis on the self as autonomous (independent self-construals).

III.   PREVALENCE OF SHYNESS: TRANSCULTURAL VARIATIONS

Although shyness is not synonymous with social anxiety, SAD and shyness share many symptoms, including avoidance of social interactions, heightened autonomic arousal in social situations (e.g., blushing, sweating) and erroneous beliefs about the extent to which symptoms of anxiety are observable to others (13). Cultural values and belief systems coupled with societal practices and social norms may influence shy behavior as well as how such behavior is viewed by others (13). In Japanese culture, it has been suggested that "shame-prone and self-effacing behavior tends to be give positive functional value and is actively promoted by society" (14). Shyness has been long believed to be an important social value in Japanese society (15).

Initial studies in Japan (16–18) found much higher rates of shyness and social anxiety disorder compared with western studies. Indeed, in cross-cultural comparisons of shyness among adolescents, the highest rates were reported in Japan and Taiwan (19). In the aforementioned study of 18- to 21-year-olds in eight countries, rates of shyness ranged from 30% in Israel to nearly 60% in Japan and Taiwan, with Mexico, Germany, India, Newfoundland, and the United States falling between these extremes. Interestingly, Chen et al. (20) reported that shy-inhibited children in Shanghai, China, were more likely to be accepted by peers, to be considered for honorary and leadership positions, and to be regarded by teachers as more competent in school compared with their peers. It has also been suggested that parental attitudes may be associated with social anxiety in some cultures. A study that examined how social anxiety related to parents' child-rearing attitudes found that American adults were more likely to have social anxiety if their parents emphasized the importance of other's opinions and used shame as a disciplinary strategy compared to Chinese/Chinese-American adults (21).

IV. PHENOMENOLOGY OF SOCIAL ANXIETY DISORDER AND TAIJIN KYOFUSHO

In eastern cultures, such as that of Japan, individuals tend to define themselves by their families and social groups, so that the self is interdependent with the group. In contrast, within the self-oriented nature of western society, an individual is defined primarily in terms of his or her ability to achieve independence and autonomy from others (22). SAD, as defined by DSM-IV, can be distinguished from taijin kyofusho (TKS), arguably the most widely described cultural variant of social anxiety and phobia, in terms of these culturally prescribed systems of independence and interdependence (23). Thus, while SAD and TKS are both constructs of social anxiety, symptom expression and distress may vary according to the social expectations of the particular culture and the way in which individuals within that culture construe themselves (24). To conceptualize this distinction, it may be useful to view SAD from a clinical-anthropological perspective (25) From this perspective; *disease* (a biomedical disorder that exist across cultures) can be distinguished from *illness* (subjective perception and experience of the disorder). A view proposed by Stein and Matsunaga (25) is that the DSM-IV construct of SAD and TKS share many phenomenological and neurobiological similarities, but that these disorders are shaped by cultural experience. For example, fear of blushing and fear of staring inappropriately are important concomitants of social interaction in SAD *and* TKS, and blushing and gaze aversion are both considered to have evolutionary and neurobiological underpinnings (26,27). These underpinnings may be shared in these disorders.

Morita first described TKS in Japan in the 1930s. Despite its origins, the syndrome is not unique to Japanese culture, and similar conditions have been reported in other East Asian countries (for example, taein-kongpo in Korea) (28). Also referred to as anthropophobia, TKS literally means the disorder (*sho*) of fear (*kyofu*) of interpersonal relations (*taijin*) (29). Two forms have been described: the "typical" type and the "offensive" type. The typical type is characterized by the "fear of being noticed" and is thought to resemble the western concept of SAD. Concerns in the typical type include gazing inappropriately at others, blushing, unpleasant body odors, and stuttering. The offensive type is characterized by a "fear of offending or embarrassing others" and is the more severe variant of typical TKS and western SAD. It is the morbid fear of offending or bringing shame upon others that results in avoidance behavior that is typically seen in TKS.

In DSM-IV nomenclature, TKS is categorized as "culture-bound" and is defined as an intense fear that the body, its parts or its functions, displease, embarrass, or are offensive to other people in appearance, odor, facial expressions, or movements (30). Several diagnostic classifications are in use, and, to date criteria for TKS have not been standardized. Table 2 shows a set of recently proposed diagnostic criteria (31) based on the work

TABLE 2   Provisional Diagnostic Criteria for TKS[a]

A. At least one of the following features:
   (1) Fear of blushing in the presence of others
   (2) Fear of stiffening of facial expressions, fear of trembling of the head, hands, feet, or voice, fear of sweating in the presence of others
   (3) Fear of physical deformities being noticed
   (4) Fear of emitting body odors
   (5) Fear of line of sight becoming uncontrollable
   (6) Fear of uncontrollable flatus in the presence of others
B. Either of the following two, because of above fear(s)
   (1) Fear of being looked at (noticed) by others
   (2) Fear of offending or embarrassing others
C. At some point during the course of disorder, the person recognizes that the fear is excessive or unreasonable.
D. The fear(s) interferes significantly with the person's normal routine, occupational (academic) functioning, or social activities or relationship, or there is marked distress about having the fear(s).
E. In individuals under age 18 years, the duration is at least 6 months.

---

[a]"Typical" type requires criterion B(1), "offensive" type requires criterion B(2).

of Kasahara (16), Takahashi (32), and Yamashita (18). According to these criteria, at least one symptom from criterion A (or "typical" symptom) is required for the diagnosis. Symptoms of "blushing" and "line-of-sight" in this category have replaced Takahashi's original descriptive terminology of "flushing" and "eye contact." To meet diagnostic criteria for the offensive subtype, the "fear of offending or embarrassing others," categorized as a criterion B symptom, must be present.

The relationship between SAD and TKS can best be defined in terms of the similarities and differences that exist between these disorders. In contrast to SAD, no systematic prevalence studies exist, however, anecdotal lines of evidence suggest a relatively higher prevalence than western SAD (33). In treatment settings, rates of 7.8% in patients with "neuroses" attending a university psychiatric outpatient clinic and rates of 45.5% in patients with neuroses attending a clinic for Morita therapy have been reported (32). SAD and TKS are both characterized by excessive fear and avoidance of social interactions and performances, and both share a similar age of onset (typically in midadolescence or early adulthood) and a male preponderance in treatment settings (32). In contrast to patients with SAD, who are more preoccupied with concerns of embarrassing themselves, concerns in TKS center on offending or embarrassing others and bringing shame on the family or social group (23). Symptoms of TKS are also most exacerbated in social situations with acquaintances, rather than with strangers or intimates, in contrast to SAD (32).

TKS resembles SAD in that patients with TKS may have a broad range of symptoms from mild social concerns in adolescence, to symptoms of SAD, to delusional beliefs about emitting unpleasant body odors, to concerns about having blemishes and physical deformities (23,32,34). This wide range of types and severity of social anxiety, including delusional forms, are considered by many Japanese psychiatrists to be forms of TKS that may be responsive to similar cognitive interventions. This suggests that the delusional subtypes of TKS may differ considerably from other delusional disorders, although this has yet to be established in clinical trials (35). Notably, in the Japanese and Korean literature, body dysmorphic disorder (BDD), characterized by a preoccupation with an imagined defect or an exaggerated distortion of a minor defect in physical appearance, is considered a form of social anxiety disorder (36). Even in the West, substantial comorbidity between BDD and generalized social anxiety disorder has been found. For example, Phillips et al. (37) reported that 97% of a cohort with BDD avoided routine social and occupational activities because of embarrassment over imagined or minimal defects in appearance. Furthermore, 50% appeared to have comorbid social anxiety disorder unrelated to BDD. Other studies have also consistently found higher rates of comorbidity with

DSM-IV classification		SAD, discrete type	SAD, generalized type	Body dysmorphic disorder Delusional disorder, somatic type
Conventional classification		TKS		
		Typical TKS		Offensive subtype of SAD [referred to as "3rd Group" (Kasahara, 1995) or "Type II" (Yamashita, 1977)]
Proposed Criteria	Normal shyness	TKS (without "fixed" delusion)		"Fixed" delusional disorder
		Type I	Type II	
		"Social anxiety spectrum disorder"		

FIGURE 1   Classification of social anxiety disorder (SAD) and taijin kyofusho (TKS). B1 and B2 refer to items 1 and 2 of the proposed criteria for TKS (Table 2).

BDD in SAD patients than in patients with other anxiety disorders (36,38,39). Similarly, a subset of patients with the offensive type of TKS may be categorized as BDD or delusional disorder (somatic type) in DSM-IV (Fig. 1).

It has also been suggested that BDD, delusional disorder (somatic type), specific SAD, generalized SAD, and offensive TKS may be more appropriately conceptualised on a spectrum of "social anxiety spectrum disorders" (this volume, chapter by Muller et al.). Arguably, there is growing evidence that these disorders overlap in their phenomenology (i.e., they are characterized by fears of embarrassing or humiliating others on account of behavior and/or appearance), age of onset, comorbidity, and preferential response to selective serotonin reuptake inhibitors (40–43).

V.   CROSS-CULTURAL ASPECTS OF TREATMENT

SAD is still poorly understood from a neurobiological perspective. Preclinical and clinical observations suggest that specific serotonergic and dopaminergic mechanisms and neuroanatomic pathways may be involved in mediating the disorder. Further, animal and human behavioral models of social affiliation, social dominance, and behavioral inhibition have become increasingly relevant to our study of social anxiety disorder and perhaps to TKS (this volume, Mathew and Coplan). Overlaps in the neurobiology and psychopharmacology of SAD and TKS have been hypothesized; however, as yet there are few direct comparative studies.

While TKS may be widely acknowledged by psychiatrists in Japan, it remains largely undertreated. This may be due to 1) the syndrome being considered as part of an individual's personality or culture rather than as a medical or psychiatric illness (44) and 2) lower levels of acceptability of social anxiety in Japan, which may account for lower levels of diagnosis and treatment of TKS. There is clearly some indication that symptoms of TKS may lessen or remit in some patients in their 30s (16,45). In Japan, psychotherapies such as Morita therapy have been a mainstay of treatment for TKS (29). In contrast to cognitive-behavioral treatment strategies for SAD, Morita therapy seeks not to reduce symptoms but to direct the individual's energy away from previous concerns, such as somatic symptoms, to allow freedom from self-preoccupation, and transcendence of the self to take on a meaningful role in relationship to others and as a member of society (29). Over the years, protocols for Morita therapy have been modified to include outpatient and group treatments (known as neo-Morita methods). It has been shown that if Morita treatment protocols are rigidly adhered to, response rates can be as high as 93.3% (46).

In at least some patients, however, pharmacological interventions may be a useful form of treatment (41). The efficacy of the selective serotonin reuptake inhibitors (SSRIs) has been well established in SAD, and they remain a first-choice pharmacotherapeutic strategy (47). To date, pharmacotherapies for TKS have not been rigorously evaluated. Nevertheless, there are a few case reports that suggest that SSRIs may be effective (41,48,49). More recently, in the largest retrospective chart review of SSRIs for TKS (41), 16 of 33 patients (48%) traditionally diagnosed with TKS who were treated with clomipramine or fluvoxamine for at least 6 months were documented to respond favorably to treatment. The most frequently reported fears in the treated sample were fears of blushing (erythrophobia), fears of appearing tense (e.g., inappropriate facial expression or observable tremor), fears of emitting an unpleasant body odor (olfactory reference), fears of a blemish or physical deformity (dysmorphophobia), and fears of staring inappropriately. All 48 patients invariably met diagnostic criteria for TKS (based on modified DSM-IV SAD criteria), 15% met criteria for the somatic type of delusional disorder (suggesting that a subset of TKS patients may lose insight into their symptoms), and 10% met criteria for body dysmorphic disorder (BDD). The preoccupation with body odor or body disfigurement may closely mirror concerns in the "offensive" subtype of TKS. In the literature, both olfactory reference syndrome (delusional disorder) and body dysmorphic disorder (including the delusional subtype with poor insight) have been shown to be responsive to SSRIs, suggesting that these agents may also be useful in TKS (42,50).

In addition to serotonin and dopamine, noradrenaline has also been implicated in SAD and possibly TKS. For example, Tancer et al. (51) demonstrated that patients with SAD, in comparison with control subjects, had a blunted growth hormone response to intravenous administration of the α_2-adrenergic agonist clonidine. Monoamine oxidase inhibitors, which increase both noradrenaline and serotonin neurotransmission and have demonstrable efficacy in SAD, have been shown to be beneficial in western patients formally diagnosed with SAD who present with TKS-like symptoms (40). However, dietary restrictions may preclude their use as first-line agents. More recently, venlafaxine (a serotonin and noradrenaline reuptake inhibitor) has demonstrated efficacy in double-blind placebo controlled studies of SAD (52); however, there are no studies of this agent in TKS. Milnacipran, an agent similar to venlafaxine that is approved for the treatment of depression in Japan, was recently assessed in a 12-week open trial in 12 patients with the offensive type of TKS (31). By the end of treatment, the mean dose of milnacipran was 110 mg/day. The presence of TKS was determined using diagnostic criteria proposed by Nagata et al. (31) (Table 2). While all patients in the sample had fears of offending or embarrassing others, the clinical presentation of TKS was not entirely consistent with what has been previously described; the majority reported a fear of blushing and a fear of eye contact becoming uncontrollable rather than a fear of emitting body odors ("offensive" TKS). Of 11 patients who completed treatment, 6 were "much improved" or "very much improved" on the Clinical Global Impression global improvement scale. The mean Liebowitz Social Anxiety Scale score and the mean TKS scale severity score (developed for the study) were significantly reduced at treatment endpoint. With regards to specific TKS symptoms, only the "fear of blushing" improved significantly compared with baseline values. Self-rated interaction anxiety and depressive symptoms did not change significantly.

VI. CONCLUSIONS

Individual differences in social anxiety may be as great as ethnic differences, and a valid starting point for the clinician is to assess and treat the individual and not the ethnic group. However, by overlooking the culture-specific symptoms of SAD, clinicians and researchers run the risk of underrecognizing and misdiagnosing SAD. SAD may be universal, but culture can have a significant impact on its prevalence, presentation, and treatment. Diagnostic criteria for SAD developed in western settings may not be sensitive to the cultural variations in symptom presentation. The challenge remains to expand these criteria by incorporating into the patient assessment symptoms of SAD that are characteristic of other cultures but which may potentially exist in our own settings, albeit at subthreshold levels.

Despite a better understanding of the variation in symptom presentation of some of the transcultural variants of SAD, such as TKS, still very little is known about their psychobiological mechanisms of causation and the usefulness of western pharmacological and psychological therapies. Conversely, it is possible that insights from the nonwestern experience may be usefully applied to treatment interventions tin western settings. These remain challenges for future research in the field.

REFERENCES

1. Kirmayer LJ. The place of culture in psychiatric nosology: taijin kyofusho and DSM-III-R. J Nerv Ment Dis 1991; 179: 19–28.
2. van Dam-Baggen R, Kraaimaat F, Elal G. Social anxiety in three western societies. J Clin Psychol 2003; 59 (suppl 6): 673–686.
3. Weissman MM, Bland RC, Canino GJ, Greenwald S, Lee CK, Newman SC, Rubio-Stipec M, Wickramaratne PJ. The cross-national epidemiology of social phobia: a preliminary report. Int Clin Psychopharmacol 1996; 11 (suppl 3): 9–14.
4. Lépine JP. Epidemiology, burden, and disability in depression and anxiety. J Clin Psychiatry 2001; 62 (suppl 13): 4–10.
5. Draguns JG, Tanaka-Matsumi J. Assessment of psychopathology across and within cultures: issues and findings. Behav Res Ther 2003; 41: 755–776.
6. Heimberg RG, Stein MB, Hiripi R, Kessler RC. Trends in the prevalence of social phobia in the United States: a synthetic cohort analysis of changes over four decades. Eur Psychiatry 2000; 15: 29–37.
7. Favarelli C, Zucchi T, Viviani B, Salmoria R, Perone A, Paionni A, Scarpato A, Vigliaturo D, Rosi S, D'Adamo D, Bartollozzi D, Cecchi C, Abrardi L. Epidemiology of social phobia: a clinical approach. Eur Psychiatry 2000; 15: 17–24.
8. Pélissolo A, Andre C, Moutard-Martin F, Wittchen HU, Lépine JP. Social phobia in the community: relationship between diagnostic threshold and prevalence. Eur Psychiatry 2000; 15: 17–24.
9. Wittchen HU, Fehm L. Epidemiology, patterns of comorbidity, and associated disabilities of social phobia. Psychiatr Clin North Am 2001; 24 (suppl 4): 617–641.
10. Stein MB, Torgrud LJ, Walker JR. Social phobia symptoms, subtypes, and severity: findings from a community survey. Arch Gen Psychiatry 2000; 57: 1046–1052.
11. Magee WJ, Eaton WW, Wittchen HU, McGonagle KA, Kessler RC. Agoraphobia, simple phobia, and social phobia in the National Comorbidity Survey. Arch Gen Psychiatry 1996; 53: 159–168.
12. Okazaki S. Sources of ethnic differences between Asian American and white American college students on measures of depression and anxiety. J Abnorm Psychol 1997; 106 (suppl 1): 52–60.
13. Henderson L, Zimbardo P. Shyness, social anxiety, and social phobia. In: Hofman SG, DiBartolo PM, eds. Social Anxiety to Social Phobia: Multiple Perspective. Needham Heights, MA: Allyn and Bacon, 2001:46–64.
14. Okano K. Shame and social phobia: a transcultural viewpoint. Bull Menninger Clin 1994; 58 (suppl 3): 323–338.

15. Benedict R. Chrysanthemum and the Sword: Patterns of Japanese Culture. Cleveland, OH: Meridian Books, 1967.

16. Kasahara Y, Fujinawa A, Sekiguchi H, Matsumoto M. Fear of eye-to-eye confrontation and fear of emitting bad odors. Tokyo: Igaku Shoin, 1972 [in Japanese].

17. Kora T. Social phobia and the Japanese historical and social environment. Kyushu Seishin-igaku 1955; 4: 125–127 [in Japanese].

18. Yamashita I. Taijin-Kyofu. Tokyo: Kanahara, 1977 [in Japanese].

19. Zimbardo PG. Shyness: what is it, what to do about it. Reading, PA: Addison-Wesley, 1977.

20. Chen X, Rubin KH, Li, B. Social and school adjustment of shy and aggressive children in China. Dev Psychopathol 1995; 7: 337–349.

21. Leung AW, Heimberg RG, Holt CS, Brunch MA. Social anxiety and perception of early parenting among American, Chinese American, and social phobic samples. Anxiety 1994; 1(2): 80–89.

22. Markus HR, Kitayama S. Culture and the self: Implications for cognition, emotion, and motivation. Psychol Rev 1991; 98: 224–253.

23. Kleinknecht RA, Dinnel DL, Kleinknecht EE. Cultural factors in social anxiety: a comparison of social phobia symptoms and taijin kyofusho. J Anxiety Disord 1997; 11 (suppl 2): 157–177.

24. Good BJ, Kleinman AM. Culture and anxiety: Cross-cultural evidence for the patterning of anxiety disorders. In: Tuna AH, Maser J, eds. Anxiety and the Anxiety Disorders. Hillsdale, NJ: Erlbaum, 1985:297–323.

25. Stein DJ, Matsunaga H. Cross-cultural aspects of social anxiety disorder. Psychiatr Clin North Am 2001; 24 (suppl 4): 773–782.

26. Trower P, Gilbert P. New theoretical conceptions of social phobia. Clin Psychol Rev 1989; 9: 19–35.

27. Emery NJ. The eyes have it: the neuroethology, function and evolution of eye gaze. Neuroscience and Biobehavioral Reviews 2000; 24: 581–604.

28. Chang SC. Social anxiety (phobia) and east Asian culture. Depression and Anxiety 1997; 5 (suppl 3): 115–120.

29. Maeda F, Nathan JH. Understanding taijin kyofusho through its treatment, Morita Therapy. Journal of Psychosomatic Research 1999; 46: 525–530.

30. American Psychiatric Association. Diagnostic and Statistical Manual of Mental Disorders. 4th ed. Washington, DC: American Psychiatric Press, 1994.

31. Nagata T, Oshima J, Wada A, Yamada H, Iketani T, Kiriike N. Open trial of milnacipran for taijin-kyofusho in Japanese patients with social anxiety disorder. International Journal of Psychiatry in Clinical Practice 2003. In press.

32. Takahashi T. Social phobia syndrome in Japan. Comprehensive Psychiatry 1989; 30: 45–52.

33. Nakamura K. A review of social phobia research and treatment: From a Morita therapist's perspective. International Bulletin of Morita Therapy 1992; 5 (suppl 1 & 2): 35–45.

34. Kasahara Y. Social phobia in Japan. Trancultural Psychiatric Research Review 1988; 25: 145–150.

35. Kirmayer LJ. Cultural variations in the clinical presentation of depression and anxiety: Implications for diagnosis and treatment. J Clin Psychiatry 2001; 62 (suppl 13): 22–28.

36. Brawman-Mintzer O, Lydiard RB, Phillips KA, Morton A, Czepowicz V, Emmanuel N, Villareal G, Johnson M, Ballenger JC. Body dysmorphic disorder in patients with anxiety disorders and major depression: a comorbidity study. Am J Psychiatry 1995; 152 (suppl 11): 1665–1667.

37. Phillips KA, McElroy SL, Keck PE Jr, Pope HG, Jr, Hudson JI. Body dysmorphic disorder: 30 cases of imagined ugliness. Am J Psychiatry, 1993; 150 (suppl 2): 302–308.

38. Wilhelm S, Otto MW, Zucker BG, Pollack MH. Prevalence of body dysmorphic disorder in patients with anxiety disorders. J Anxiety Disord 1997; 11 (suppl 5): 499–502.

39. Zimmerman M, Mattia JI. Body dysmorphic disorder in psychiatric outpatients: recognition, prevalence, comorbidity, demographic, and clinical correlate. Compr Psychiatry 1998; 39 (suppl 5): 265–270.

40. Clarvit SR, Schneier FR, Liebowitz MR. The offensive subtype of taijin-kyofusho in New York City: the phenomenology and treatment of social anxiety disorder. J Clin Psychiatry 1996; 57: 523–527.

41. Matsunaga H, Kiriike N, Matsui T, Iwasaki Y, Stein DJ. Taijin kyofusho: a form of social anxiety disorder that responds to serotonin reuptake inhibitors. Int J Neuropsychopharmacol 2001; 4: 231–237.

42. Phillips KA, Albertini RS, Rasmussen SA. A randomized placebo-controlled trial of fluoxetine in body dysmorphic disorder. Arch Gen Psychiatry 2002; 59 (suppl 4): 81–388.

43. Tada K, Kojima T. The relationship of olfactory delusional disorder to social phobia. J Nerv Ment Dis 2002; 190 (suppl 1): 45–47.

44. Tajima O. Mental health care in Japan: recognition and treatment of depression and anxiety disorders. J Clin Psychiatry 2001; 62 (suppl 13): 39–44.

45. Russell JG. Anxiety disorders in Japan: a review of the Japanese literature on shinkeishitsu and taijin kyofusho. Cult Med Psychiatry 1989; 13 (suppl 4): 391–403.

46. Morita S. The therapeutic result of special treatment for shinkeishitsu. In: Kora T, eds. Morita Shoma Zenshu. Vol 3. Tokyo: Hakuyosha 1974:67–71 [in Japanese].

47. Blanco C, Antia SX, Liebowitz MR. Pharmacotherapy of social anxiety disorder. Biol Psychiatry 2002; 51: 109–120.

48. Kizu A, Miyoshi N, Yoshida Y, Miyagishi T. A case with fear of emitting body odour resulted in successful treatment with clomipramine. Hokkaido Igaku Zasshi 1994; 69: 1477–1480.

49. Asakura S, Tsukishima T, Kitagawa N, Denda K, Koyama T. A clinical study of one's bodily odors phobia. Jpn J Clin Psychiatry 2000; 29: 313–320 [in Japanese].

50. Stein DJ, Le Roux L, Bouwer C, van Heerden B. Is olfactory reference syndrome on the obsessive-compulsive spectrum? Two cases and a discussion. J Neuropsychiatr Clin Neurosci 1998; 10: 96–99.

51. Tancer ME, Stein MB, Uhde TW. Growth hormone response to intravenous clonidine in social phobia: comparison to patients with panic disorder and healthy volunteers. Biol Psychiatry 1993; 34 (suppl 9): 591–595.

52. Stein MB, Mangano R. Long-term treatment of generalized social anxiety disorder with venlafaxine XR. Poster Presentation, ADAA Annual Conference, Toronto, Canada, 2003.

53. Hwu HG, Yeh EK, Chang L. Prevalence of psychiatric disorders in Taiwan defined by the Chinese Diagnostic Interview Schedule. Acta Psychiatr Scand 1989; 79 (suppl 2): 136–147.

54. Lépine JP, Lellouch J. Classification and epidemiology of social phobia. Eur Arch Psychiatr Clin Neurosci 1995; 244 (suppl 6): 290–296.

55. Degonda M, Angst J. The Zurich study: XX: Social phobia and agoraphobia. Eur Arch Psychiatr Clin Neurosci 1993; 243 (suppl 2): 95–102.

56. Favarelli C, Guerrini Degl'Innocenti B, Giardinelli L. Epidemiology of anxiety disorders in Florence. Acta Psychiatr Scand 1989; 79 (suppl 4): 308–312.

57. Wittchen HU, Essau CA, von Zerssen D, Krieg JC, Zaudig M. Lifetime and six-month prevalence of mental disorders in the Munich Follow-Up Study. Eur Arch Psychiatr Clin Neurosci 1992; 241 (suppl 4): 247–258.

58. Stefansson JG, Lindal E, Bjornsson JK, Guomundsdottir A. Lifetime prevalence of specific mental disorders among people born in Iceland in 1931. Acta Psychiatr Scand 1991; 84 (suppl 2): 142–149.

59. Wells JE, Bushnell JA, Hornblow AR, Joyce PR, Oakley-Browne MA. Christchurch Psychiatric Epidemiology Study: Part I. Methodology and lifetime prevalence for specific psychiatric disorders. Aust N Z J Psychiatry 1989; 23 (suppl 3): 15–326.

9

The Role of Environmental Factors in the Etiology of Social Anxiety Disorder

Borwin Bandelow, Aicha Charimo Torrente, and Eckart Rüther
University of Göttingen,
Göttingen, Germany

I. INTRODUCTION

Social anxiety disorder (SAD) is a common and often disabling condition with an etiology that has yet to be established. Environmental, genetic, and neurobiological factors have been discussed as possible causes contributing to the development of social phobia.

Environmental influences likely to be involved in the development of social anxiety include traumatic experiences in childhood, unfavorable parental rearing styles, modeling, and traumatic conditioning experiences. Identifying possible risk factors, such as childhood adversities, is vital in developing prevention programs and enabling care providers to predict which individuals are most likely to develop the disorder. Psychotherapeutic interventions that are based on detection and compensation of early developmental trauma can only be regarded as rational if investigations show that the impact of early traumatic events is substantial.

Knowledge on environmental factors is solely based on retrospectives studies, which are subject to recall biases. The research to date is limited by the relatively small number of studies that sample clinical populations of individuals with SAD.

In this chapter, the literature on the influence of environmental factors in the etiology of SAD is reviewed, and a recent study on early traumatic life events, child-rearing styles, and other risk factors is presented in detail.

A. Traumatic Childhood Experiences

The influence of developmental trauma has not yet been investigated exhaustively. Stein et al. (1) compared childhood physical or sexual abuse in 125 patients with anxiety disorders (panic disorder, SAD, or obsessive-compulsive disorder) with a healthy control group. Fifty-five of their patients had SAD, but the rates of childhood adversities were not reported separately for SAD patients. Childhood physical abuse was higher among patients with anxiety disorders than among comparison subjects, and sexual abuse was higher among women with anxiety disorders than among comparison women. Another comparison with a control group also reported higher rates of childhood trauma in anxiety patients, but the sample included only 13 patients with "pure" social anxiety disorder (2). Our own study (3), which is described later in this chapter, was the first detailed investigation of traumatic childhood experiences in a sample of patients with pure social anxiety disorder. In this study, higher rates of childhood adversities were also reported.

In a nonclinical sample of subjects identified as having social anxiety disorder in a representative survey, higher rates of traumatic childhood experiences were observed by Chartier et al. (4). Tweed et al. (5) also investigated a nonclinical sample and did not find an association between SAD and parental death or separation.

Available studies provide conflicting data about whether the influence of childhood adversities is specific for certain psychiatric diagnoses or rather represents a general risk factor. In the study by Stein et al. (1), the rate of childhood abuse was higher in women with panic disorder than in those with SAD or obsessive compulsive disorder (OCD). In a comparison to patients with panic disorder, Safren et al. (6) found significantly lower rates of past childhood physical or sexual abuse in patients with SAD. They did not compare their results with a healthy control group. In contrast, David et al. (2) showed that patients with SAD had a significantly higher prevalence of childhood trauma than those who met criteria for panic disorder and agoraphobia.

Other studies did not find a specific association of childhood adversities with particular psychiatric disorders. Mancini et al. (7) found no difference in the incidence of childhood sexual abuse in patients with SAD, panic disorder, generalized anxiety disorder, or OCD. Kessler et al. (8), using data from the National Comorbidity Survey, examined the association between several childhood adversities and a number of mental disorders, including SAD. The adversities showed little specificity.

B. Unfavorable Parental Child-Rearing Styles

The clinical impression that SAD patients perceive their parents as being uncaring or overprotective has been investigated in a number of studies.

In a study of 81 patients with phobias and a control group, those assigned to the SAD group scored both parents as less caring and as overprotective, while those assigned to an agoraphobia group differed from controls only in reporting less maternal care (9). Higher SAD scores were associated with greater maternal care and greater maternal overprotection. In another comparison of perceived parental rearing practices and attitudes of subjects with SAD, agoraphobia, height phobia, and nonpatient normal controls, those with SAD and height phobia scored both parents not only as lacking in emotional warmth but also as having been rejective and overprotective. Agoraphobia reported both parents as having lacked emotional warmth but only their mothers as being rejecting. The perception of negative rearing practices of parents appeared to be stronger in height phobia than in either social phobia or agoraphobia (10). In a subsequent study, these findings obtained with outpatients were replicated with inpatients. Inpatients with SAD rated both their parents as having been rejective, having lacked emotional warmth, and having been overprotective (11). In our own study, described below, SAD patients also reported significantly more unfavorable child-rearing styles than control subjects.

In a representative community sample of nonclinical adolescents, the perceived parenting style (overprotection and rejection) was associated with the development of SAD (12).

However, in these retrospective studies, subjects' opinions of their parents' rearing styles may have been distorted by subjective interpretations, as socially anxious subjects may be oversensitive to such parental behaviors as rejection and criticism.

C. Model Learning

Earlier family and twin studies converge to support an underlying genetic component to SAD (this volume, chapter by M. Stein et al.). When children exhibit the same socially anxious behavior as their parents, these traits may have been transmitted genetically but also via model learning (13). When a son observes his father being shy in social situations, he may later imitate this behavior. Family studies cannot disentangle the relative contributions of genetic and environmental influences.

A number of retrospective studies investigated the possible transmission of socially anxious behavior via model learning. Adults with SAD as compared with those with agoraphobia perceived their parents as seeking to isolate them, as overemphasizing the opinions of others, and as deemphasizing family sociability (14,15). Caster et al. (16), who found that adolescents reporting higher levels of social anxiety also perceived their parents as socially anxious, interviewed the parents of their subjects. They observed that parent perceptions of child-rearing styles and family environment did not differ between parents of socially anxious and non–socially anxious adolescents. Rapee and Melville (17) also investigated the agreement of the reports of patients with panic disorder or SAD and the reports of their mothers. The mothers provided mixed results, disagreeing on a more standard measure but showing agreement on a more operationalized measure.

There is only one study that directly observed that an anxious cognitive style may be mediated by family processes (18). Anxious, oppositional, and nonpatient children were asked to provide plans of action to ambiguous scenarios. Anxious children predominantly chose avoidant solutions, whereas the oppositional children chose aggressive solutions. After discussing these solutions within their families, both the anxious children's avoidant plans of action and the oppositional children's aggressive plans increased. In summary, the evidence for transmission of socially anxious behavior via modeling is still limited.

D. Traumatic Conditioning Experiences

Conditioning theories suggested that repeated exposure to social-evaluative situations in which subjects experienced embarrassing interactions—such as being repeatedly berated, criticized, or otherwise devalued—may play a role in the development of SAD (19). Persistent social anxiety was conceptualized as the effect of pairing social stimuli (e.g., being scrutinized by others) with negative experiences (e.g., being embarrassed or laughed at). However, for the development of other phobias, such as agoraphobia or specific phobias, conditioning experiences seem less probable as an etiological explanation. While two-thirds of subjects with dog phobias reported a negative experience with a dog, so did an equivalent number of those without dog fear (20). Similarly, only 11.5% of persons with height phobia were classified as directly conditioned cases (21).

The evidence for a role of conditioning experiences in the development of SAD is weak. In a survey of individuals with SAD, 58% of the respondents reported the onset of social fear after a traumatic event (22). However, this rate was not compared with that in a control group. In a controlled study, 68 individuals with specific or generalized SAD and 25 normal controls were assessed for presence of traumatic conditioning experiences. Only patients with the specific but not with the generalized subtype, the more severe form of SAD, reported a significantly higher frequency of traumatic conditioning episodes than nonfearful subjects (23).

II. A STUDY OF EARLY TRAUMATIC EXPERIENCES, PARENTAL CHILD-REARING STYLES, FAMILY HISTORY OF MENTAL DISORDERS, AND BIRTH-RISK FACTORS IN PATIENTS WITH SOCIAL ANXIETY DISORDER

In this section, we summarize the findings of a recent study of patients with SAD that investigated early traumatic experiences (such as separations from parents), parental child-rearing styles (e.g., overcontrolling), familial factors (i.e., first-degree relatives with anxiety disorders), and birth risk factors (such as premature birth, low birth weight, or others). The study is described elsewhere in detail (3). To our knowledge, this was the first extensive investigation of childhood adversities in a sample of "pure" SAD patients.

Fifty patients with SAD were interviewed in person after confirming the diagnoses by using the SCID (Structured Clinical Interview for DSM-IV) (24). A total of 120 subjects who were free of psychiatric disorders according to a SCID interview were taken from a pool of 155 healthy controls in order to match patients and control subjects for age and sex.

Subjects were interviewed in person or by telephone using a standardized questionnaire with 203 questions already used in an earlier study with panic disorder patients (25). The questionnaire contained items concerning: 1) traumatic life events during childhood until the age of 15, 2) parental child-rearing styles and attitudes towards the subjects, 3) psychiatric disorders in family members, and 4) birth risk factors.

Patients with SAD reported significantly more separations from the parents (e.g., due to hospitalizations or because they were raised by persons other than their parents), parents' marital discord, or prolonged illness of the child. There was a significantly higher degree of violence in the families (e.g., violence directed by the father against the children or their mother). Sexual abuse, including forced sexual acts with penetration, was also more common in the patient group.

To determine whether not only single events but rather a combination of multiple severe traumatic life events was associated with SAD, scoring was listed on a "severe trauma scale," which included separation from the parents, severe physical handicap of the subject during childhood, parents' marital problems, alcohol abuse by one or both parents, severe psychiatric illness of parents, violence in the family, and sexual abuse. On this 10-point scale, patients had significantly more severe traumatic events (mean score 2.0; SD 1.28) than control subjects (0.82; SD 1.1; $p < 0.0001$). Only 6 (12%) of the SAD patients but 63 (52.5%) of the controls did not report any severe traumatic events at all ($\chi^2 = 24.0$; $p < 0.0001$).

These rates can be compared with results obtained with the same questionnaire in patients with panic disorder (25) or borderline personality disorder (26). In all three disorders, significantly higher scores were found than in the control groups, with patients with SAD having an intermediate position between borderline personality disorder and panic disorder (Fig. 1).

In general, patients reported more unfavorable parental child-rearing styles than controls. They reported to a significantly higher extent that

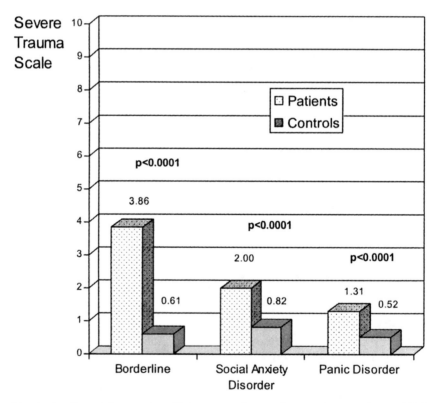

FIGURE 1   Comparisons of multiple severe traumatic experiences during childhood in adult patients with borderline personality disorder, social anxiety disorder, and panic disorder. Mean scores on a 0 to 10 "Severe Trauma Scale."

punishment by their parents was inadequate; that their fathers were short-tempered and dominant, restricting their children's autonomy and being less caregiving and that their mothers, who also restricted their autonomy and were less caregiving.

SAD patients reported higher rates of first-degree relatives with any mental disorder, any anxiety disorder, panic disorder, SAD, generalized anxiety disorder, or suicidality. They also reported a higher degree of alcohol abuse by their fathers. However, this study was not conducted by interviewing the other family members directly. It is questionable whether subjects were fully informed about their relatives' psychiatric problems and how reliable interviewers' classifications of the family members' psychiatric disorders were on the basis of the patients' reports.

There were no significant differences between the two groups regarding birth risk factors, including age of mother or father over 35 years at childbirth, premature birth, low birth weight, cesarean section, perinatal complications, or congenital defects.

A. Interaction of Environmental and Genetic Factors

Complex interdependencies exist among the various environmental and biological risk factors for psychiatric disorders. A correlative association between risk factors and outcomes does not prove causation, because these associations can sometimes be explained by latent, or moderator, variables. For example, alcohol abuse is highly correlated with lung cancer, but only through the moderator variable smoking, which is highly correlated with both alcohol drinking and lung cancer.

If we examine a certain risk factor in an isolated way, we run the risk of suspecting a causal relationship between this risk factor and the development of SAD that is in fact nonexistent or at least relatively small. When patients with SAD report that their parents demonstrated significantly more overprotection than parents of healthy control subjects, we cannot simply conclude that overprotection is the main cause for developing SAD, as this correlation may be solely due to other variables that have a much stronger etiological contribution.

When we have identified a number of possible risk factors for SAD, which is the one that shows the strongest contribution? Let us consider an example of a father and his son, both of whom have SAD. The father is an alcoholic, is frequently absent from home, is unhappy in his marriage, and beats wife and children. When his son develops SAD, is this mainly due to his father's alcoholism or to familial violence, frequent separation from the father, or to the parents' marital discord? Or did the son simply inherit social anxiety from his father and can all other observed associations be explained by the interdependency of social anxiety and alcohol abuse? It becomes clear that risk factors should not be examined independently but rather in an integrative model.

To determine the relative contribution of the investigated risk factors, we performed a logistic regression analysis with the data obtained in our study of childhood adversities in SAD. Logistic regression is a statistical method that may be able to identify the "true" contribution of a certain risk factor to a certain outcome by separating out moderator variables. This kind of analysis is often used to investigate the relationship between a criterion and a set of ordinal explanatory variables. It can identify events that are directly associated with the criterion, i.e., being a member of the SAD or the control group, and to filter out events that are only indirectly associated via latent variables. Based on assumptions in the literature, we analyzed a number of risk factors by using logistic regression, including: 1) separation from parents, 2) childhood sexual abuse, 3) violence in the family, 4) birth risk factors, 5) unfavorable parental child-rearing styles, and 6) first degree relatives with a history of anxiety disorders (including panic disorder, generalized anxiety disorder, and SAD).

The highest odds ratio was found for familial anxiety disorders (Table 1). Separation from parents also had a significant but smaller influence. There was only a trend toward a statistically significant contribution of childhood sexual abuse. Violence in the family, unfavorable parental attitudes, and birth risk factors did not contribute significantly. Thus, although inadequate child-rearing styles were significantly reported more often in the patient group, this risk factor seemed not be directly associated with the etiology of SAD.

TABLE 1   Logistic Regression—Risk Factors Associated with Social Anxiety Disorder

Variable	Odds ratio	Confidence intervals	p value
First degree relatives with anxiety disorder	127.6	28.0–581.3	<0.0001
Separation from parents	3.5	1.8–6.7	0.0001
Childhood sexual abuse	4.3	0.8–23.8	0.092 (trend)
Violence in family	3.8	0.6–24.3	0.16 (N.S.)[a]
Unfavorable parental rearing styles	1.00	0.9–1.1	0.76 (N.S.)
Birth risk factors	1.23	0.6–2.5	0.56 (N.S.)

[a]N.S. = not significant.

III. CONCLUSION

In studies of childhood adversities in adults with SAD, higher rates of separation from parents, marital problems, violence, and sexual abuse in the families of SAD patients were found. Our controlled study was the first to confirm these results in a sample with "pure" SAD patients. However, like all other studies in this field, this study has certain limitations, such as recall biases due to its retrospective nature.

It is possible that not only specific single emotional stress events but rather multiple ones are associated with the anxiety disorder. An analysis of combinations of multiple severe traumatic events demonstrated significantly higher scores in the patients' group than in healthy controls. Childhood adversities seemed to be less frequent than in patients with borderline personality disorder but more frequent than in panic disorder patients.

In our study, parental rearing styles also were rated as more unfavorable by the social anxiety disorder patients, which confirmed the results of earlier investigations. However, not only adverse environments, but also a family history of psychiatric disorders, in particular anxiety disorders, were associated with social anxiety disorder in this study. Indeed, in a logistic regression model, familial anxiety disorders were identified by far as the most relevant risk factor among the ones investigated. Separation from parents also showed a significant, but much weaker contribution. For childhood sexual abuse, only a trend towards a statistically significant association was found. In the case of multifactorial etiology, logistic regression may be able to identify the "true" contribution of a certain risk factor.

The role of other possible environmental factors still requires confirmation. These include the familial transmission via modeling or the triggering of social anxiety through traumatic conditioning experiences. Even these factors may be mediated by neurobiology and genetics, so that future studies need to integrate environmental and neurobiological variables.

REFERENCES

1. Stein MB, Walker JR, Anderson G, Hazen AL, Ross CA, Eldridge G, Forde DR. Childhood physical and sexual abuse in patients with anxiety disorders and in a community sample. Am J Psychiatry 1996; 153:275–277.
2. David D, Giron A, Mellman TA. Panic-phobic patients and developmental trauma. J Clin Psychiatry 1995; 56:113–117.
3. Bandelow B, Charimo Torrente A, Wedekind D, Broocks A, Hajak G, Rüther E. Early traumatic life events, parental rearing styles, family history of psychiatric disorders, and birth risk factors in patients with social anxiety disorder. Eur Arch Psychiatry Clin Neurosci (accepted for publication).

4. Chartier MJ, Walker JR, Stein MB. Social phobia and potential childhood risk factors in a community sample. Psychol Med 2001; 31:307–315.
5. Tweed JL, Schoenbach VJ, George LK, Blazer DG. The effects of childhood parental death and divorce on six-month history of anxiety disorders. Br J Psychiatry 1989; 154:823–828.
6. Safren SA, Gershuny BS, Marzol P, Otto MW, Pollack MH. History of childhood abuse in panic disorder, social phobia, and generalized anxiety disorder. J Nerv Ment Dis 2002; 190:453–456.
7. Mancini C, Van Ameringen M, MacMillan H. Relationship of childhood sexual and physical abuse to anxiety disorders. J Nerv Ment Dis 1995; 183:309–314.
8. Kessler RC, Davis CG, Kendler KS. Childhood adversity and adult psychiatric disorder in the US National Comorbidity Survey. Psychological Medicine 1997; 27:1101–1119.
9. Parker G. Reported parental characteristics of agoraphobics and social phobics. Br J Psychiatry 1979; 135:555–560.
10. Arrindell WA, Emmelkamp PM, Monsma A, Brilman E. The role of perceived parental rearing practices in the aetiology of phobic disorders: a controlled study. Br J Psychiatry 1983; 143:183–187.
11. Arrindell WA, Kwee MG, Methorst GJ, van der Ende J, Pol E, Moritz BJ. Perceived parental rearing styles of agoraphobic and socially phobic inpatients. Br J Psychiatry 1989; 155:526–535.
12. Lieb R, Wittchen HU, Hofler M, Fuetsch M, Stein MB, Merikangas KR. Parental psychopathology, parenting styles, and the risk of social phobia in offspring: a prospective-longitudinal community study. Arch Gen Psychiatry 2000; 57:859–866.
13. Bandura A. Analysis of modeling behavior. In: Bandura A, ed. Psychological Modeling: Conflicting Theories. Chicago: Aldine, 1971:71–99.
14. Bruch MA, Heimberg RG. Social phobia and perceptions of early parental and personal characteristics. Anxiety Res 1989; 2:57–65.
15. Bruch MA, Heimberg RG. Differences in perceptions of parental and personal characteristics between generalized and nongeneralized social phobics. J Anxiety Dis 1994; 8:155–168.
16. Caster JB, Inderbitzen HM, Hope D. Relationship between youth and parent perceptions of family environment and social anxiety. J Anxiety Disord 1999; 13:237–251.
17. Rapee RM, Melville LF. Recall of family factors in social phobia and panic disorder: comparison of mother and offspring reports. Depress Anxiety 1997; 5:7–11.
18. Barrett PM, Rapee RM, Dadds MM, Ryan SM. Family enhancement of cognitive style in anxious and aggressive children. J Abnorm Child Psychol 1996; 24:187–203.
19. Rachman S. The conditioning theory of fear-acquisition: a critical examination. Behav Res Ther 1977; 15:375–387.
20. DiNardo PA, Guzy LT, Jenkins JA, Bak RM, Tomasi SF, Copland M. Etiology and maintenance of dog fears. Behav Res Ther 1988; 26:241–244.

21. Menzies RG, Clarke JC. The Etiology of acrophobia and its relationship to severity and individual-response patterns. Behav Res Ther 1995; 33:795–803.
22. Öst LG. Age of onset in different phobias. J Abnorm Psychol 1987; 96:223–229.
23. Stemberger RT, Turner SM, Beidel DC, Calhoun KS. Social phobia: an analysis of possible developmental factors. J Abnorm Psychol 1995; 104:526–531.
24. First MB, Spitzer RL, Gibbon M, Williams JBW. Structured Clinical Interview for DSM-IV Axis I Disorders, Clinician Version (SCID-CV). Washington, DC: American Psychiatric Press, 1996.
25. Bandelow B, Späth C, Álvarez Tichauer G, Broocks A, Hajak G, Rüther E. Early traumatic life events, parental attitudes, family history, and birth risk factors in patients with panic disorder. Compr Psychiatry 2002; 43:269–278.
26. Bandelow B, Krause J, Wedekind D, Broocks A, Hajak G, Rüther E. Early traumatic life events, parental attitudes, family history, and birth risk factors in patients with borderline personality disorder and healthy controls. Psychiatr Res. In press.

10

Cognitive Theories of Social Phobia

Deborah A. Roth

University of Pennsylvania,
Philadelphia, Pennsylvania, U.S.A.

I. INTRODUCTION

In 1985, Liebowitz and colleagues (1) called social phobia (SP) the "neglected anxiety disorder" (p. 729). While research into this most prevalent anxiety disorder (2) certainly accelerated in the late 1980s and early 1990s, the development of cognitive models to explain the maintenance of social phobia served to further spur research into the nature of this disorder as well as how to treat it. In this chapter, cognitive models of social phobia are described and research evidence supporting them is reviewed. While cognitive behavioral treatments are reviewed elsewhere (this volume, chapter by Heimberg), the ways in which the cognitive models have informed current approaches to treatment is also briefly discussed.

II. BASIC CONCEPTS: THE COGNITIVE MODELS

A. Clark and Wells's Cognitive Model (1995)

The first cognitive model of social phobia was proposed by Clark and Wells (3). The model serves not to explain the etiology of social phobia but rather to explain why social avoidance and distress are typically maintained over time in the absence of treatment. The model starts with the socially anxious individual entering a social situation, at which time assumptions about the social world and oneself as a social being are activated. Clark and Wells propose that three main kinds of beliefs are activated when socially anxious individuals find themselves in social situations. First, they hold excessively high standards for themselves. For example, during a casual conversation, they might expect to have no pauses at all; or during a speech or presentation, they might expect never to stumble over even one word. Second, they hold conditional beliefs about themselves with respect to these standards, such as "If I pause during the conversation, the other person will think I'm an idiot" or "If I stumble over a word during my presentation, I'll lose my job." These two kinds of assumptions are reflective of both an overestimation of the likelihood of negative outcomes in social situations as well as their cost were they to occur. Finally, in a broader sense, individuals with social phobia also hold unconditional beliefs about themselves. Regardless of any specific behavior, they might see themselves as being odd, or losers, or unlikable.

Taken together, these kinds of beliefs lead individuals with social phobia to perceive danger in the social world and, not surprisingly, when they are in social situations, they begin to experience a range of cognitive, physiological, and behavioral symptoms. This "anxiety program," as it has been termed by Clark and Wells, leads to a shift in focus of attention, such that socially anxious individuals begin to process the self as a social object. Rather than focusing on the social situation at hand, SPs focus on how they are feeling and, most importantly, on how they are coming across to others.

This tendency to process the self as a social object can have many negative consequences. The experience of physiological symptoms and negative cognitions about the self are taken as further evidence that the social world is threatening and that the socially anxious individual cannot function in it (e.g., "Since I'm blushing, I must be making a fool of myself"). Physiological symptoms can also spur further physiological symptoms. For example, when a person notices his heart racing, he might become anxious, causing his heart to race even faster. Excessive self-focus can also interfere with the processing of social information. By paying so much attention to themselves, individuals with social phobia can miss out on important information in the social environment that could serve to disconfirm their negative beliefs. Furthermore, self-focus can make people come across as unfriendly or as lacking social skills, thus increasing the likelihood that individuals with social phobia really will have negative experiences in the social realm, serving as further evidence for their already negative beliefs.

Clark and Wells propose a number of factors that prevent individuals with social phobia from acquiring information that would serve to disconfirm these negative beliefs. As already suggested, the major factor is self-focused attention and the tendency to see oneself as a social object. Since self-focus gets in the way of the processing of social information, individuals with social phobia tend to draw conclusions about how they came across in social situations from their "felt sense" of how they did. For example, a person might leave a social situation thinking, "I felt nervous, so everyone must have seen how nervous I was." Unfortunately, these conclusions are based on faulty information, and the next time they enter feared situations, the same faulty beliefs are activated, again increasing self-focus.

Another factor that serves to maintain social phobia is the use of safety behaviors. While social phobia is associated with avoidance of social and performance situations, few individuals with the disorder are completely socially isolated. Either by choice or necessity, SPs do enter social situations, but feel that they need to engage in subtle avoidance strategies [also referred to as safety behaviors (4)] to make these situations more manageable and prevent feared outcomes from occurring. Safety behaviors are logically connected to the feared outcomes of SPs. An individual with social phobia who worries about bringing up topics in casual conversation that will not interest people might not speak at all. Similarly, an individual with social phobia who fears spilling her drink at a cocktail party might hold her glass with two hands, grip it very tightly, and lower her head to the glass so that she will not risk spilling as she raises the glass to her mouth. When feared outcomes do not occur, SPs incorrectly attribute their nonoccurrence to the use of safety behaviors, denying themselves the opportunity to see that such outcomes are unlikely to occur even without safety behaviors. Furthermore, they deny themselves the opportunity to see that even if feared outcomes did occur, they would be far less costly than expected. For example, adults do not commonly spill their drinks, and when they do, it rarely has terribly negative consequences.

Individuals with social phobia also fail to recognize that safety behaviors can have a paradoxical effect, actually increasing the likelihood that their feared outcomes will occur. An individual who fears spilling her drink might grip her glass so tightly than she actually causes her arms to shake, increasing the likelihood that she will spill. Some safety behaviors can also make people come across less well than if they had exhibited the feared behavior. A person might be judged more negatively for sitting silently in a social situation than if he had brought up a topic that was not of interest to everyone.

The final factor that serves to maintain social phobia over time occurs not during social situations but rather in anticipation of them and also once they are over. Before entering social situations, SPs experience significant anticipatory anxiety. They end up entering social situations expecting the worst. This can have two detrimental effects. When SPs expect the worst, they feel that it is very important to monitor how they are coming across and to try to prevent negative outcomes, thereby increasing self-focused attention and the use of safety behaviors. In addition, when we expect the worst, we tend to be on the lookout for information that will confirm these beliefs. As such, when in social situations, SPs selectively attend to negative cues, causing them to miss out on positive ones.

When SPs leave social situations, they tend to engage in what Clark and Wells have termed the "postmortem." They mentally review what they have said and how they believe that they came across to others. For some SPs, this process can occupy hours of thought. Very strong memories of social failure are encoded, and these inaccurate memories are activated the next time the socially anxious person enters a social situation, again leading to self-focused attention and a bias to picking up on the negative to the exclusion of the positive.

B. Rapee and Heimberg's Cognitive Behavioral Model of Social Phobia (1997)

The other major model of social phobia was proposed by Rapee and Heimberg (5). Their model of social phobia begins with the assumption that individuals with social phobia place a great deal of importance on making a desirable impression on others and, furthermore, view others as being highly critical. When individuals with social phobia anticipate being in social situations or actually are in social situations, they form a mental representation of themselves as seen by the audience. This representation is formed from various sources, including information stored in long-term memory (e.g., memories of how they felt that they performed in that same situation in the past), current experience (e.g., physical symptoms like racing heart or sweating), as well as external cues (e.g., reaction from the audience when giving a speech or reaction from a person with whom they are chatting). When individuals with social phobia find themselves in social situations, their attentional resources are dedicated to these sources of information, which will help them to form this mental representation of how they are coming across to others.

This self-generated mental representation is then compared to the perceived expectations of the audience. In other words, individuals with social phobia assess the discrepancy between their perceived behavior and the standard that they believe is held for them by the audience. The degree of this discrepancy helps SPs to determine the probability that they will be negatively evaluated by the audience. If they perceive this probability to be high, further anxiety is experienced. This can include physical symptoms, negative beliefs about the self and the social world, as well as behavioral changes. These physical, cognitive, and behavioral symptoms are then used to further confirm the negative mental representation that the individual with social phobia holds for himself. Focusing on internal signs of anxiety as well as external signs of negative evaluation precludes SPs from picking up on evidence in the environment that could serve to disconfirm their beliefs about their ability to function in the social world. Furthermore, generating negative images of themselves as social objects certainly has a negative impact on SPs the next time they think about entering, or actually enter, a social situation.

III. COMMONALITIES OF THE COGNITIVE MODELS

The models proposed by Clark and Wells (3) and Rapee and Heimberg (5) have common features. Both models propose that when individuals with social phobia enter social situations, assumptions about the self and the social world are activated. Clark and Wells propose that these assumptions lead to a shift in focus, such that SPs see themselves as social objects. Similarly, Rapee and Heimberg propose that SPs develop a mental representation of themselves as they think they are seen by the audience.

Both of the models suggest that there are two main kinds of consequences of this shift in focus. First, there are behavioral consequences. Most notably, SPs begin to engage in safety behaviors or subtle avoidance strategies to try to increase the likelihood that they will make a desired impression and that feared outcomes will not occur. Both the shift in self-focus and behavioral changes then influence the way that information is processed. Attention, memory, and interpretations are all skewed in the direction of the negative, effectively maintaining negative beliefs about the self and one's ability to function in the social world. In the following section of the chapter, the empirical evidence for these features is reviewed and attention is paid to the role that each plays in the maintenance of social phobia.

IV. EMPIRICAL SUPPORT FOR THE COGNITIVE MODELS

A. Assumptions About the Self and the Social World

When anticipating social events and when actually in them, a number of beliefs about oneself and the social world are activated for people with social phobia. As noted, Clark and Wells (3) suggest that there are three categories of assumptions: excessively high standards for social performance, conditional beliefs concerning the consequences of performing in a certain way, and unconditional negative beliefs about the self (6). Similarly, Rapee and Heimberg (5) suggest two general assumptions: that people are critical and that it is extremely important to be judged positively by others.

There is ample evidence to support the notion that individuals with social phobia set very high standards for themselves. Perhaps the most convincing evidence comes from studies examining perfectionism in people with social phobia. As compared to people without the disorder, those with social phobia have greater concern over the consequences of making mistakes and experience more doubts about the right course of action to take in situations (7–9). Furthermore, individuals with social phobia strongly endorse the experience of socially prescribed perfectionism, suggesting that they are very sensitive to what they think is expected of them by others (7,10).

Further evidence for the high standards held by SPs comes from studies that ask patients to participate in various social tasks and then to rate their own behavior. Other participants in these mock social situations (usually experimental confederates) and/or objective observers are also asked to make similar ratings, allowing for a comparison between how socially anxious people judge themselves and how they are judged by others. Studies consistently show that individuals with social phobia rate themselves more harshly than they are rated by others (11–14).

While no studies have yet explored whether people with social phobia view others as more critical or judgmental than do people without the disorder, there is evidence to suggest that individuals with social phobia are very attuned to cues in the environment that could be interpreted as signs of criticism or negative evaluation. The face-in-the crowd paradigm has been used to see how quickly SPs notice a discrepant face in an array of faces that all exhibit the same facial expression. Gilboa-Schechtman and colleagues (15) found that individuals with social phobia and nonclinical controls were both quicker at finding an angry face in a crowd of neutral faces than they were at finding a happy face in a crowd of neutral faces. However, this discrepancy was particularly pronounced in individuals with social phobia. Two studies, both in nonclinical samples, have shown that individuals who score high on a measure of social anxiety are more likely than individuals who score low on a measure of social anxiety to notice signs of negative feedback and are less likely to notice signs of positive feedback while making a speech to an audience (16,17). Finally, studies have shown that SPs have better memory (both recognition and recall) for negative, critical faces than for faces that exhibit positive or neutral facial expressions (18,19).

B. Shift in Self-Focus and Subsequent Use of Safety Behaviors

At this point, the individual with social phobia has entered a social situation, activating beliefs about the self as social object and about the social world. Specifically, SPs set high standards for themselves and pick up on cues in the environment that are suggestive of criticism and negative evaluation by others, leading them to perceive a large discrepancy between how they think they are coming across and what they think is expected of them by the audience (20,21). Given this large discrepancy, SPs then tend to overestimate the likelihood that negative outcomes will occur for them in social situations (as is reviewed in greater detail later in the chapter).

With these kinds of beliefs activated, a few crucial things happen. Since SPs have identified a discrepancy between how they think they are coming across and how they believe they should be coming across, they are motivated to engage in behaviors that will narrow this discrepancy. This is where the notion of safety behaviors fits into the picture of social phobia. As already noted, safety behaviors are logically connected to the outcomes that SPs fear and can be conceptualized as a way of bringing behavior in line with what SPs believe is expected of them by the audience.

The superordinate problem, however, is that in order to evaluate this discrepancy and attempt to correct it, individuals with social phobia need to be focused on the self. In fact, research has shown that when in social situations, SPs tend to take an "observer perspective," seeing themselves as they think they are seen by others. In effect, individuals with social phobia tend to "spectator" on themselves, rather than taking a "field perspective" in which people view situations through their own eyes (22). Wells and co-workers (23) found that when people with social phobia and nonclinical controls were asked to imagine themselves in nonsocial situations, both groups tended to take a field perspective; but when asked to imagine themselves in social situations, SPs were more likely than nonclinical controls to take the observer perspective. Wells and Papageorgiou (22) further explored perspective-taking in people with social anxiety disorder, agoraphobia, blood-injection-injury phobias, as well as nonclinical controls. The findings from this study revealed that the shift from observer to field perspective in social versus nonsocial situations was unique to SPs. When imagining both social and nonsocial situations, individuals with agoraphobia were found to consistently take an observer perspective while individuals with blood-injection-injury phobias and nonclinical controls were found to consistently take a field perspective. Findings from a study by Hackmann et al. (24) are consistent with Wells's studies. In that study, individuals with social phobia were more likely than nonclinical controls to take an observer perspective when asked to describe images of themselves in social situations. Furthermore, as compared to controls, the images of people with social phobia were more likely to be negative and distorted.

As already noted, when people enter social situations, past experiences can be used as a means of predicting how they will come across to others. For individuals with social phobia, memories of themselves in social situations also seem to be encoded from an observer perspective. Coles et al. (25) also examined memory perspective in patients with social phobia. In their study, participants with social phobia were asked to recall and imagine themselves in social situations in which they had experienced low, medium, or high social anxiety. As the degree of anxiety associated with memories increased, people with social phobia were more and more likely to take an observer perspective, while nonclinical controls were slightly more likely to take a field perspective. The tendency to take the observer perspective most commonly occurred during performance/public speaking events, suggesting that external sources of feedback during this type of event may be difficult or ambiguous to read. Therefore, individuals may rely more on internal sources of information as a means of evaluating their performance (and to determine how they think others evaluate their performance) in these situations. Coles et al. (26) further explored memory perspective in patients with social phobia who completed two behavior tests, making a speech and having a casual conversation. Immediately after the behavior tests as well as 3 weeks later, SPs recalled the role-plays from a more observer/less field perspective than did the nonclinical controls. In fact, over time, this observer/field discrepancy actually became more pronounced for the SPs.

Hirsch and colleagues (27) recently explored the impact that holding a negative self-image might have on individuals with social phobia. In their study, SPs were asked to have two casual conversations, one while picturing a very negative self-image (as they typically would during social interactions) and one while picturing a neutral self-image. Holding a negative self-image in one's mind had very detrimental effects on the conversation. While in the negative self-image condition, SPs reported feeling more anxious, believed that their anxiety symptoms were more visible, and rated their performance more poorly. These ratings were mirrored by blind raters who gave more negative ratings of behavior in the negative self-image condition than in the neutral image condition.

C. Effects on Information Processing

When individuals with social phobia are self-focused and engaging in safety behaviors, their ability to accurately process information in the social environment deteriorates. Researchers have explored attentional bias, memory bias, and judgment bias in social phobia, not only to demonstrate that these biases exist but also to show how they contribute to the maintenance of social anxiety over time.

1. Attentional Bias

There is ample evidence to suggest that SPs selectively attend to social threat–relevant information in the environment. SPs tend to dwell on words relevant to social threat, as indicated by both Stroop studies (9,28–30) and a study using the dot-probe paradigm (31). Complex results have been reported for studies that made use of a modified dot-probe paradigm in which participants are presented with faces rather than words. These studies are premised on the assumption that faces are more externally valid markers of feedback from others than are mere words. The general finding from modified dot-probe studies is that SPs quickly notice faces and then seem to divert their attention away from them, indicative of a vigilance-avoidance pattern of processing (32). What is unclear is whether SPs are sensitive to all faces (33) or sensitive only to those that are emotionally valenced (34). It is interesting to note that Chen et al. (33) employed a clinical sample, while Mansell et al. (34) employed a nonclinical sample. The greater severity of social anxiety experienced by participants in the Chen et al. study seems to have made all faces seem threatening, even those that showed no emotion at all. Clearly, more research is needed to see if these interesting differences between individuals with social phobia and those who are socially anxious are robust.

It is interesting to consider how the tendency to divert attention away from faces might facilitate maintenance of social anxiety. First, people who do not attend to facial expressions might come across as lacking social skills. While speech certainly drives conversations, facial expressions play an important role as well, and by not attending to them, socially anxious individuals might miss out on important cues that would make the conversation flow. Similarly, by not looking at faces, socially anxious individuals fail to make eye contact with the people to whom they are speaking. A fascinating article recently investigated visual scanning patterns in patients with social phobia (35). In this study, patients with social phobia and nonclinical controls were shown photos of an individual exhibiting a positive, negative, or neutral expression. While the visual scanpath of the non-clinical controls followed a normal inverted triangular shape (indicating that they focus primarily on the eyes but also on the nose and mouth), the visual scanpaths of SPs show a "hyperscanning" strategy. Their eye movements "dart" all over the face and also are directed away from the face, fixating only for very short periods of time on the eyes, nose, and mouth. This tendency to hyperscan was particularly pronounced for negative and neutral faces (as compared to positive faces), and the tendency to avoid the eye area was most pronounced with negative faces.

How might this diversion of eye contact and general pattern of scanning impact on the social interactions of SPs? As already noted, avoiding eye contact can most certainly make people look as if they lack skill or as if they are disinterested. Furthermore, having a conversation with someone who fails to make eye contact can be uncomfortable even for people who are not socially anxious. This general focus of attention away from faces can result in negative social interactions for socially anxious individuals, serving to confirm their negative beliefs. Similarly, by diverting attention away from faces, socially anxious individuals can also miss out on positive cues, likes smiles or nods, that could serve to disconfirm their beliefs.

2. Memory Bias

It is clear that socially anxious individuals selectively attend to socially threatening information in their environments. Once they have attended to it, however, do they have a better memory for it than for neutral information or for information that might be threatening but not socially relevant? This question has been difficult to answer. In contrast to the research on attentional bias, studies on memory bias have been less consistent. Studies using paradigms borrowed from cognitive science have shown mixed results, with some finding evidence of memory bias (36) and the majority failing to find such evidence (37,38).

Studies that have used more externally valid stimuli do suggest that a memory bias might exist in social phobia. Specifically, studies have shown that SPs have an enhanced memory for critical faces (18,19). It is interesting to note that data collected from nonclinical samples of socially anxious individuals suggest that they also experience some memory impairments in social situations. For example, highly socially anxious individuals seem to retain less social information of a nonthreatening nature (e.g., information about the interests, appearance, and background of a conversational partner) than do less socially anxious individuals (39–43).

These findings fit very nicely with the concept of self-focused attention. When SPs find themselves in potentially evaluative situations, they become very concerned with how they come across to others. After social interactions, it seems that they remember information about exactly this (e.g., critical faces) while missing out on other information in the environment. This can have a negative impact on SPs in numerous ways. If people come away from social situations most clearly recalling criticism (as is the case with the "postmortem"), they might be inclined to avoid social interactions in the future. If they do participate in subsequent social interactions, they might not remember important things like the names of people they have met before or important information about them. This might make them seem unskilled or aloof, increasing the likelihood that they will actually have negative interactions with others, and thus serving to confirm their already negative beliefs.

3. Judgment and Interpretation Biases

SPs also exhibit judgment and interpretation biases that influence their perceptions of themselves and of the social world. As was already noted, individuals with social phobia tend to be their own worst critics, judging themselves more negatively than they judge others and also judging themselves more negatively than they are judged by others (11–14). SPs also view the social world in a very negative way. They expect negative outcomes in social situations (44–46), they assign very negative interpretations to ambiguous social situations (47) and to mildly negative social situations (48), and they tend to see negative social events as extremely costly and catastrophic (44,45,48). It makes sense that such biases could contribute to the maintenance of social anxiety. If people expect negative outcomes (and costly ones at that), it is reasonable for them to want to avoid social situations. By failing to actually engage in social situations, socially anxious individuals deny themselves the opportunity to gather disconfirmatory evidence. An added complication, of course, is that when socially anxious individuals gain some evidence that *could* be used to disconfirm their beliefs, they tend to interpret it in a negative light anyway.

V. HOW HAVE THE COGNITIVE MODELS INFORMED TREATMENT?

To summarize, the cognitive models proposed by Clark and Wells and by Rapee and Heimberg paint a very similar portrait of the individual with social phobia and illuminate how this disorder is maintained over time. This understanding of the factors that maintain social phobia has informed approaches to treatment.

The major task in treatment for social phobia is correcting the faulty assumptions held by individuals with social phobia. Both cognitive and behavioral strategies are helpful in this regard. Some treatment programs, such as cognitive behavioral group therapy (CBGT) (49), target cognitive errors directly very early on in treatment. It is assumed that with more rational beliefs, patients will be more willing to enter feared social situations and will be more likely to pick up on information when in them that could be used to further disconfirm their faulty beliefs.

The core component of most treatment programs for social phobia (including Heimberg's CBGT) however, is exposure to social situations that are feared and/or avoided. In fact, dismantling studies (50) and metaanalyses (51–54) have suggested that exposure is the most effective component of CBT for social phobia. Exposures, while behavioral in nature, impact not only the anxiety and avoidance associated with social phobia but also the cognitive dysfunction associated with the disorder. Successful treatment for social phobia is associated with improvements in quality of life (55) and with improvements in the information processing deficits described earlier in this chapter. With successful treatment, individuals with social phobia are less likely to expect negative outcomes in social situations and come to see these outcomes as less costly were they to occur (44,46).

Perhaps the greatest advances in CBT for social phobia in recent years have been changes in the way that exposures are carried out. When patients hear about the exposure component of treatment, many query why their social phobia has persisted despite the fact that they regularly engage in social interactions. The research on focus of attention and safety behaviors suggests that it is not enough for patients to simply *be* in social situations. Rather, patients must come to recognize the importance of shifting the focus of attention and dropping safety behaviors, thus facilitating their *engagement* in social situations, rather than just being present.

This suggests that the way in which instructions are provided to patients prior to doing exposures is of tantamount importance, as is the way that the exposure experience is processed once it is over. The importance of instructions for exposure is best demonstrated by Wells and Papageorgiou (56). In this study, SPs engaged in a number of tasks based on their individual fear and avoidance hierarchy (exposures included eating and drinking with other people, making conversation with strangers, and being in a seminar) either under a control condition where no specific instructions were given, after having been given the rationale for doing exposures (based on the habituation model), and after having been instructed to take an external perspective rather than focusing inward on the self. Being told to take an external perspective resulted in greater decrements in anxiety and negative beliefs about the self as compared to simply being provided with the rationale for exposures.

In addition to setting up exposures in a very specific way, clinicians who work with SPs need to ensure that their patients do not sabotage successful exposures once they are over. As already noted, Clark has suggested that SPs come away from situations making judgments based on how they *felt* in the situation rather than on what actually occurred. This felt sense is taken as evidence of how others perceive them in social situations. Another important advance in the treatment of social phobia is helping patients to see themselves as they are seen by others, demonstrating for them that their felt sense is inaccurate. Clark and his colleagues have used a technique called video feedback as a means of correcting these negative self-images. Patients are videotaped while engaging in a social or performance situation and are then instructed to watch the video as an objective observer would—in other words, to try to see themselves as they are viewed by others. Again, the nature of the instructions for the exercise are crucial. In a study by Harvey and co-workers (57), half of the participants were simply asked to view a tape of themselves giving a speech. The other half were asked about their expectations of what they would see before the tape was played. This manipulation, termed "cognitive preparation," was meant to illuminate for patients the discrepancy between their felt sense of how they looked during the speech and how they actually looked. While all participants rated their performance more positively after they had seen the tape than before, this difference was in fact significantly greater for participants who had received cognitive preparation.

Helping patients to shift their focus of attention and drop safety behaviors is the hallmark of the cognitive therapy for social phobia developed by Clark and colleagues (6). Very positive effects for this approach to treatment have been reported in a single-case study (58), with a series of 15 consecutively referred patients (6), and in a controlled trial comparing cognitive therapy to fluoxetine (59). Other studies have also provided support for the importance of helping patients to shift focus of attention (60,61) and drop safety behaviors (4,62) during treatment for social phobia. By making these essential changes, SPs dedicate less attention to information that confirms their negative beliefs (e.g., physiological symptoms, negative cognitions, etc.) and place more attention on information that serves to disconfirm their beliefs (e.g., positive feedback from others, etc.). Furthermore, by being more engaged and picking up on more positive feedback, SPs come to see that social situations can be actually be pleasant and enjoyable. These shifts in behavior and beliefs break the pattern of social avoidance and distress that is the hallmark of social phobia.

REFERENCES

1. Liebowitz MR, Gorman JM, Fyer AJ, Klein DF. Social phobia: review of a neglected anxiety disorder. Arch Gen Psychiatry 1985; 42:729–735.
2. Kessler RC, McGonagle KA, Zhao S, Nelson CB, Hughes M, Eshleman S, Wittchen H-U, Kendler KS. Lifetime and 12-month prevalence of DSM-III-R psychiatric disorders in the United States: Results from the National Co-morbidity Survey. Arch Gen Psychiatry 1994; 51: 8–19.
3. Clark DM, Wells A. A cognitive model of social phobia. In: Heimberg RG, Liebowitz MR, Hope DA, Schneier FR, eds. Social Phobia: Diagnosis, Assessment, and Treatment. New York: Guilford Press, 1995:69–93.

4. Wells A, Clark DM, Salkovskis P, Ludgate J, Hackmann A, Gelder MG. Social phobia: the role of in-situations safety behaviors in maintaining anxiety and negative beliefs. Behav Ther 1995; 26: 153–161.

5. Rapee RM, Heimberg RG. A cognitive-behavioral model of anxiety in social phobia. Behav Res Ther 1997; 35:741–756.

6. Clark DM. A cognitive perspective on social phobia. In: Crozier WR, Alden LE, eds. International Handbook of Social Anxiety: Concepts, Research and Interventions Relating to the Self and Shyness. New York: Wiley, 2001:405–430.

7. Antony MM, Purdon CL, Huta V, Swinson RP. Dimensions of perfectionism across the anxiety disorders. Behav Res Ther 1998; 36:1143–1154.

8. Juster HR, Heimberg RG, Frost RO, Holt CS. Social phobia and perfectionism. Personality Indiv Diff 1996; 21:403–410.

9. Lundh LG, Öst LG. Stroop interference, self-focus, and perfectionism in social phobics. Personality Indiv Diff 1996; 20:725–731.

10. Bieling PJ, Alden LE. The consequences of perfectionism for patients with social phobia. Br J Clin Psychol 1997; 36:387–395.

11. Alden LE, Wallace ST. Social phobia and social appraisal in successful and unsuccessful social interactions. Behav Res Ther 1995; 33:497–505.

12. Rapee RM, Lim L. Discrepancy between self- and observer ratings of performance in social phobics. J Abnorm Psychol 1992; 101:728–731.

13. Rapee RM, Hayman K. The effects of video feedback on the self-evaluation of performance in socially anxious subjects. Behav Res Ther 1996; 34:315–322.

14. Stopa L, Clark DM. Cognitive processes in social phobia. Behav Res Ther 1993; 31:255–267.

15. Gilboa-Schechtman E, Foa EB, Amir N. Attentional biases for facial expressions in social phobia: The face-in-the-crowd paradigm. Cognition Emotion 1999; 13:305–318.

16. Perowne S, Mansell W. Social anxiety, self-focused attention, and the discrimination of negative, neutral and positive audience members by their nonverbal behaviours. Behav Cogni Psychother 2002; 30: 11–23.

17. Veljaca K, Rapee RM. Detection of negative and positive audience behaviors by socially anxious subjects. Behav Res Ther 36:311–321.

18. Foa EB, Gilboa-Schechtman E, Amir N, Freshman M. Memory bias in generalized social phobia: remembering negative emotional expressions. J Anxiety Disord 2000; 14:501–519.

19. Lundh LG, Öst LG. Recognition bias for critical faces in social phobics. Behav Res Ther 1996; 34: 787–794.

20. Strauman TJ. Self-discrepancies in clinical depression and social phobia: Cognitive structures that underlie emotional disorders? J Abnorm Psychol 1989; 98:14–22.

21. Weilage M, Hope DA. Self-discrepancy in social phobia and dysthymia. Cogn Ther Res 1999; 23: 637–650.

22. Wells A, Papageorgiou C. The observer perspective: Biased imagery in social phobia, agoraphobia, and blood/injury phobia. Behav Res Ther 1999; 37:653–658.

23. Wells A, Clark DM, Ahmad S. How do I look with my minds eye: Perspective taking in social phobic imagery. Behav Res Ther 1998; 36:631–634.

24. Hackmann A, Surawy C, Clark DM. Seeing yourself through others' eyes: A study of spontaneously occurring images in social phobia. Behav and Cogn Psychother 1998; 26:3–12.

25. Coles ME, Turk CL, Heimberg RG, Fresco DM. Effects of varying levels of anxiety within social situations: Relationship to memory perspective and attributions in social phobia. Behav Res Ther 2001; 39:651–665.

26. Coles ME, Turk CL, Heimberg RG. The role of memory perspective in social phobia: Immediate and delayed memories for role-played situations. Behav Cogn Psychother 2002; 30:415–425.

27. Hirsch CR, Clark DM, Mathews A, Williams R. Self-images play a causal role in social phobia. Behav Res Ther 2003; 41:909–921.

28. Hope DA, Rapee RM, Heimberg RG, Dombeck MJ. Representations of the self in social phobia: vulnerability to social threat. Cogn Ther Res 1990; 14: 177–189.

29. Maidenberg E, Chen E, Craske M, Bohn P, Bystritsky A. Specificity of attentional bias in panic disorder and social phobia. J Anxiety Disord 1996; 10: 529–541.

30. Mattia JI, Heimberg RG, Hope DA. The revised Stroop color-naming task in social phobics. Behav Res Ther 1993; 31:305–313.

31. Asmundson GJG, Stein MB. Selective processing of social threat in patients with generalized social phobia: evaluation using a dot-probe paradigm. J Anxiety Disord 1994; 8:107–117.

32. Mogg K, Mathews A, Weinman J. Memory bias in clinical anxiety. J Abnorm Psychol 1987; 96:94–98.

33. Chen YP, Ehlers A, Clark DM, Mansell W. Patients with generalized social phobia direct their attention away from faces. Behav Res Ther 2002; 40:677–687.

34. Mansell W, Clark DM, Ehlers A, Chen YP. Social anxiety and attention away from emotional faces. Cognition Emotion 1999; 13:673–690.

35. Horley K, Williams LM, Gonsalvez C, Gordon E. Social phobics do not see eye to eye: a visual scanpath study of emotional expression processing. J Anxiety Disord 2003; 17: 33–44.

36. Amir N, Foa EB, Coles, ME. Implicit memory bias for threat-relevant information in generalized social phobia. J Abnorm Psychol 2000; 109: 713–720.

37. Lundh LG, Öst LG. Explicit and implicit memory bias in social phobia: the role of subdiagnostic type. Behav Res Ther 1997; 35: 305–317.

38. Rapee RM, McCallum SL, Melville LF, Ravenscroft H, Rodney JM. Memory bias in social phobia. Behav Res Ther 1994; 32:89–99.

39. Bond CF, Omar AS. Social anxiety, state dependence, and the next-in-line effect. J Exp Social Psychol 1990; 26:185–198.

40. Daly JA, Vangelisti AL, Lawrence SG. Self-focused attention and public speaking anxiety. Personality Indiv Diff 1989; 10: 903–913.

41. Hope DA, Heimberg RG, Klein JF. Social anxiety and the recall of interpersonal information. J Cogn Psychother 1990; 4:185–195.

42. Hope DA, Sigler KD, Penn DL, Meier V. Social anxiety, recall of interpersonal information, and social impact on others. J Cogn Psychother 1998; 12: 303–322.
43. Kimble CE, Zehr HD. Self-consciousness, information load, self-presentation, and memory in a social situation. J Soc Psychol 1982; 118:39–46.
44. Foa EB, Franklin ME, Perry KJ, Herbert JD. Cognitive biases in generalized social phobia. J Abnorm Psychol 1996; 105:433–439.
45. Gilboa-Schechtman E, Franklin ME, Foa EB. Anticipated reactions to social events: differences among individuals with generalized social phobia, obsessive-compulsive disorder, and nonanxious controls. Cogn Ther Res 2000; 24:731–746.
46. Lucock MP, Salkovskis PM. Cognitive factors in social anxiety and its treatment. Behav Res Ther 1988; 26:297–302.
47. Amir N, Foa EB, Coles ME. Negative interpretation bias in social phobia. Behav Res Ther 1998; 36:959–970.
48. Stopa L, Clark DM. Social phobia and interpretation of social events. Behav Res Ther 2000; 38:273–283.
49. Heimberg RG, Becker RE. Cognitive-Behavioral Group Therapy for Social Phobia. Basic Mechanisms and Clinical Strategies. New York: Guilford Press, 2002.
50. Hope DA, Heimberg RG, Bruch MA. Dismantling cognitive behavioral group therapy for social phobia. Behav Res Ther 1995; 33:637–650.
51. Fedoroff IC, Taylor S. Psychological and pharmacological treatments of social phobia: A meta-analysis. J Clin Psychopharmacol 2001; 21: 311–324.
52. Feske U, Chambless DL. Cognitive behavioral versus exposure only treatment for social phobia: a meta-analysis. Behav Ther 1995; 26: 695–720.
53. Gould RA, Buckminster S, Pollack MH, Otto MW, Yap L. Cognitive-behavioral and pharmacological treatment for social phobia: a meta-analysis. Clin Psychol Sci Pract 1997; 4:291–306.
54. Taylor S. Meta-analysis of cognitive-behavioral treatment for social phobia. J Behav Ther Exp Psychiatry 1996; 27:1–9.
55. Eng W, Coles ME, Heimberg RG, Safren SA. Quality of life following cognitive behavioral treatment for social anxiety disorder: preliminary findings. Depression Anxiety 2001; 13:192–193.
56. Wells A, Papageorgiou C. Social phobia: Effects of external attention on anxiety, negative beliefs, and perspective taking. Behav Ther 1998; 29:357–370.
57. Harvey AG, Clark DM, Ehlers A, Rapee RM. Social anxiety and self-impression: cognitive preparation enhances the beneficial effects of video feedback following a stressful social task. Behav Res Ther 2000; 38:1183–1192.
58. Bates A, Clark DM. A new cognitive treatment for social phobia: a single case study. J Cogn Psychother 1998; 12:289–302.
59. Clark DM, Ehlers A, McManus F, Hackmann A, Fennell M, Campbell H, Flower T, Davenport C, Louis B. Cognitive therapy vs fluoxetine in generalized social phobia: a randomized placebo controlled trial. J Consult Clin Psychol. In press.

60. Hofmann SG. Self-focused attention before and after treatment of social phobia. Behav Res Ther 2000; 38:717–725.
61. Woody SR, Chambless DL, Glass CR. Self-focused attention in the treatment of social phobia. Behav Res Ther 1997; 35:117–129.
62. Morgan H, Raffle C. Does reducing safety behaviors improve treatment response in patients with social phobia? Aust NZ J Psychiatry 1999; 33: 503–510.

11

Animal Models of Social Anxiety

Sanjay J. Mathew
New York State Psychiatric Institute,
Columbia University College of Physicians
and Surgeons,
New York, New York, U.S.A.

Jeremy D. Coplan
State University of New York, Downstate,
and New York State Psychiatric Institute,
New York, New York, U.S.A.

I. INTRODUCTION

Animal models of human social anxiety have become invaluable tools for understanding basic concepts in neural circuitry, behavioral pharmacology, receptor function, and attachment behavior. Models ranging from rodent anxiety tests to mouse genetic knockouts have provided important data in the quest for potential anxiolytics and targets for drug development. More challenging, however, has been the development and validation of animal models that homologously model human social anxiety. Since impairments in social interaction form the cornerstone of many psychiatric illnesses beyond social anxiety disorder—including autism, schizophrenia, and schizotypal personality—it is likely that the most cogent animal models of social anxiety will have broad applicability to a variety of human illnesses. In that respect, it has been suggested that animal models for psychiatric illnesses should be judged by their relevance to the specific questions they are being used to address rather than their disease homology (1).

A recent consensus conference sponsored by the Anxiety Disorders Association of America identified several of the key challenges regarding the study of animal models of anxiety (2):

- Improve understanding of social context and tests of social interaction in animal models
- Study "adaptive" responses to adversity to provide an avenue toward identifying novel therapeutic strategies
- Show that knockout and overexpression of the same gene have opposite and reliable effects on anxiety phenotype
- Identify genes in humans that are linked to anxiety disorders and manipulate them in animal models ("top-down" approach)
- Perform gene expression studies in animal models to identify possible targets for drug development ("bottom-up" approach)
- Identify neurodevelopment of anxiety-relevant circuits and evaluate the effect of drugs at different stages of development

Because of the particular salience of primate social behavior for understanding social anxiety in humans, this chapter focuses on nonhuman primate models of social anxiety. Like humans, primates are particularly dependent upon social relationships, and laboratory-based behavioral observations can be readily conducted. Specifically, this chapter discusses several theory-driven and mechanistic models relevant to social anxiety that aim to address some of the challenges listed above. For a discussion of the extensive literature in genetic animal models relevant to anxiety, the reader is referred to a recent review (3).

II. USING PRIMATE MODELS TO DEVELOP A FUNCTIONAL NEUROANATOMY OF SOCIAL BEHAVIOR

A. Neuroanatomical Correlates of Social Behavior: Corpus Striatum

Nonhuman primate models are particularly useful in developing anatomical hypotheses regarding the brain's fear circuitry and might allow for differentiation of social anxiety from other forms of anxiety and "distress disorders" (4). While recognizing that social behavior across species results from a complex orchestration of different neurocircuits in multiple brain regions, it has been useful nonetheless to focus on circuitry in several specific regions. The corpus striatum, a key component of the basal ganglia, has emerged as a leading brain region implicated in human social anxiety disorder and thus is a region under investigation in primate models. The striatum receives projections from neurons of the entire cerebral cortex and thalamus as well as dopaminergic projections from the substantia nigra compacta and serotonergic fibers from the dorsal raphe nuclei of the midbrain (5). In addition, several types of interneurons exist within the striatum, with varied neurotransmitter and neuropeptide expression (6).

Recent high-spatial-resolution positron emission tomography (PET) studies have enabled delineation of striatal subregions in human (7,8) and nonhuman primates (9). The anteroventral striatum (AVS) is composed of the nucleus accumbens, ventromedial caudate, and anteroventral putamen and the dorsal striatum (DS) is composed of dorsal caudate and putamen. The AVS is innervated by the amygdala and the prefrontal cortical (PFC) regions involved in reward-related and emotional processing (processes most relevant to social anxiety), while the DS primarily receives afferent connections from cortical areas involved in sensorimotor function. Distinguishing across distinct striatal subregions has enabled recent understanding about the relationships between regional dopaminergic tone and euphoria (9) and cognitive functioning (10), with implications for social behavioral regulation.

The anatomical overlap between the AVS and the nucleus accumbens, a region implicated in brain reward mechanisms and the reinforcing aspects of drugs of abuse, suggests mechanisms related to the baseline differences in social affiliation across members of the same species. A prominent view is that the neural substrates of social affiliation and attachment are those pathways which couple social recognition (as manifested by olfactory, auditory, and visual stimuli) with the neural pathways for reinforcement, primarily the dopaminergic projections from the ventral tegmental area to the nucleus accumbens and prefrontal cortex (11). Pathological conditions associated with impaired social dexterity and contingently appropriate social responses have been hypothesized to be related to dopaminergic dysfunction. In patients with social anxiety disorder, at least two single photon emission computed tomography (SPECT) studies have found deficits of dopaminergic innervation into the striatum (12,13), while an early proton magnetic resonance spectroscopy (MRS) study reported abnormalities in striatal subregions (14).

In summary, the corpus striatum appears to play a pivotal role in mediating reward-related processing of social stimuli, and impaired dopaminergic neurotransmission in this region appears to be implicated in some studies. Primate neuroimaging investigations of striatum, combined with neurochemical assays, can offer models of brain structure and function that reliably map onto observed social behavior under baseline and social stress conditions.

B. Primate Amygdala and Its Implications for Understanding Social Anxiety

The amygdala is a complex of nuclei in the anterior temporal lobe that has long been implicated in the mediation of emotional and species-typical social behavior (16). Recent studies in rhesus monkeys have served to highlight the specific social-contextual fear role of the amygdala versus other kinds of fear behavior (17). In a series of experiments, amygdalectomized monkeys demonstrated increased social affiliation, decreased anxiety, and increased confidence compared to control monkeys, particularly in early encounters (18). Amaral has characterized these monkeys as lacking the "behavioral brake," or usual wariness regarding social interactions (17). The suggestion from these studies is that the amygdala functions as the protective "brake" on engagement of objects or organisms while an evaluation of potential threat is carried out (17). In this respect, social anxiety (and, more broadly, aberrant social affiliativeness) might represent a dysfunction of the amygdala's social-evaluative function. These recent findings contrast with historical lesion studies, suggesting that amygdalectomy produced a decrease in social interaction and increased aggression from conspecifics (19,20). An important limitation of the early studies, however, was the lack of anatomical specificity of the amygdala lesions.

Primate investigations of neurodevelopmental aspects of amygdalar function related to social anxiety have emerged in the past few years. Amygdalar lesions in 2-week-old macaque monkeys were found to produce less fear than controls of novel objects such as rubber snakes but more fear behavior during dyadic social interactions (21). Importantly, this finding suggests that in the neonatal brain, regions beyond the amygdala regulate social fear reactions generally subsumed by the amygdala in mature primates. Further evidence of the importance of neurodevelopment comes from longitudinal studies of monkeys in which bilateral amygdalectomies were conducted soon after birth (22). These monkeys were observed to have long-term severely impaired affiliative and social behavior. In summary, anatomically precise lesion studies in primate amygdala continue to offer valuable data about the role of this structure in modulating social anxiety.

C. Role of Primate Prefrontal Cortex in Social Anxiety: Focus on Anterior Cingulate

While much of the neuroanatomical investigation in social anxiety has been in corpus striatum and amygdala, PFC regions play pivotal roles in affective processing and emotional regulation (23). A neuronal substrate of emotional regulation, represented by the Papez circuit, involves the anterior thalamus, anterior cingulate gyrus, parahippocampal gyrus, hippocampus, fornix, mammillary bodies, and thalamus. The anterior cingulate cortex has emerged as being particularly relevant to affective and emotional regulation (24). The anterior cingulate cortex seems to contain certain specialized cells called "spindle cells" that appeared late in the evolution of our species (24). In human infants, these cells cannot be discerned at birth, and their emergence at the age of four months coincides with the infant's capacity to hold its head steady, smile spontaneously, and visually track and reach for external objects.

Social anxiety disorder's clinical features resemble many of the anxiety-like behavioral traits observed in nonhuman primates reared in our laboratory under variable foraging demand (VFD). In VFD rearing, social groups of nursing bonnet macaque (*Macaca radiata*) mother-infant dyads confront conditions for a few months in which the mother's food, while always ample, occasionally requires more time and effort to obtain, alternating with periods of essentially ad libitum feeding. Studies have found VFD-reared infants, even years later, to be more fearful and more easily distressed by fear-inducing stimuli (see full discussion of abnormalities in VFD in Sec. III.C, below). We conducted cross-sectional proton MRS in subgenual anterior cingulate in adult VFD-reared and control primates on a 1.5-tesla MRI system (25). MRS is a neuroimaging modality that permits in vivo ascertainment in a regionally specific manner of several important neurotransmitters—e.g., γ-aminobutyric acid (GABA) and glutamate-glutamine (Glx) as well as neurometabolites relevant to neuronal density and integrity (N-acetyl-aspartate, NAA). Neuroimaging investigations in VFD primates offer several advantages over clinical social anxiety populations in developing a functional anatomy of social anxiety: 1) the potential for repeated longitudinal neuroimaging and social-behavioral assessments, which can be controlled over the primate's lifetime; 2) the absence of confounding influences of medication, disease comorbidity, substance abuse, and family history (controlled for by random assignment to rearing groups) on measures of neuronal structure and integrity; and 3) the potential for guided post-mortem studies that would enable correlations of developmental brain imaging findings, behavior, and neuropathology. Indeed, terminal neuropathological investigations of VFD primates—including analyses of neurogenesis, glial proliferation, and hippocampal mossy fiber sprouting—have the potential to offer important histological correlates of in vivo neuroimaging findings with broad applicability to many neurological and psychiatric conditions.

In anterior cingulate, adult male VFD-subjects displayed significantly decreased NAA resonance and significantly increased glutamate-glutamine-GABA (Glx) resonance when compared to age- and sex-matched controls (25). That is, VFD primates even 10 years after exposure to the rearing stress paradigm displayed abnormalities in measures of neuronal integrity and Glx function in anterior cingulate. The NAA deficits noted in our VFD primates in anterior cingulate suggest that early socially adverse rearing results in long-term trait-like shifts in neuronal function in PFC regions. Inasmuch as Glx predominately comprises glutamate/glutamine, elevations of VFD Glx resonance are also consistent with the reduced anterior cingulate GABA observed in other animal early-life-stress models, in that diminished medial PFC GABA inhibition in VFDs might be permissive of glutamatergic neurotoxicity in this region, resulting in lowered neuronal viability (NAA). The MRS findings in our model suggest important neurodevelopmental aspects to anterior cingulate function in that the social stressor was applied early in life but had long-term pernicious consequences for both behavior and neurobiology. These MRS findings support the view of Amaral and colleagues regarding the relevance of neurodevelopment in anatomically specific hypotheses of social function.

III. ANIMAL MODELS OF THE NEUROCHEMISTRY OF SOCIAL ANXIETY: FOCUS ON CORTICOTROPIN RELEASING FACTOR (CRF)

A. CRF Secretion and Neuropathological Consequences

One of the major limitations of the human social anxiety literature is the cursory understanding of the role of stress-related neuropeptides such as CRF in disorder pathophysiology. CRF is a 41–amino acid peptide involved in integrating the behavioral, autonomic, and hormonal responses to stress in the mammal, and CSF CRF has been found to be elevated in patients with posttraumatic stress disorder (PTSD) and subtypes of mood disorders although not in social anxiety disorder (26). The supposition that early-life increases in CSF CRF may in fact be neurotoxic, independent of the effects of glucocorticoids, remains understudied. Hypersensitivity of central glucocorticoid negative-feedback systems has been invoked to account for the hippocampal tissue loss or compromised functional integrity of the hippocampus in PTSD subjects (27). It is curious that such effects occur within the context of normal to low cortisol levels that have been reported in PTSD. Certainly the facilitative effect of amygdaloid CRF on glutamatergic neurotransmission can be clearly quantified in the locus ceruleus region of the brainstem (28), suggesting that CRF may independently mediate neurotoxic effects via enhancement of the glutamatergic system.

To address the impact of excessive exposure to CRF early in life, Brunson et al. (29) administered CRF centrally to young rats and followed them into adulthood. Upon analysis of their hippocampus in adulthood, these subjects showed progressive loss of CA3 pyramidal layer cells, upregulation of CRF receptors in the CA3 region, and exuberant growth or sprouting of mossy fibers from the dentate gyrus to the CA3 region. The synapses of the hippocampal CA3 region are prominently glutamatergic, and the alterations resulting from the heightened CRF may promote a hyperglutamatergic state and excitotoxicity in this region. The finding of hippocampal CA3 cell loss in rodents developmentally exposed to CRF is one potential key in understanding the neurobiological impact of adverse early rearing and its impact on phenotypic social anxiety. Corroborative studies are still required to fully characterize the role of exuberant mossy fiber sprouting as a possible source of hyperglutamatergic activity leading to hippocampal cell loss.

B. Primate Model of Intracerebroventricular Infusion of CRF

Monkey models have recently been used to examine the relationship between CRF, behavior, brain metabolism, and neurochemistry (30). Integrating PET with behavioral observations in the laboratory, it was found that CRF infusion (intracerebroventricular) increased glucose metabolism in amygdala and hippocampus, and increased depressive-like behaviors only in socially housed monkeys (30). This landmark study verified the idea that CRF has different behavioral effects in different social contexts, and that individual response to elevated CRF tone may depend on such socially mediated factors such as social group, support network, and social dominance hierarchies. The authors conclude: "if we are to continue studying the role of CRF in the pathophysiology of human psychiatric conditions using animal models, we must do so under the appropriate social contexts" (Ref. 30, p. 15754). The implications for the study of human social anxiety disorder are clear: the difficulty in demonstrating abnormal hypothalamic-pituitary-adrenal (HPA) axis activity might reflect the fact that studies in social anxiety have generally been performed in the resting, unchallenged state. Having the patient encounter a socially stressful situation, with concurrent neurochemical assessments, might be more likely to yield the expected HPA-axis abnormalities.

C. The VFD Model: Neurochemical Abnormalities Derived from an Early Social Stressor

For the past 30 years, our primate behavioral laboratory has studied the bonnet macaque (*Macaca radiata*), a strongly gregarious species that exhibits stable adult and maternal-infant relationships, demonstrates both cooperative and competitive interactions, and manifests playful interactions throughout infancy and adolescence (31). By imposition of environmental stressors, systematic behavioral change has been observed in these primates (32–34), whose mediating neurobiology is experimentally accessible. The VFD model has potential relevance to human psychiatric disorders marked by fearful avoidance of social interaction, separation anxiety, and depressive affect, and is potentially useful in its suggestion that early insecure maternal attachment may shift behavior and neurobiology toward a trait-like socially anxious and timid profile.

Rosenblum and colleagues (34) developed this model by exposing nursing mothers to unpredictable foraging demand conditions and experimentally inducing unstable attachment patterns to their infants. Genetically random, group-living, mother-infant dyads live in environments in which the mother is confronted with alternating 2-week periods in which ample food is readily obtainable with little or no effort (low foraging demand, LFD), or in which food, while still ample, requires considerably more time and effort to obtain (high foraging demand, HFD). Control subjects face only LFD conditions throughout a comparable period, and both groups are on ad libitum feeding before and after the experimental conditions. Six to eight 2-week alterations in foraging demand in the VFD subjects provide a level of salient environmental uncertainty which alters normal maternal response patterns, with profound consequences for the offspring. All subjects are permanently separated from their mother and maintained in peer groups at 1 year of age.

Grown primates raised under VFD conditions, in comparison to predictably reared comparison subjects, showed stable increases in levels of social timidity—e.g., social subordination, avoidance of agonistic encounters, and decreased species-typical huddling. Other disturbances evident in VFD subjects at various stages of development include: 1) greater expression of depressive episodes upon maternal separation; 2) diminished autonomous functioning; and 3) decreased exploratory behavior when challenged by novel stimuli. Investigation of the brain neurochemistry in VFD-reared subjects has revealed specific abnormalities in biological systems important in stress responsivity and affect regulation. VFD-reared subjects showed sustained elevations in cisternal cerebrospinal fluid (CSF) CRF concentrations into young adulthood (35), replicating earlier findings from the same subjects in juveniles (36). Moreover, significant within-group stability of CRF over a 30-month period was noted within the longitudinally assessed VFD-reared group (35). Despite high levels of juvenile CSF CRF, these VFD subjects showed lower CSF cortisol levels (36). Elevations of CSF CRF in juvenile VFD subjects were positively correlated with contemporaneous levels of CSF somatostatin, as well as the metabolites of serotonin (5-hydroxyindoleacetic acid [5-HIAA]) and dopamine (homovanillic acid [HVA]) (37). Finally, VFD subjects displayed exaggerated behavioral responses to the noradrenergic probe yohimbine and blunted behavioral responses to the serotonin probe m-chlorophenylpiperazine (38). The overall suggestion from these neurochemical and neurohormonal data is that early rearing disturbances in nonhuman primates produce enduring changes in biogenic amines and components of the HPA axis, resembling many of the abnormalities seen in humans who suffer from pathological anxiety disorders. See Table 1 for a summary of VFD abnormalities.

In summary, the VFD model is useful in its suggestion that early environmental stress, particularly of an affective nature, may shift behavior and neurobiology towards a trait-like socially anxious profile. The altered dopaminergic metabolites in the CSF in VFD-reared primates parallels the numerous dopaminergic abnormalities observed in social anxiety disorder patients. The increased Glx resonance in anterior cingulate of VFDs is consonant with clinical hypotheses in social phobia suggesting glutamate-GABA imbalances in prefrontal and limbic brain regions. Behaviorally, the VFD-reared primates resemble what Kagan et al. (39) described in a group

TABLE 1   Summary of Abnormalities Observed in Variable-Foraging-Demand Primates

1. Stable behavioral and neurobiological abnormalities analogous to those found in mood and anxiety disorders in humans.
2. Even years after rearing, VFD subjects appear to be less gregarious and display a diminished stress repertoire to fearful stimuli.
3. VFD-reared monkeys show persistent dysregulation of the HPA axis, as indicated by elevations in CSF of the stress-related neuropeptide CRF and by alterations in their cortisol response to stress.
4. Alterations have also been found in a number of other biological systems in VFD-reared monkeys, including their growth hormone response to clonidine challenge.
5. Impaired immunological responses to stress, as reflected in circulating levels of transforming growth factor β_1.
6. Abnormal central levels of monoamine metabolites and somatostatin.
7. A VFD offspring cohort reared with a late postpartum onset of VFD produced low levels of CSF CRF and high cortisol levels. CSF CRF was inversely correlated with CSF 5-HIAA, while plasma cortisol correlated with the anti-inflammatory cytokine transforming growth factor β1. This latter set of studies emphasized the importance of critical periods or "developmental windows" in molding the neurodevelopmental trajectory.

Key: VFD, variable foraging demand; HPA, hypothalamic-pituitary-adrenal; CSF, cerebrospinal fluid; CRF, corticotropin releasing factor; 5-HAA, 5-hydroxyindoleacetic acid.

of young children who manifested characteristics of "behavioral inhibition to the unfamiliar." These children exhibit exaggerated heart rate acceleration to stress, high early morning salivary cortisol levels, and levels of behavioral inhibition (BI) correlated with high total norepinephrine activity. Longitudinal biobehavioral studies in VFD primates thus offer salient mechanistic models to understand developmental antecedents of social anxiety disorder.

IV. OTHER PRIMATE MODELS RELEVANT TO SOCIAL ANXIETY

A. Social Subordination Stress

Nonhuman primates live in complex, highly organized social groups marked by stable and hierarchical relationships among individuals who engage in complex modes of social communication (17). Shively (40) conducted critical non-human primate studies in social subordination and dominance in laboratory-housed cynomolgus female monkeys. Behavioral observations indicated that subordinates spent more time alone fearfully scanning their social environment than dominants. Neurochemical investigations of these subordinates revealed evidence of HPA axis hyperactivity, impaired serotonergic functioning, and impaired dopaminergic neurotransmission. Upon challenge with ACTH, social subordinates hypersecreted the stress hormone cortisol. After the fenfluramine challenge test (a serotonin releaser), laboratory-housed cynomolgus macaques exhibited a blunted prolactin response, suggesting diminished central serotonergic activity. The monkeys with a blunted prolactin response were more socially withdrawn and spent less time in passive body contact than those showing a high prolactin response (41). Using a haloperidol challenge test, a dopamine antagonist which enhances prolactin secretion through tubero-infundibular dopamine pathways, reduced prolactin responses were observed in subordinates (41). This result suggested that subordinates had lowered sensitivity of postsynaptic dopamine receptors in this pathway. Consistent with the neuroendocrine data, a PET study (42) of subordinates showed decreased striatal D2 receptor binding, suggesting abnormal central dopaminergic neurotransmission. This finding closely resembles a SPECT study in humans with social anxiety disorder, discussed previously (12).

Studies of socially subordinate baboons in the wild have revealed other neuroendocrine abnormalities that mimic findings in socially anxious human subjects. Hypercortisolemia, as well as resistance to feedback inhibition by dexamethasone, has also been reported by Sapolsky et al. (43) in baboons. Subordinate male baboons were found to have lower insulinlike growth factor I (IGF-I) levels than dominants (44). This finding might explain the observed association between short stature and social anxiety disorder found in one study (45).

There are several important limitations of subordination models as they apply to patients with social anxiety disorder. First, there is minimal to no evidence of a HPA axis disturbance in social anxiety disorder. Second, the prolactin response to fenfluramine differs in subordinate models versus patients with social anxiety disorder (46). Thus, the major correlative finding in the primate subordination stress model with social anxiety disorder is striatal dopaminergic dysfunction. Whether this dysfunction is a by-product of social stress or a feature of social subordinance per se is unclear from these studies.

B. Attachment Models

Historically, the rich animal literature in attachment biology has been relatively neglected in understanding social anxiety disorder, as compared to its integral contribution in understanding autistic spectrum disorders. However, emerging genetic links between autism and social anxiety disorder suggest a reexamination of attachment neurobiology in social anxiety (48,49). Numerous neurotransmitter systems—most notably the serotonin, opioid, and oxytocin systems—have been investigated clinically in autism and preclinically in primate models of attachment. Raleigh and colleagues showed that enhancement of serotonergic function resulted in improved social affiliativeness in primates, while low serotonin levels promoted avoidance (50). In separate but related work, free-ranging primates with low levels of CSF 5-HIAA showed less social competence and were more likely to emigrate at a younger age from their social groups than primates with higher levels of CSF 5-HIAA (51).

The brain opioid system has been implicated as a regulator of attachment behaviors in primates and other species for many years. In one study of non-human primates, 10 juvenile macaques living in a stable social group with their mothers and other group companions were administered the opiate antagonist naloxone (52). The primates receiving naloxone made more grooming solicitations and received more grooming, and increased their proximity with their mothers. Kalin studied reunion of nonhuman primate infants following separations from their mother, and demonstrated that both infants and mothers who were administered the opiate morphine showed a significant reduction in clinging behaviors, while those given naltrexone (an opiate antagonist) increased clinging behaviors (53). Finally, there is evidence of complex interrelationships between endogenous opioid activity and other proaffiliative neurotransmitter systems. For example, it was

TABLE 2 Nonhuman Primate Models Relevant to Social Anxiety Disorder

Model	Neurobiological alterations	Brain regions	Clinical correlation
Subordination stress	Reduced 5-HT activity	Prefrontal cortex, raphe nuclei	Blushing
	Decreased striatal D2 binding	Corpus striatum, nucleus accumbens, VTA (midbrain)	Increased substance abuse
	HPA axis activation	Hippocampus, amygdala	Anxiety and fear
VFD	Increased cerebrospinal fluid levels of CRF, HVA, 5-HIAA, and lower cortisol; blunted GH response to clonidine	Hippocampus, amygdala, prefrontal cortex	Comorbid PTSD behavioral inhibition
		Hypothalamic neurons of nucleus arcuatus, paraventricular CRF neurons	Comorbid anxiety and depression
Attachment	Serotonin dysregulation	Prefrontal cortex, raphe nuclei	Social incompetence
	Oyxtocin	Prefrontal cortex, limbic areas, posterior pituitary	Autistic/schizoid relational patterns
	Opiate dysregulation	Diffuse regions of prefrontal cortex, periaqueductal gray	Increased social anxiety in opioid abusers

Key: 5-HT, serotonin; CRF, corticotropin releasing factor; HVA, homovanillic acid; GH, growth hormone; VTA, ventral tegmental area; PTSD, posttraumatic stress disorder.

demonstrated that opiate activity was increased by oxytocin injections in the rat (54). A noteworthy clinical correlate of this line of research is the evidence that opioid abusers have high rates of social anxiety (55).

The neurohormone oxytocin is well established in the initiation but not the maintenance of maternal behavior and pair bonding (11), as well as in social interactions in nonhuman primates (56). As one example, a genetically engineered mouse lacking oxytocin emitted few isolation calls and had reduced social interactions (11). Although incomplete in explaining the varied cognitive misappraisals observed in patients with social anxiety disorder, primate attachment models provide a useful construct for the aberrant social affiliativeness seen in social anxiety disorder, and provide guides for future investigations of the clinical neurobiology of the disorder. See Table 2 (adapted from Ref. 26) for a summary of selected preclinical models of social anxiety disorder with their respective clinical correlations.

V. FUTURE DIRECTIONS IN PRIMATE MODELS OF SOCIAL ANXIETY: DEMONSTRATION OF NEUROGENESIS

One of the seminal recent findings in neurobiology is the accumulating evidence for the remarkable plasticity of the brain and the development of neurogenesis in diverse brain regions such as the cortex, hippocampus, cerebellum, and olfactory bulb (57). Gould et al. (58) demonstrated altered neuroplasticity in tree shrews in an enduring dominant-subordinate relationship derived from a social dominance paradigm (59). Specifically, there was a rapid decrease in the number of new cells produced in the dentate gyrus of hippocampus of subordinate tree shrews compared to those unexposed to a stressful experience (58). This finding was more recently replicated in marmoset monkeys using a resident intruder paradigm, a psychosocial stress model similar to that of the dominant-subordinate models for the tree shrews (60). At this time, we do not know the nature of neuroplastic changes in the brains of human infants with early signs and symptoms of social anxiety; thus, the clinical implications of stress-induced decreases in granule cell production in animal models is unknown. However, recent studies show that granule neurons are potentially involved in hippocampal-dependent learning tasks (61), and that consequent decreases in the number of granule neurons are likely to alter the adult hippocampal formation (61). Socially stressful experiences, which increase levels of circulating glucocorticoids and stimulate hippocampal glutamate release (62), might thus inhibit granule cell neurogenesis. Several other factors have been found to impede hippocampal neurogenesis, including stress, inflammation, CRF, glucocorticoids, glutamate and N-methyl-D-aspartate (NMDA) receptor agonists, and opiates. Other factors stimulate and enhance neurogenesis: electroconvulsive shock, lithium and anticonvulsants, antidepressants and other 5-HT$_{1A}$ receptor agonists, brain-derived neurotrophic factor (BDNF), and the anti-apoptotic gene Bcl-2. In adult social anxiety disorder, we have hypothesized that excessive glutamatergic transmission in hippocampal and cortical regions might be a key component of the dysfunctional circuitry, and successful treatments might serve to prevent the inhibition of neurogenesis while modifying glutamatergic neurotransmission (26). As most of the work to date relating neurogenesis to social stressors has been performed in rodent and subprimate species, future primate investigations of neurogenesis are needed.

VI. CONCLUSIONS

Much work remains to be done to understand the biological bases of social anxiety in humans, and primate models offer useful avenues for investigation. A better understanding of the developmental neurobiology of the primary brain regions discussed—striatum, amygdala, PFC—and their interactions with key neurotransmitter systems (CRF, dopamine, serotonin, glutamate) is necessary. Where primate research might prove particularly fruitful is in targeting susceptibility genes for the broad social anxiety phenotype. It is clear there is a limited understanding of the interaction between genetic vulnerability and stress exposure in socially anxious persons. In that respect, cross-fostering paradigms in which primates raised under socially stressful conditions (e.g., VFD, subordination stress) are randomly assigned to the offspring of either socially withdrawn or socially competent mothers, might help to answer the question of whether stress exposure has a more deleterious effect on genetically susceptible individuals. Ultimately, a more refined understanding of these processes would offer insights not only into social anxiety disorder but into other disorders with impairments in social functioning.

ACKNOWLEDGMENTS

The authors wish to thank Shirne Baptiste, B.A., Christen Kidd, A.B., Leonard Rosenblum, Ph.D., and Eric Smith, Ph.D., for their valuable contributions to this work.

REFERENCES

1. McKinney WT. Overview of the past contributions of animal models and their changing place in psychiatry. Semin Clin Neuropsychiatry 2001; 6(1): 68–78.
2. Anxiety Disorders Association of America. Conference on novel treatment approaches for treatment refractory anxiety. Landsdowne, VA. June 16–17, 2003.

3. Finn DA. Genetic animal models of anxiety. Neurogenetics 2003; 4(3): 109–135.
4. Cuthbert BN. Social anxiety disorder: trends and translational research. Biol Psychiatry 2002; 51: 4–10.
5. Gonzalo N, Moreno A, Erdozain MA, et al. A sequential protocol combining dual neuroanatomical tract-tracing with the visualization of local circuit neurons within the striatum. J Neurosci Methods 2001; 111(1): 59–66.
6. Kawaguchi Y, Wilson CJ, Augood SJ, et al. Striatal interneurones: chemical, physiological and morphological characterization. Trends Neurosci 1995; 18: 527–535.
7. Kegeles LS, Martinez D, Kochan LD, et al. NMDA antagonist effects on striatal dopamine release: positron emission tomography studies in humans. Synapse 2002; 43: 19–29.
8. Drevets WC, Gautier C, Price JC, et al. Amphetamine-induced dopamine release in human ventral striatum correlates with euphoria. Biol Psychiatry 2001; 49: 81–96.
9. Drevets WC, Price JC, Kupfer DJ, et al. PET measures of amphetamine-induced dopamine release in ventral versus dorsal striatum. Neuropsychopharmacology 1999; 21(6): 694–709.
10. Mozley LH, Gur RC, Mozley PD, et al. Striatal dopamine transporters and cognitive functioning in healthy men and women. Am J Psychiatry 2001; 158(9): 1492–1499.
11. Insel TR, Winslow JT. The neurobiology of social attachment. In: Charney DS, Nestler EJ, Bunney BS, eds. Neurobiology of Mental Illness. New York: Oxford University Press, 1999: 880–890.
12. Schneier FR, Liebowitz MR, Abi-Dargham A, et al. Low dopamine D2 receptor binding potential in social phobia. Am J Psychiatry 2000; 157: 457–459.
13. Tiihonen J, Kuikka J, Bergstrom K, et al. Dopamine reuptake site densities in patients with social phobia. Am J Psychiatry 1997; 154: 239–242.
14. Davidson JR, Krishnan KR, Charles HC, et al. Magnetic resonance spectroscopy in social phobia: preliminary findings. J Clin Psychiatry 1993; 54(Dec suppl): 19–25.
15. Kampe KK, Frith CD, Dolan RJ, et al. Reward value of attractiveness and gaze. Nature 2001; 413(6856): 589.
16. Kling AS, Brothers L. The amygdala and social behavior. In: Aggleton JP, ed. The Amygdala: Neurobiological Aspects of Emotion, Memory and Mental Dysfunction. New York: Wiley-Liss, 1992: 353–378.
17. Amaral DG. The primate amygdala and the neurobiology of social behavior: implications for understanding social anxiety. Biol Psychiatry 2002; 51: 11–17.
18. Emery NJ, Capitanio JP, Mason WA, Machado CJ, Mendoza SP, Amaral DG. The effects of bilateral lesions of the amygdala on dyadic social interactions in rhesus monkeys (*Macaca mulatta*). Behav Neurosci 2001; 115(3): 515–544.
19. Rosvold HE, Mirsky AF, Pribram KH. Influence of amygdalectomy on social behavior in monkeys. J Comp Physiol Psychol 1954; 47: 173–178.
20. Kluver H, Bucy PC. Preliminary analysis of functions of the temporal lobes in monkeys. Arch Neurol Psychiatry 1939; 42: 979–1000.

21. Prather MD, Lavenex P, Mauldin-Jourdain ML, Mason WA, Capitanio JP, Mendoza SP, Amaral DG. Increased social fear and decreased fear of objects in monkeys with neonatal amygdala lesions. Neuroscience 2001; 106(4): 653–658.

22. Bachevalier J, Malkova ML, Mishkin M. Effects of selective neonatal temporal lobe lesions on socioemotional behavior in infant rhesus monkeys (*Macaca mulatta*). Behav Neurosci 2001; 115: 545–559.

23. Davidson RJ. Anxiety and affective style: role of prefrontal cortex and amygdala. Biol Psychiatry 2002; 51: 68–80.

24. Allman JM, Hakeem A, Erwin JM, Nimchinsky E, Hof P. The anterior cingulate cortex. The evolution of an interface between emotion and cognition. Ann N Y Acad Sci. 2001; 935:107–117.

25. Mathew SJ, Shungu DC, Mao X, Smith ELP, Perera GM, Kegeles LS, Perera T, Lisanby SH, Rosenblum LA, Gorman JM, Coplan JD. A magnetic resonance spectroscopic imaging study of adult nonhuman primates exposed to early-life stressors. Biol Psychiatry 2003; 54(7): 727–735.

26. Mathew SJ, Coplan JD, Gorman JM. Neurobiological mechanisms of social anxiety disorder. Am J Psychiatry 2001; 158(10): 1558–1567.

27. Yehuda R, Boisoneau D, Lowy MT, Giller EL Jr. Dose-response changes in plasma cortisol and lymphocyte glucocorticoid receptors following dexamethasone administration in combat veterans with and without posttraumatic stress disorder. Arch Gen Psychiatry 1995; 52: 583–593.

28. Valentino RJ, Rudoy C, Saunders A, Liu XB, Van Bockstaele EJ. Corticotropin-releasing factor is preferentially colocalized with excitatory rather than inhibitory amino acids in axon terminals in the peri-locus coeruleus region. Neuroscience 2001; 106: 375–384.

29. Brunson KL, Eghbal-Ahmadi M, Bender R, Chen Y, Baram TZ. Long-term, progressive hippocampal cell loss and dysfunction induced by early-life administration of corticotropin-releasing hormone reproduce the effects of early-life stress. Proc Natl Acad Sci USA 2001; 98: 8856–8861.

30. Strome EM, Wheler GHT, Higley JD, Loriaux DL, Suomi SJ, Doudet DJ. Intracerebroventricular corticotropin-releasing factor increases limbic glucose metabolism and has social context-dependent behavioral effects in nonhuman primates. Proc Natl Acad Sci USA 2002; 99(24): 15749–15754.

31. Coplan JD, Rosenblum LA, Gorman JM. Primate models of anxiety: longitudinal perspectives. Psychiatr Clin North Am 1995; 18(4): 727–743.

32. Andrews MW, Rosenblum LA. Dominance and social competence in differentially reared bonnet macaques, In: Ehara A, ed. Primatology Today: XIIIth Congress of the International Primatological Society. Amsterdam, Elsevier, 1991: 347–350.

33. Andrews MW, Rosenblum LA. Attachment in monkey infants raised in variable- and low-demand environments. Child Dev 1991; 62: 686–693.

34. Rosenblum LA, Paully GS. The effects of varying environmental demands on maternal and infant behavior. Child Dev 1984; 55: 305–314.

35. Coplan JD, Smith ELP, Altemus M, Scharf BA, Owens MJ, Nemeroff CB, Gorman JM, Rosenblum LA. Variable foraging demand: sustained elevations

in cisternal cerebrospinal fluid corticotropin releasing factor concentrations in adult primates. Biol Psychiatry 2001; 50: 200–204.

36. Coplan JD, Andrews MW, Rosenblum LA, Owens MJ, Friedman S, Gorman JM, Nemeroff CB. Persistent elevations of cerebrospinal fluid concentrations of corticotropin-releasing factor in adult nonhuman primates exposed to early-life stressors: implications for the pathophysiology of mood and anxiety disorders. Proc Natl Acad Sci USA 1996; 93: 1619–1623.

37. Coplan JD, Trost RC, Owens MJ, Cooper TB, Gorman JM, Nemeroff CB, Rosenblum LA. Cerebrospinal fluid concentrations of somatostatin and biogenic amines in grown primates reared by mothers exposed to manipulated foraging conditions. Arch Gen Psychiatry 1998; 55: 473–477.

38. Rosenblum LA, Coplan JD, Friedman S, et al. Adverse early experiences affect noradrenergic and serotonergic functioning in adult primates. Biol Psychiatry 1994; 35: 221–227.

39. Kagan J, Reznick JS, Snidman N. The physiology and psychology of behavioral inhibition in children. Child Dev 1987; 58: 1459–1473.

40. Shively CA. Social subordination stress, behavior, and central monoaminergic function in female cynomolgus monkeys. Biol Psychiatry 1998; 44(9): 882–891.

41. Botchin MB, Kaplan JR, Manuck SB, Mann JJ. Low versus high prolactin responders to fenfluramine challenge: marker of behavioral differences in adult male cynomolgus macaques. Neuropsychopharmacology 1993; 9(2): 93–99.

42. Grant KA, Shively CA, Nader MA, Ehrenkaufer RL, Line SW, Morton TE, Gage HD, Mach RH. Effect of social status on striatal dopamine D2 receptor binding characteristics in cynomolgus monkeys assessed with positron emission tomography. Synapse 1998; 29(1): 80–83.

43. Sapolsky RM, Alberts SC, Altmann J. Hypercortisolism associated with social subordinance or social isolation among wild baboons. Arch Gen Psychiatry 1997; 54(12): 1137–1143.

44. Sapolsky RM, Spencer EM. Insulin-like growth factor I is suppressed in socially subordinate male baboons. Am J Physiol 1997; 273 (4 Pt 2): R1346–1351.

45. Stabler B, Tancer ME, Ranc J, Underwood LE. Evidence for social phobia and other psychiatric disorders in adults who were growth hormone deficient during childhood. Anxiety 1996; 2(2): 86–89.

46. Tancer ME, Mailman RB, Stein MB, Mason GA, Carson SW, Golden RN. Neuroendocrine responsivity to monoaminergic system probes in generalized social phobia. Anxiety 1994–1995; 1(5): 216–223.

47. Raleigh MJ, McGuire MT, Brammer GL, Yuwiler A. Social and environmental influences on blood serotonin concentrations in monkeys. Arch Gen Psychol 1984; 41: 405–410.

48. Smalley SL, McCracken AJ, Tanguay P. Autism, affective disorders, and social phobia. Am J Med Genet 1995; 60: 19–26.

49. Piven J, Palmer P. Psychiatric disorder and broad autism phenotype: evidence from a family study of multiple-incidence autism families. Am J Psychiatry 1999; 156: 557–563.

50. Raleigh MJ, Brammer GL, McGuire MT. Male dominance, serotonergic systems, and the behavioral and physiological effects of drugs in vervet monkeys (*Cercopithecus aethiops sabaeus*). In: Miczek KA, ed. Ethopharmacology: Primate Models of Neuropsychiatric Disorders. New York: Liss, 1983.

51. Mehlman PT, Higley JD, Faucher I, Lilly AA, Taub DM, Vickers J, Snomi SJ, Linnoila M. Correlation of CSF 5-HIAA concentration with sociality and the timing of emigration in free-ranging primates. Am J Psychiatry 1995; 152: 907–913.

52. Schino G, Troisi A. Opiate receptor blockade in juvenile macaques: effect on affiliative interactions with their mothers and group companions. Brain Res 1992; 576(1): 125–130.

53. Kalin NH, Shelton SE, Lynn DE. Opiate systems in mother and infant primates coordinate intimate contact during reunion. Psychoneuroendocrinology 1995; 20 (7): 735–742.

54. Uvnas-Moberg K. Oxytocin may mediate the benefits of positive social interaction and emotions. Psychoneuroendocrinology 1998; 23 (8): 819–835.

55. Grenyer BF, Williams G, Swift W, Neill O. The prevalence of social-evaluative anxiety in opioid users seeking treatment. Int J Addict 1992 Jun; 27(6):665–673

56. Winslow JT, Insel TR. Social status in pairs of squirrel monkeys determines the behavioral response to central oxytocin administration. J Neurosci 1991; 11(7): 2032–2038.

57. Gould E, Tanapat P. Stress and hippocampal neurogenesis. Biol Psychiatry 1999; 46: 1472–1479.

58. Gould E, McEwen BS, Tanapat P, Galea LAM, Fuchs E. Neurogenesis in the dentate gyrus of the adult tree shrew is regulated by psychosocial stress and NMDA receptor activation. J Neurosci 1997; 17: 2492–2498.

59. Von Holst D. Social stress in the tree-shrew: its causes and physiological and ethological consequences. In: Martin RD, Doyle GA, Watlker AC, eds. Prosimian Biology. Philadelphia: University of Pittsburgh, 1972.

60. Gould E, Tanapat P, McEwan BS, Flugge G, Fuchs E. Proliferation of granule cell precursors in the dentate gyrus of adult monkeys is diminished by stress. Proc Natl Acad Sci USA 1998; 95: 3168–3171.

61. Gould E, Reeves AJ, Fallah M, Tanapat P, Fuchs E. Hippocampal neurogenesis in adult Old World primates. Proc Natl Acad Sci USA 1999; 96: 5263–5267.

62. Moghaddam B, Bolinao M. Stein-Behrens B, Sapolsky R. Glucocorticoids mediate the stress induced extracellular accumulation in the hippocampus. J Neurochem 1994; 63: 596–602.

63. Stewart J, Kolb B. The effects of neonatal gonadectomy and prenatal stress on cortical thickness and asymmetry in rats. Behav Neural Biol 1988; 49: 344–360.

64. Schoups AA, Elliott RC, Friedman WJ, Black IB. NGF and BDNF are differentially modulated by visual experience in the developing geniculocortical pathway. Dev Brain Res 1995; 86: 326–334.

65. Nibuya M, Nestler EJ, Duman RS. Chronic antidepressant administration increases the expression of cAMP response element binding protein (CREB) in rat hippocampus. J Neurosci 1996; 16(7): 2365–2372.
66. Duman RS, Heninger GR, Nestler EJ. A molecular and cellular theory of depression. Arch Gen Psychiatry 1997; 54: 597–606.

12

The Promise of Neurobiology in Social Anxiety Disorder

Michael Van Ameringen
and Catherine Mancini
McMaster University,
Hamilton, Ontario, Canada

I. INTRODUCTION

In spite of the high prevalence rate of social anxiety disorder (SAD) in the general population (1), little is known about its pathophysiology or neurobiology. Neurobiological investigation of SAD has used a variety of approaches, reviewed in this chapter, including chemical and neuroendocrine challenges, evaluations of neurotransmitter functioning, and structural and functional neuroimaging studies.

A. Challenge Studies

Challenge studies use exogenous chemical agents to induce the individual's naturally occurring anxiety symptoms. They tend to confirm an underlying biological mechanism of the disorder. Researchers have challenged patients with SAD with a variety of agents including lactate (2), caffeine (3), CO_2 (4–6), cholecystokinin (CCK) (7), pentagastrin [a synthetic analogue of the cholecystokinin tetrapeptide (CCK4)] (8), and the benzodiazepine antagonist flumazenil (9). These substances have been successfully used to induce panic attacks in individuals with panic disorder. However, with the exception of pentagastrin or high concentrations of CO_2, these challenges have not shown consistent panicogenic effects in SAD patients compared to controls. Flumazenil induced panic attacks in panic disorder patients (10) but failed to do so in a group of SAD patients (9). Gorman administered 35% CO_2 to patients with panic disorder and SAD as well as normal controls. In this study, all subjects experienced increased anxiety and ventilation rates. The individuals with SAD showed an intermediate response between that of the controls and panic disorder patients (4). In a further similar study, Caldirola and colleagues gave 35% CO_2 to patients with panic disorder, SAD and comorbid panic disorder, SAD alone, and as well as healthy controls. Both the panic disorder and SAD patients showed similar increased anxiogenic reactions to 35% CO_2 compared to normal controls. Those with comorbid panic disorder and SAD experienced similar reactions to those seen in patients with either disorder alone (6). These studies indicate that both social SAD and panic disorder patients have a similar hypersensitivity to high-dose CO_2 (35%) and therefore may share a common underlying biological vulnerability.

Van Vliet et al. demonstrated that SAD patients were more sensitive to pentagastrin infusions than normal controls, although the result did not reach significance (8). In a larger study, McCann and colleagues evaluated the response of patients with SAD and panic disorder as well as normal controls to pentagastrin infusion (11). A social interaction test was also included as part of the pentagastrin challenge. Both patient groups had similar rates of pentagastrin-induced panic attacks, implying that SAD and panic disorder patients may share a common pathophysiologic mechanism. However, the anxiety experienced by patients with SAD was not the same as that experienced in anxiety-provoking social situations, a finding that is reported in other studies. Overall, the results of the challenge studies do not support any specific underlying neurobiological abnormality although patients with SAD and panic disorder may share some common, unidentified vulnerability.

B. Neuroendocrine Assessments

Neuroendocrine assessments have been used in psychiatry in order to compare baseline and/or dynamic neuroendocrine measures in psychiatric patients and controls. Elevations in plasma cortisol have long been associated with stress in both animals and humans. Studies to date suggest that patients with SAD do not have any significant hyperactivity of the hypothalamic-adrenal-pituitary (HPA) axis when compared to normal controls (12,13). Similarly, no abnormalities in the hypothalamic-pituitary-thyroid (HPT) axis have been found in patients with SAD, with the exception of an exaggerated pressor effect following thyroid hormone (TRH) stimulation (14,15).

C. Serotonin Functioning

While the efficacy of the selective serotonin reuptake inhibitors (SSRIs) provides, perhaps, the best evidence for a role of the serotonergic system in SAD (16), other evidence also exists suggesting that SAD is, at least in part, due to a serotonergic disturbance. Serotonin appears to play an important role in social dominance and affiliative behavior in monkeys (17–20). Research evidence regarding the role of serotonin in human social behavior is reminiscent of the primate work (21). Dominant social status seems to be associated with high serotonin levels, while low serotonin levels are often associated with subordinate status. Additionally, dominant social status seems to be achieved at least partly by affiliative behavior. The administration of 5-HT reuptake blockers, such as fluoxetine or tryptophan, promoted social dominance acquisition in monkeys (19).

Peripheral measures of serotonin include the measurement of the binding capacity of the platelet serotonin transporter or platelet serotonin $5-HT_2$ receptor. Stein et al. (22) found no differences in platelet ^{3}H-paroxetine binding (a measure of the serotonin uptake) in SAD as compared to individuals with panic disorder and healthy controls. Shlik and colleagues evaluated the neuroendocrine and behavioral responses to the SSRI citalopram in 18 SAD patients compared with controls and found no differences (23). In another neuroendocrine challenge study, Tancer and colleagues (24) performed a double-blind placebo-controlled study using probes for the noradrenergic (clonidine), serotonergic (fenfluramine), and dopaminergic (levodopa) systems. Both patients with SAD and controls showed a similar neuroendocrine profile except for an elevated cortisol response to fenfluramine in SAD, suggesting a selective supersensitivity to the postsynaptic serotonergic receptors (24).

Condren et al. (25) evaluated prolactin response to a buspirone challenge in 14 patients with generalized SAD and 14 healthy controls. SAD patients had a greater prolactin response than controls suggesting an increased sensitivity of central 5-Hydroxytryptophan 1A (5-HT1A) receptors in generalized SAD.

These studies are suggestive of the role of serotonin in social behavior and social anxiety that may be involved in SAD. However, serotonin and the serotonergic system are unlikely the whole story.

D. Dopamine Functioning

Several lines of evidence suggest dopaminergic dysfunction in SAD. For example, drugs that enhance dopamine, such as the monoamine oxidase inhibitors (MAOIs), are effective in treating this disorder. Mikkelson and colleagues (26) reported the development of SAD symptoms after treatment with dopamine blocking agents such as haloperidol. In addition, high rates of SAD have been reported in patients with Parkinson's disease (27). In depressed patients, low cerebral spinal fluid (CSF) dopamine was found to correlate with measures of introversion (28) although it is unclear whether the lowered CSF dopamine is a consequence or a mediator of anxiety. Low levels of CSF homovanillic acid (HVA), a dopamine metabolite, have been found in patients with SAD and comorbid panic disorder (29). However, the levodopa challenge test, which assesses central dopaminergic function, showed no difference in response between patients with SAD and controls (24).

E. Adrenergic Functioning

Levin and colleagues reported elevations in heart rate and blood pressure in the face of a public speaking task in individuals with SAD; these were similar to those of healthy controls (30). Stein and colleagues reported that patients with SAD had a greater mean change in diastolic blood pressure on standing as compared to normal controls as well as higher resting and 5-minute plasma norepinephrine (NE) levels following an orthostatic challenge (31). In a further study, Stein and colleagues employed a variety of challenges to the autonomic nervous system (ANS) and reported that patients with SAD showed an increased blood pressure response to the Valsalva maneuver, an exaggerated vagal withdrawal in response to exercise, but normal heart rate, blood pressure, and plasma NE levels (32). Coupland et al. reported a smaller decrease in blood pressure immediately after an orthostatic challenge in SAD patients compared to normal controls, suggesting sympathetic hyperactivity (33). However, they did not find the higher plasma levels of NE before and after the challenge as in previous studies.

The alpha-2 (α_2) adrenergic antagonist yohimbine has been reported to increase social anxiety in patients with SAD and is associated with increased plasma 3-methoxy-4-hydroxyphenylglycol concentrations (34). Tancer and colleagues (35) have reported mixed results in growth hormone response to the α_2 agonist clonidine. They reported a reduced growth hormone (GH) response to intravenous but not oral clonidine. The blunted GH response to clonidine is also found in individuals with panic disorder, major depression, and generalized anxiety disorder and may reflect reduced postsynaptic adrenergic α_2 receptor functioning due to NE overactivity. In summary, patients with SAD may have some abnormalities in noradrenergic reactivity, which may be somewhat different than those found in other anxiety disorders.

F. CRF and Tachykinins

It appears that the release of CRF is closely associated with activation of the noradrenergic system and to the nonspecific stress response (36). Although there is little information available about the new CRF receptor antagonists, they may prove to be effective treatments for SAD. Similarly, the potential role and efficacy of new agents that affect the tachykinins (e.g., substance P, Neurokinin (NK) A, and NK B receptor antagonists) is unknown. However, Stein and colleagues (37) and Rapaport and Stein (38) reported no differences in neuropeptide Y levels and serum interleukin-2 or soluble interleukin-2 receptors in patients with SAD compared to normal controls.

II. GABA

Gamma-aminobutyric acid (GABA) is the main inhibitory neurotransmitter of the brain. There is a growing body of research implicating the potential use of GABAergic pharmacological agents in the treatment of SAD. For example, gabapentin is an anticonvulsant that acts to increase central GABA as well as having activity at voltage-sensitive Na^+ and Ca^{2+} channels. In a study by Pande and colleagues (39), it has been reported to effectively reduce SAD symptoms. The anticonvulsant pregabalin is a structural analogue of GABA that appears to bind to a subunit of voltage-dependent calcium channels (40). In a randomized double-blind study of 135 patients with SAD treated with pregabalin or placebo, Feltner and colleagues (41) found that the pregabalin group had a significant reduction in SAD symptoms compared to the placebo group.

Other pharmacological agents considered to be effective treatments for SAD also appear to affect the GABA system. The MAOI phenelzine has been reported to enhance neurological concentrations of GABA (42). Benzodiazepines such as clonazepam are known to reduce anxiety by boosting the sensitivity of GABA receptors (43). Evidence from animal literature has shown that neuroactive steroids can modulate the GABA/benzodiazepine receptor complex. Heydari and Le Melledo (44) studied 12 generalized social phobics and 12 controls and found that concentrations of the neuroactive steroid pregnenolone sulfate were significantly lower in patients with SAD than in controls. The authors suggested that the decreased level of pregnenolone sulfate may be reflective of a homeostatic attempt to decrease anxiogenic activity through a lesser negative modulation of the $GABA_A$/BZD receptor and a lesser positive modulation of the NMDA receptor. Condren et al. (45) administered baclofen to 15 individuals with SAD and 15 controls and measured subsequent growth hormone (GH) response. GH response was significantly reduced in SAD subjects compared to controls, suggesting central dysregulation of $GABA_B$ receptor function. Given the preliminary evidence of a dysregulation in the GABA system and the effect of GABAergic agents in reducing social anxiety (46), the role of GABA in SAD requires further elucidation.

In the quest to understand the brain mechanisms that may be involved in SAD, researchers have turned to the relatively new technology of brain imaging. Brain imaging techniques allow for a noninvasive method of evaluating structural abnormalities as well as brain activity in specific areas of the brain, often through the induction of anxiety while the subject is performing a particular task.

A. Electroencephalography (EEG)

In the only EEG study of SAD published to date, Davidson and colleagues (47) compared SAD patients to controls prior to and immediately following a public speaking task. They found that those with SAD had a significant selective activation of the right frontal alpha power, which was highly correlated with their change in subjective anxiety levels.

III. STRUCTURAL AND FUNCTIONAL IMAGING

A. Magnetic Resonance Spectroscopy (MRS)

In a magnetic resonance spectroscopy (MRS) study, Davidson et al. reported a reduction in choline and creatine in both thalamic and caudate areas, suggesting lower central nervous system (CNS) metabolic activity in the basal ganglia area, white matter, and other cortical and noncortical gray areas in patients with SAD (48).

Potts et al. (49) were unable to replicate these results, finding a significant age-dependent decrease in putamen volumes. The authors hypothesized that age may be associated with a decrease in putamen volume and possibly functionality in SAD. In another MRS study using more advanced technology, Tupler et al. (50) found elevated levels of choline and myo-inositol in the cortical gray matter, possibly reflecting abnormalities in second-messenger and cellular membrane functioning.

B. Single-Photon-Emission Computed
Tomography (SPECT)

In the first SPECT study, Stein and Leslie (51) compared individuals with SAD with matched controls but were unable to find differences in regional blood flow. A SPECT study by Tiihonen et al. (52) found markedly reduced striatal presynaptic dopamine reuptake site densities in SAD subjects as compared to controls, suggesting reduced dopamine functioning in SAD.

Li et al. (53), using another D_2 radioligand, found that striatal post-synaptic D_2 receptor binding was associated with symptom severity as measured by the Liebowitz Social Anxiety Scale.

Using the D_2 radioligand ^{123}I-IBZM, Schneier et al. (54) found a significantly lower mean D_2 receptor binding in SAD patients relative to controls, a result that is consistent with the hypothesis of decreased dopamine activity in SAD.

Schneier and colleagues (55) recently examined the availability of the dopamine transporter and found no significant difference in the striatal dopamine transporters between unmedicated generalized SAD individuals and controls. This did not replicate their previous findings.

Van der Linden and colleagues (56) performed a SPECT study on 15 individuals with SAD before and after an 8-week trial of citalopram. Citalopram treatment led to a significant reduction in activity in the anterior and lateral part of the left temporal cortex; the anterior, lateral, and posterior part of the left midfrontal cortex; and the left cingulum. These findings suggest that SSRI treatment may alter temperolimbic and medial frontal functioning.

C. Functional Magnetic Resonance Imaging (fMRI)

Birbaumer and colleagues (57) reported on an fMRI study where SAD patients and healthy controls were presented with two slides of neutral faces and exposed to an aversive odor and a neutral air puff. Aversive odors elicited more bilateral activation in the amygdala in all participants, whereas neutral faces elicited amygdalar activity in the individuals with SAD but not in the controls. Those with SAD also responded to the faces with significantly more bilateral amygdalar activation. It was hypothesized that in patients with SAD, the amygdala is involved in the processing of potentially fear-related objects such as human faces.

In another, similar fMRI study, Schneider et al. (58) studied 12 patients with SAD and 12 controls who were exposed to either a neutral air puff or an aversive odor along with slides of neutral human faces. The presentation of neutral faces with the negative odor led to increased activation in the amygdala and hippocampus in SAD individuals but not in controls. These authors suggested that conditioning to aversive stimuli is processed in subcortical regions with differing patterns of response in individuals with SAD as compared to controls.

Stein and colleagues (59) studied 15 generalized SAD patients and 15 controls who were presented with 60 colored photographs from a standardized set of human facial expressions and asked to identify the gender of the person in the photograph. When compared to controls, SAD patients produced a significantly greater percentage of blood oxygen level–dependent signal changes in the left allocortex. This effect was observed for contemptuous compared to happy faces and for angry compared to happy faces. The authors suggested that there may be a role for differential amygdalar functioning in generalized SAD, particularly in the processing of disorder-salient stimuli.

D. Positron Emission Topography (PET)

In a symptom provocation study, Malizia et al. (60) gave SAD subjects an autobiographical script describing a situation they feared and a controlled script describing a neutral situation. The authors observed that socially anxious subjects showed increased activation in the right dorsolateral prefrontal cortex and in the left parietal cortex. This pattern of activation was not observed in anticipatory anxiety in the healthy volunteers (61).

Using ^{15}O-PET, Reiman (62) had 7 SAD patients sing the alphabet song, either alone or while being observed. Significantly increased rCBF (regional cerebral blood flow) was found in the thalamus, midbrain, lateral prefrontal, midcingulate, sensorimotor, and anterior temporal cortices in the observed condition.

Van Ameringen et al. (63) continued the investigation of rCBF using ^{15}O-PET in a social anxiety provocation paradigm. Six male subjects with SAD were asked to watch a video of themselves giving an impromptu talk while in the presence of several "communication experts" (the exposure condition). In the baseline condition, subjects viewed a video of a socially competent individual giving a speech. PET scans of subjects in the exposure condition showed deactivations in the visual and medial frontal cortices.

Kelsey et al. (64) performed PET scans in SAD subjects before and after open-label nefazodone treatment. Prior to nefazodone treatment, subjects were instructed in an imagery script designed to induce feelings of social and performance anxiety. They were asked to rate the degree of anxiety they experienced while listening to a tape of the imagery script while inside the PET scanner. Social anxiety was correlated positively with rCBF in the bilateral cortex, as well as in the right middle temporal gyrus, caudate, frontal pole, and lateral orbital frontal cortex. There was a significant negative correlation between rCBF localized in the executive regions in the midfrontal gyrus and self-reported levels of anxiety. In postnefazodone scans, social anxiety related rCBF involved areas of positive correlation in the right medial orbital frontal cortex and anterior cingulate gyrus.

Furmark et al. (65) furthered investigations using a 5-HTP the radiotracer in SAD subjects and controls, finding an attenuated uptake of [beta-^{11}C] 5-HTP in limbic/paralimbic areas, including the periamygdaloid and rhinal cortices of the SAD individuals. The authors suggested that there may be a suppressed 5-HTP synthesis within neural pathways involved with fear and anxiety regulation, further implicating serotonin in the neurobiology of SAD. Tillfors (66) used ^{15}O-PET in SAD subjects and a group of matched controls while giving a 2-1/2-minute speech while alone or observed. The public speaking task yielded enhanced rCBF in the amygdaloid complex and decreased cortical activation in individuals with SAD versus controls. The authors suggested that SAD symptom activation was more associated with increased subcortical activity, while the controls had an increase in cortical activation.

Furmark et al. (67) had individuals with SAD undergo ^{15}O-PET while performing a public speaking task and being observed by a silent audience. Patients were randomized to one of 3 conditions: the SSRI citalopram, group cognitive behavioral therapy (CBGT), or a waiting list control group. Scans were repeated after nine weeks of either treatment. Symptom improvement was found to be equal in both the citalopram and CBGT groups. Regardless of treatment approach, responders were found to have a decreased rCBF response to public speaking bilaterally in the amygdala, hippocampus, and periamygdaloid, rhinal and parahippocampal cortices.

Kent et al. (68), using PET, evaluated a SSRI transporter (SERT) radiotracer to determine paroxetine occupancy of SERT in SAD. After 3 to 6 months of paroxetine treatment, there was greater than 80% occupancy in all brain regions measured, implicating the involvement of the serotonin system in SAD.

IV. SUMMARY

Despite the use of a wide range of strategies investigating the neurobiology of SAD, our review revealed no clearly defined biological abnormalities in SAD. The majority of the studies described were exploratory in nature and not driven by any theoretical model of SAD. The inconclusive findings could be attributed to methodological problems with these studies, including lack of placebo controls; the use of single-blind designs; and inclusion of subjects who had comorbidity, were on medication, or had not been differentiated by subtype (generalized versus nongeneralized) or symptom cluster (presence or absence of panic attacks).

Pharmacological probes and challenge studies to date seem to suggest that in comparison to panic disorder, SAD sits somewhere between panic disorder and normal controls. Neuroimaging studies have described differences in regional brain functioning in generalized SAD (this volume, chapter by Fredrikson and Furmark). Although a variety of brain areas have been implicated with neuroimaging techniques, there is little consistency between studies and the results are inconclusive. However, with the accumulated reports to date, brain structures—including basal ganglia, amygdala, as well as various cortical regions—have been implicated as playing a role in SAD.

It has been postulated that SAD is a multidetermined disorder that may involve the amygdala as well as the dopaminergic and serotonergic systems. Much of the research mentioned above also found a correlation between symptoms of social anxiety and increased blood flow to the amygdalohippocampal regions of the brain. This increased blood flow to the phylogenetically older areas of the brain is most often paired with a decrease in blood flow to the more cognitive regions of the brain.

Different systems may be involved in different subtypes of patients. At present, our subtyping of SAD is quite rudimentary—i.e., generalized versus nongeneralized SAD and SAD with and without panic attacks. In order to better understand the neurobiology and treatment response of SAD, we will likely have to develop more sophisticated typologies of SAD based on research with animal models, psychiatrically healthy and shy individuals, and ever more sophisticated imaging and labeling techniques. It is likely that as we learn more about dominance, affiliation, behavioral inhibition, and behavioral approaches, we will be better able to understand the neurobiology of different subtypes of SAD as well as predictors of treatment response (69).

One of the nonspecific effects of stress is a dysregulation in dopaminergic functioning. However, social status in monkeys is reflected in dopamine D_2 striatal differences (70). In addition, the ascending dopamine system has been found to play an important role in the control of approach motivation and behavior in animals and humans (71–76). Such results may help to understand both the findings of dopamine abnormalities in SAD and the importance ascribed to avoidance.

Gray (77) argues that the behavioral activation (BA) system and the behavioral inhibition (BI) system are the two primary systems that guide all behavior. The BI system is sensitive to cues of punishment and assists the organism in avoiding punishment. The BA system, on the other hand, is sensitive to cues for reward and guides the organism toward reinforcers. As we have seen, dopamine has been closely associated with approach motivation (Gray's BA system), while serotonin has been implicated in avoidance (Gray's BI system) (78,79). Perhaps the best way to understand the role of dopamine and serotonin is to view the BA (dopamine) and BI (serotonin) systems as mutually antagonistic systems that regulate social and affiliative behaviors. Current treatment strategies may work by reducing avoidance (Gray's BI system) through manipulation of the serotonergic system. Attempts to increase the incentive value of social interaction (Gray's BA system) through manipulations of the dopaminergic system may also be advantageous. Indeed, it may be that, at least for some social SAD patients, the most important effect of serotonergic agents are their downstream effects on dopaminergic systems (80).

REFERENCES

1. Kessler RC, McGonagle KA, Zhao S, Nelson CB, Hughes M, Eshleman S, Wittchen HU, Kendler KS. Lifetime prevalence of DSM-II-R psychiatric disorders in the United States: results from the National Cormorbidity Survey. Arch Gen Psychiatry 1994; 51:8–19.
2. Liebowitz MR, Fyer AJ, Gorman JM, Dillan D, Davies S, Stein JM, Cohen BS, Klein DF. Specificity of lactate infusions in social phobia versus panic disorders. Am J Psychiatry 1985,142:947–950.
3. Tancer ME, Stein MB, Uhde TW. Lactate response to caffeine in panic disorder; a replication using an "anxious control group." Biol Psychiatry 1991, 29:57.
4. Gorman JM, Papp, LA, Martinez J. Goetz RR, Hollander E, Liebowitz MR, Jordan F. High-dose carbon dioxide challenge test in anxiety disorder patients. Biol Psychiatry 1990; 28:743–757.
5. Papp LA, Klein DF, Martinez J, Schneier F, Cole R, Liebowitz, MR, Hollander G, Fyer AT, Jordan F, Gorman JM. Diagnostic and substance specificity of carbon dioxide induced panic patients. Am J Psychiatry 1993; 150:250–257.
6. Caldirola D, Perna G, Arancio, C, Bertani A, Bellodi L. The 35% carbon dioxide challenge test in patients with social phobia. Psychiatry Res 1997; 71: 41–48.
7. Bradwijn J. CCK. British Association for Psychopharmacology Summer Meeting, Cambridge, UK, July 1997.
8. Van Vliet IM, Westenberg HGM, Slaap BR, den Boer JA, Ho Pian KL. Anxiogenic effects of pentagastrin in patients with social phobia and health controls. Biol Psychiatry 1997; 42(1):76–78.
9. Coupland NJ, Bell C, Potokar JP, Dorkins E, Nutt DJ. Flumazenil challenge in social phobia. Depress Anxiety 2000; 11(1):27–30.
10. Nutt DJ, Glue P, Lawson C, Wilson S. Flumazenil provocation of panic attacks: evidence for altered benzodiazepine receptor sensitivity in panic disorder. Arch Gen Psychiatry 1990; 47:917–925.
11. McCann UD, Slate SO, Geraci M, Roscow-Terril D, Udhe TW. A comparison of the effects of intravenous pentagastrin on patients with social phobia, panic disorder, and healthy controls. Neuropsychopharmacology 1997; 16(3): 229–237.
12. Uhde TW, Taner ME, Gelernter CS, Vittone BJ. Normal urinary free cortisol and postdexamethasone cortisol in social phobia: comparison to normal volunteers. J Affect Disord 1994; 30(3):155–161
13. Potts NLS, Davidson JRT, Krishnan KRR, Doraiswamy PM, Ritchie JC. Levels of urinary free cortisol in social phobia. J Clin Psychiatry 1991; 52 (11 suppl): 41–42.

14. Tancer ME, Stein MB, Gelernter CS, Uhde TW. The hypothalamic-pituitary-thyroid axis in social phobia. Am J Psychiatry 1990; 147(7): 929–933.

15. Tancer ME, Stein MB, Uhde TW. Effects of tyrotropin-releasing hormone on blood pressure and heart rate in phobic and panic patients: results of a pilot study. Biol Psychiatry 1990; 27(7):781–783.

16. Van Ameringen M, Mancini C, Farvolden P, Oakman J. Pharmacotherapy for social phobia: What works, what might work, and what does not work at all. CNS Spectrums 1999; 4(11):61–68.

17. Highley JD, King ST Jr, Hasert MF, Champux M, Suomi SJ, Linnoila M. Stability of interindividual differences in serotonin function and its relationship to severe aggression and competent social behavior in rhesus macaque females. Neuropsychopharmacology 1996; 14:67–76.

18. Raleigh MJ, Brammer GL, Yuwiler A,Flannery JW, McGuire MT, Geller E. Serotonergic influences on the social behavior of vervet monkeys (*Cercopithecus aethiops sabaeus*). Exp Neurol 1980; 68:322–334.

19. Raleigh MJ, Brammer GL, McGuire MT, Yuwiler A. Dominant social status facilitates the behavioral effects of serotonergic agonists. Brain Res 1985; 348: 274–282.

20. Westergaard GC, Mehlman PT, Suomi SJ, Higley JD. CSF 5-HIAA and aggression in female macaque monkeys: species and interindividual differences. Psychoparmacology 1995; 146:440–446.

21. Knutson B, Wolkowitz OM, Cole SW, Chan T, Moore EA, Johnson RC, Terpstra J, Turner RA, Reus VI. Selective alteration of personality and social behavior by serotonergic intervention. Am J Psychiatry 1998; 155:373–379.

22. Stein MB, Delaney SM, Chartiet M. 3H paroxetine binding to platelets of patients with social phobia: comparison to patients with panic disorder and health volunteers. Biol Psychiatry 1995; 37:224–228.

23. Shilk J, Maron E, Aluoja A, Vasar V, Toru I. Citalopam challenge in social anxiety disorder. 15th ECNP Congress, Barcelona, Spain, October 5–9, 2002. Eur Neuropsychopharmacol 2002; 12(suppl 3): S339.

24. Tancer ME, Mailman RB, Stein MB, Mason GA, Carson SW, Golden RN. Neuroendocrine responsivity to monoaminergic system probes in generalized social phobia. Anxiety 1994–1995; 1(5):216–223.

25. Condren RM, Dinan TG, Thakore JH. A preliminary study of buspirone stimulated prolactin release in generalized social phobia: evidence for enhanced serotonergic responsivity? Eur Neuropsychopharmacol 2002; 12:349–354.

26. Mikkelson EJ, Deltor J, Cohen DJ. School avoidance and social phobia triggered by haloperididol in patients with Tourette's syndrome. Am J Psychiatry 1981; 138:1572–1576.

27. Richard IH, Schiffer RB, Kurlan R. Anxiety and Parkinson's disease. J Neuropsychiatr Clin Neurosci 1996; 8:383–392.

28. King R, Mefford I, Wang C, Murchison A, Caligari EJ, Berger PA. CSF dopamine levels correlate with extraversion in depressed patients. Psychiatr Res 1986; 19:305–310.

29. Johnson M, Lydiard R, Zealberg J, Fossey MD, Ballenger JC. Plasma and CSF HVA levels in panic patients with comorbid social phobia. Biol Psychiatry 1994; 36:425–427.

30. Levin AP, Saoud J, Struaman T, Gorman JM, Fyer AJ, Crawford R, Liebowitz MR. Responses of generalized and discrete social phobics during public speaking. J Anxiety Disord 1993; 7:207–221.

31. Stein MB, Tancer ME, Uhde TW. Heart rate and plasma norepinephrine responsivity to arthostatic challenge in social anxiety disorder: comparison of patients with panic disorder and social phobia and normal control subjects. Arch Gen Psychiatry 1992; 49:311–317.

32. Stein MB, Asmundson G, Chartier M. Autonomic responsivity in generalized social phobia. J Affect Disord 1994; 31:211–221.

33. Coupland NY, Bailey JE, Potokar JP. Abnormal cardiovascular responses to standing in panic disorder and social phobia. J Psychopharmacol 1995; 9(suppl 3): A73.

34. Potts NL, Book S, Davidson JR. The neurobiology of social phobia. Int Clin Psychopharmacol 1996; 11(suppl3):43–48.

35. Tancer ME, Stein MB, Uhde TW. Growth hormone response to IV clonidine in social phobia: comparison to patients with panic disorder and healthy volunteers. Biol Psychiatry 1994; 34:252–256.

36. Koob GF. Corticotropin-releasing factor, norepinephrine, and stress. Biol Psychiatry 1999; 46:1167–1180.

37. Stein MR, Hauger HL, Dhalla KS, Chartier MJ, Asmundson GJ. Plasma neuropeptide Y in anxiety disorders: finding in panic disorder and social phobia. Psychiatry Res 1996; 5(9):183–188.

38. Rapaport MH, Stein MD. Serum interlukin-2 and soluble interleukin-2 receptor levels in generalized social phobia. Anxiety 1994; 1;50–53.

39. Pande AC, Davidson JR, Jefferson JW, Janney CA, Katzelnick DJ, Weisler RH, Greist JH, Sutherland SM. Treatment of social phobia with gabapentin: a placebo-controlled study. J Clin Psychopharmacol 1999; 19(4):341–348.

40. Field MJ, Oles RJ, Sing L. Pregabalin may represent a novel class of anxiolytic agents with a broad spectrum of activity. Br J Pharmacol 2001; 132:1–3.

41. Feltner DE, Davidson JRT, Pollack MH, Stein MB, Futterer R, Jefferson JW, Lydiard RB, Duboff E, Robinson P, Phelps M, Slomkowski M, Werth JL, Pande AC. A placebo-controlled, double-blind study of pregabalin treatment of social anxiety disorder: outcomes and predictors of response. 39th Annual Meeting of the American College of Neuropsychopharmacology, Puerto Rico, Dec 1–14, 2000.

42. Baker GB, Wong JT, Yeung JM, Coutts RT. Effects of the antidepressant phenelzine on brain levels of gamma-amino butynic acid (GABA). J Affect Disord 1991; 21:207–211.

43. Robow LE, Russek SJ, Farb DH. From ion currents to genomic analysis: recent advances in $GABA_A$ receptor research. Synapse 1995;19:149–177.

44. Heyardi B, Le Melledo JM. Low pregnenolone sulphate plasma concentrations in patients with generalized social phobia. Psychol Med 2002; 32:929–933.

45. Condren RM, Lucey JV, Thakore JH. A preliminary study of baclofen-induced growth hormone release in generalized social phobia. Hum Psychopharmacol Clin Exp 2003; 18:125–130.

46. Davidson JRT, Potts NS, Richichi E, Krishnan R, Ford SM, Smith R, Wilson WH. Treatment of social phobia with clonazepam and placebo. J Clin Psychopharmacol 1993; 13:423–428.

47. Davidson RJ. Marshall JR, Tomarken AJ. Henriques JB. While a phobic waits: regional brain electrical and autonomic activity in social phobics during anticipation of public speaking. Biol Psychiatry 2000:47:85–95.

48. Davidson JRT, Krishnan KRR, Charles HC, Boyko O, Potts NL, Ford SM, Patterson L. Magnetic resonance spectroscopy in social phobia: preliminary findings. J Clin Psychiatry 1993,54(12 suppl):19–25.

49. Potts NL, Davidson JRT, Krishnan KR, Doraiswamy PM. Magnetic resonance imaging in social phobia. Psychiatry Res 1994, 52:35–42.

50. Tupler LA, Davidson JRT, Smith RD, Lazeras F, Charles HC, Krishnan KRR. A repeat proton magnetic resonance spectroscopy study in social phobia. Biol Psychiatry 1997; 2:419–424.

51. Stein MB, Leslie WD. A brain single photon-emission computed tomography (SPECT) study of generalized social phobia. Biol Psychiatry 1996; 39:825–828.

52. Tiihonen J, Kuikka J, Bergstrom K, Lepola U, Koponen H, Leinonen E. Dopamine reuptake site densities in patients with social phobia. Am J Psychiatry 1997; 154:239–242.

53. Li DM, Chokka P, McEwan AJB, Logus W, Mantei S, Hanson J, Tibbo P. The relationship of striatal dopamine with social phobia a gender: a SPECT study. Biological Psychiatry Meeting, Washington, DC, 1999.

54. Schneier FR, Liebowitz MR, Abi-Dargham A, Zea-Ponce Y, Lin SH, Laruelle M. Low dopamine D_2 receptor binding potential in social phobia. Am J Psychiatry 2000, 157:457–459.

55. Schneier FR, Martinez, PM, Zhu Z, Liebowitz MR. Dopamine transporter binding in social phobia. 156th Annual Meeting of the American Psychiatric Association, San Francisco, CA, May 17–22, 2003.

56. van der Linden GJ. Stein DJ. van Balkom AJ. The efficacy of the selective serotonin reuptake inhibitors for social anxiety disorder (social phobia): a meta-analysis of randomized controlled trials. Int Clin Psychopharmacol 2000, 15 (suppl 2):S15–S23.

57. Birbaumer N, Grodd W, Diedrich O, Klose U, Erb M, Lotze M, Schneider F, Weiss U, Flor H. f-MRI reveals amygdala activation to human faces in social phobics. Neuroreport 1998; 9:1223–1226.

58. Schneider F, Weiss U, Kessler C, Muller-Gartner HW, Posse S, Salloum J, Grodd W, Himmelmann F, Gaebel W, Birbaumer N. Subcortical correlates of differential classical conditioning of aversive emotional reactions in social phobia. Biol Psychiatry 1999; 45:863–871.

59. Stein MB, Goldin PR, Sareen J, Eyler Zorrilla LT, Brown GG. Increased amygdala activation to angry and contemptuous faces in generalized social phobia. Arch Gen Psychiatry 2002; 59:1027–1034.

60. Malizia AL, Wilson SJ, Bell CM, Nutt DJ, Grasby PM. Neural correlates of anxiety provocation in social phobia. Neuroimage 1997; 5:S301.
61. Malizia AL. PET studies in experimental and pathological anxiety. J Psychopharmacol 1997; 11(3): A88.
62. Reiman EM. The Application of positron emission tomography to the study of normal and pathologic emotions. J Clin Psychiatry 1997; 58 (suppl 16):4–12.
63. Van Ameringen M, Mancini C, Oakman JM, Kamath M, Nahmias C, Szechtman, H. A pilot study of PET in social phobia. Biol Psychiatry 1998; 43:31S.
64. Kelsy JE, Selvig AL, Knight BT, et al. Treatment of generalized social phobia with the 5HT2 antagonist nefazodone. Anxiety Disorders of America's 20th Annual Conference. Washington DC, March 23–26, 2000.
65. Furmark T. Social phobia: from epidemiology to brain function. In: Comprehensive Summaries of Uppsala Dissertations from the Faculty of Social Sciences. Uppsala, Sweden: Acta Universitatis Upsaliensis, 2000.
66. Tillfors M, Furmark T, Marteinsdottir I, Fischer H, Pissiota A, Langstrom B, Fredrikson M. Cerebral blood flow in subjects with social phobia during stressful speaking tasks: a PET study. Am J Psychiatry 2001; 158:1220–1226.
67. Furmark T, Tillfors M, Marteinsdottir I, Fisher H, Pissiota A, Langstrom B, Fredrikson M. Common changes in cerebral blood flow in patients with social phobia treated with citalopram or cognitive behavioral therapy. Arch Gen Psychiatry 2002 59:425–433.
68. Kent JM, Coplan JD, Lombardo I, Hwang DR, Huang Y, Mawlawi O, Van Heertum RL, Slifstein M, Abi-Dargham A, Gorman JM, Laruelle M. Occupancy of brain serotonin transporters during treatment with paroxetine in patients with social phobia: a positron emission tomography study with [^{11}C]McN 5652. Psychopharmacology 2002; 164:341–348.
69. Oakman J, Van Ameringen M, Mancini C, Farvolden P. Challenges in the treatment of social phobia. In: Crozier WR, ed. Shyness. London: Routledge, 2000.
70. Grant KA, Shively CA, Nader MA, Ehrenkaufer RL, Line SW, Morton TE, Gage D, Mach RH. Effect of social status on striatal dopamine D2 receptor binding characteristics in cynomolgus monkeys assessed with positron emission tomography. Synapse 1998, 29:80–83.
71. Cohen JD, Braver TS, O'Reilly RC. A computational approach to prefrontal cortex, cognitive control and schizophrenia: recent developments and current challenges. Philos Trans R Soc Lond. Ser B: Biol Sci 1996, 351:1515–1527.
72. Depue RA, Luciana M, Arbisi P, Collins P, Leon A. Dopamine and the structure of personality: Relation of agonist-induced dopamine activity to positive emotionality. J Personality Soc Psychol 1994; 67:485–498.
73. Egelman DM, Person C, Montague PR. A computational role for dopamine delivery in human decision-making. J Cogn Neurosci 1998; 10:623–630.
74. Contreras-Vidal JL, Schultz, W. A predictive reinforcement model of dopamine neurons for learning approach behavior. J Comp Neurosci 1999; 6:191–214.

75. Koob GF. Hedonic valence, dopamine and motivation. Mol Psychiatry 1996; 1:186–189.
76. Schultz, W. Predictive reward signal of dopamine neurons. J Neurophysiol 1998; 80:1–27.
77. Gray JA. The Neuropsychology of Anxiety. Oxford, UK: Oxford University Press, 1982.
78. Deakin JFW, Graeff FG. 5-HT and mechanisms of defense. J Psychopharmacol 1991; 5:305–315.
79. Hansenne M, Ansseau M. Harm avoidance and serotonin. Biol Psychiatry 1999; 51:77–81.
80. Dubovsky SL. Beyond the serotonin reuptake inhibitors: rationales for the development of new serotonergic agents. J Clin Psychiatry 1994; 55(2 suppl): 34–44.

13

Genetics of Social Anxiety Disorder and Related Traits

Murray B. Stein
University of California San Diego,
San Diego, California, U.S.A.

Joel Gelernter
Yale University School of Medicine,
New Haven, Connecticut, U.S.A.

Jordan W. Smoller
Massachusetts General Hospital,
Boston, Massachusetts, U.S.A.

I. GENETIC EPIDEMIOLOGY OF SOCIAL ANXIETY AND RELATED TRAITS

A. Introduction

Among the anxiety disorders, social anxiety disorder has garnered increased attention in recent years, owing in part to the demonstration of its high prevalence and marked impact on functioning (1,2). Social anxiety disorder is associated with numerous adverse psychosocial and socioeconomic outcomes, including early dropout from school, reduced job earnings, increased direct and indirect health care costs, and poor health-related quality of life

(3–5) (this volume, Baldwin and Buis). The study of social anxiety disorder from a genetic perspective is particularly compelling for several reasons. First, social anxiety disorder is heritable (6,7), particularly in its more severe form, generalized social phobia (GSP) (8). Second, GSP is an early-onset disorder, with over 90% of cases occurring by the early teen years (9); this makes it possible to study young adults with a very low risk of phenotypic misclassification. Third, the relationship between certain heritable quantitative traits (e.g., social interactional anxiety) and GSP has been sufficiently well studied that this provides an additional opportunity to find linkage to a phenotype that may be closer to biological reality than that provided by the fourth edition of the *Diagnostic and Statistical Manual of Mental Disorders* (DSM-IV) (10,11). For all these reasons, further exploration of the genetic bases for social anxiety disorder and related traits will be a worthwhile endeavor. In this chapter, we review the available evidence for the heritability of social anxiety disorder and characterological traits that may underlie this disorder. We also consider possible candidate genes for social phobia. Finally, we review the very small but growing literature implicating particular genes or genomic regions as susceptibility factors for social anxiety disorder and related traits.

B. Evidence for Heritability

1. Twin Studies of Shyness and Other Social Anxiety-Related Traits

a. Shyness and Social Anxiety. Twin studies have long shown that shyness is a strongly heritable trait (12,13). In a study of childhood anxiety comprising 326 same-sex twin pairs (174 monozygotic and 152 dizygotic pairs), higher correlations were found for social anxiety symptoms in monozygotic than dizygotic twin pairs, leading to the conclusion that these symptoms are genetically influenced (14).

Negative evaluation fears figure prominently in the cognitive psychology of patients with social anxiety disorder. In a recent study, we examined the heritability of negative evaluation fears using a twin sample (7). We also examined the relationships between negative evaluation fears and personality dimensions relevant to social anxiety disorder. Scores on the brief version of the Fear of Negative Evaluation Scale (Brief-FNE) (15) were examined in a sample of 437 (245 monozygotic and 192 dizygotic) twin pairs. Biometrical model-fitting was conducted using standard statistical methods. Genetic and environmental correlations with personality dimensions from the Dimensional Assessment of Personality Pathology-Basic Questionnaire (DAPP-BQ) (16,17) were also calculated. In this study, broad heritability estimate of the Brief-FNE was 48%. Additive genetic effects and unique environmental effects emerged as the primary influences on negative evaluation fears. Genetic correlations between Brief-FNE scores and the Submissiveness, Anxiousness, and Social Avoidance facets of the DAPP-BQ were high (r_g ranging from 0.78 to 0.80). These observations lead us to conclude that a cognitive dimension central to the phenomenology (and perhaps etiology) of social anxiety disorder, the fear of being negatively evaluated, is moderately heritable. Moreover, the same genes that influence negative evaluation fears appear to influence a cluster of anxiety-related personality characteristics.

It is generally believed that avoidant personality disorder, a Cluster C personality disorder in DSM-IV with a prevalence rate of approximately 1.8% in a community sample (18), is an alternate manifestation (actually an alternate categorization) of severe GSP (19). As noted earlier, we found in our twin study that fear of negative evaluation is strongly genetically correlated to avoidant personality traits (7). These observations strengthen the likelihood that such traits form part of the characterological template for GSP and offer clues to a personality "endophenotype" that may be fruitfully investigated in future genetic studies.

   b.   Behavioral Inhibition to the Unfamiliar.   Behavioral inhibition to the unfamiliar (BI) is a temperamental profile, observed in approximately 20% of young Caucasian children, defined by a stable tendency to be avoidant, quiet, and behaviorally restrained in unfamiliar situations (20,21). Twin studies show that BI has a strong genetic etiology, with heritability estimates as high as 50 to 70% (22,23). These findings support the view that BI may be an intermediate phenotype of certain anxiety disorders such as GSP, which is more amenable to genetic dissection than are the clinical disorders themselves (24). It has recently been shown that adults who had been designated with BI in childhood show a heightened amygdala response to novelty as demonstrated with functional magnetic resonance imaging (fMRI) (25,26). It may soon be possible to consider this an even more proximate phenotype (or "endophenotype") than BI and to use functional neuroimaging in combination with genetic techniques to uncover susceptibility factors for social anxiety disorder and related disorders.

2.   Twin Studies of Social Anxiety Disorder

Twin studies conducted using older definitions of social phobia suggest that a modest portion of the familial resemblance is heritable (27–29). Kendler et al. reported heritability data for social phobia based on a population-based study of female twins, with two assessments 8 years apart (30); heritability of social phobia was estimated as 51% (corrected for unreliability). Kendler et al. reported heritability of 24% for social phobia based on a sample of male twins (without correction for unreliability) (31). Together, these studies support a moderate role for genetic influences on susceptibility to social phobia (6). In an adolescent female twin sample, Nelson et al. estimated sharing of genetic and environmental vulnerability between social phobia and comorbid disorders (32). Although, in contrast to other studies, they found a very low heritability rate for social phobia, they did find strong genetic correlations between social phobia and major depression. These observations point to the possibility that there may be considerable overlap in the genes influencing social phobia and major depression, suggesting that the high comorbidity seen between these two disorders may have a strong genetic basis.

3.   Family Studies

   a.   Family Studies of Shyness and Behavioral Inhibition.   A recent study examining the mothers of shy children strongly supports an etio-pathological relationship between shyness and SP (33). In this study, 867 four-year-old preschoolers were screened by having their mothers complete a shyness scale. Using established norms, the investigators identified 108 children (12.5%) with shyness, 43 of whom they were able to contact for further study. They also included a group of 56 nonshy, behaviorally disturbed children and 26 with no disturbance. The investigators conducted standardized psychiatric interviews with the children's mothers, who were blind to the group status of their children. They found that mothers of children who were "purely shy" (i.e., had shyness but no other behavioral disturbance) had significantly higher rates of anxiety disorders in general and social phobia in particular (odds ratio 7.6) than the mothers of nonshy children.

   Evidence from longitudinal and high-risk family studies have demonstrated that BI is a developmental and familial risk factor for anxiety disorders, including social phobia and panic disorder (34–36). Schwartz and colleagues examined the longitudinal relationship between early-childhood behavioral inhibition and adolescent anxiety disorders (37). Seventy-nine children who were classified as inhibited or uninhibited at age 2 were reassessed with a structured diagnostic interview at age 13. Being inhibited at age 2 approximately doubled the odds for having generalized social anxiety disorder at age 13. Interestingly, the relationship was specific, in that childhood behavioral inhibition did not increase the odds for specific phobia, separation anxiety, or performance anxiety. These results are consistent with studies documenting increased rates of social anxiety disorder among parents of behaviorally inhibited children (38,39) and speak to the shared familial nature of these constructs.

b. Familial Aggregation of Social Anxiety Disorder. Martin et al. examined anxiety and depressive disorders in the mothers and fathers of children with anxious school refusal (40). They tested for the existence of differences in familial aggregation between children suffering from school refusal related to separation anxiety disorder and those suffering from phobic disorder–based school refusal. Using blind interviews, they looked at lifetime parental disorders for the two groups. They found an increased prevalence of panic disorder (with or without agoraphobia) among the parents of school refusers with separation anxiety disorder and an increased prevalence of simple and/or social anxiety disorder among the parents of phobic school refusers. This observation of significant differences in familial aggregation considering the subgroups of anxious school-refusing children attests to the probable specificity of transmission of these syndromes.

Social anxiety disorder has consistently been found to aggregate in families of adult probands with social anxiety disorder, with the strongest evidence of familial aggregation seen for GSP (8,32,41). Children of patients with social anxiety disorder also have high rates of this disorder (42). One study suggested that social anxiety disorder aggregates independently of other phobic disorders (43). A metaanalysis reported a summary odds ratio for the familiality of phobic disorders including social anxiety disorder of 4.1 (95% CI: 2.7 to 6.1) (6). Based on data available from family studies of social anxiety disorder, the recurrence risk ratio for first-degree relatives (λ_1) appears to be in the range of 2 to 6. These data suggest that social anxiety disorder should be considered among the group of neuropsychiatric disorders (e.g., bipolar disorder, schizophrenia, panic disorder) potentially amenable to genetic mapping using linkage strategies.

c. Familial Aggregation of Social Anxiety and Related Traits. Many psychiatric nosologists agree that it would be extremely surprising if nature and DSM-IV concurred and that mental disorders were inherited according to DSM-IV–defined phenotypes (44,45). Instead, they hypothesize that what may be inherited is a set of temperamental traits that serve as susceptibility factors for these disorders. In this regard, we examined a number of potential risk factors for social phobia in a family study of GSP (10). We found that first-degree relatives of GSP probands scored significantly higher than first-degree relatives of comparison subjects on measures of social anxiety as well as on the anxiety-related personality trait of harm avoidance. A single factor, accounting for 84% of the variance, was strongly associated with being a relative of a GSP proband. We concluded that one or more of these quantitative traits might be a more proximate phenotype for what is genetically transmitted in this complex disorder. This study suggests that opportunities to detect linkage may lie not only with well-defined qualitative

DSM phenotypes (e.g., GSP) but also with well-characterized related traits (e.g., social interactional anxiety, behavioral inhibition, neuroticism, and extraversion).

C. Clues from Other Disorders

1. Autism

Autism is a behavioral syndrome characterized by impairment in communication and reciprocal social interaction in conjunction with stereotyped repetitive patterns of behavior (46,47). Several studies have documented elevated rates of social phobia among first-degree relatives of autistic probands (48,49). The genetic etiology of autism, like that of many neuropsychiatric disorders, is thought to be complex, and the disorder itself (which may extend to Asperger's syndrome as a less severe phenotype) is likely to be genetically heterogeneous. In the past few years, a number of large-scale linkage studies have identified numerous potential risk loci for autism (50–53). Other studies have identified polymorphisms associated with autism that may be relevant to social anxiety, such as the gamma-aminobutyric acid type-A receptor beta3 subunit gene (*GABRB3*) (54) and the gene coding for the arginine vasopressin 1a receptor (*AVPR1A*) (55). Given the apparent aggregation of social anxiety disorder in at least some families with autism, the measurement of autism-related traits [e.g., deficits in reciprocal social behavior (56,57)] in families with social anxiety might lead to the discovery of a more homogenous subtype of social anxiety disorder that lends itself more readily to genetic linkage analysis. Furthermore, some of the genes already highlighted as potential risk factors for autism may, in fact, be worth exploring as risk factors for social anxiety disorder.

2. Selective Mutism

Selective mutism, the refusal to speak in front of unfamiliar people, has been found to occur in 0.18 to 0.71% of children (58–62). First-degree family members of children with selective mutism have increased rates of social phobia and parents have an increase in social anxiety-related traits (61,63,64). Case reports of monozygotic twin concordance for selective mutism (65) and of an association with fragile X syndrome in some cases (66) indicate a possible genetic basis for selective mutism. If, as some investigators believe, selective mutism is a severe, early-onset form of social phobia (63,67), it may be fruitful to conduct linkage and/or family-based association studies in this disorder, and such studies may be informative with regard to genetic susceptibility factors for social phobia.

II. MOLECULAR GENETICS OF SOCIAL ANXIETY DISORDER AND RELATED TRAITS

A. Linkage Studies in Social Anxiety Disorder

In earlier work, we were able to provide evidence excluding linkage of GSP to the serotonin transporter, serotonin$_{2A}$ receptor, and a series of DA receptor genes (68,69). These studies, which were designed in the early 1990s, had power only to detect major susceptibility loci, a situation we now know to be unrealistic for a complex disease or trait (70,71). Most recently, as part of a study of genetics of anxiety disorders in families ascertained through probands with panic disorder [previous linkage results published for panic disorder and agoraphobia (72) and simple phobia (73)], we have conducted a genomewide linkage analysis at 10 cM resolution for social phobia in a set of extended pedigrees (approximately 160 individuals) (74). Multipoint lod score and Zlr analysis were completed using ALLEGRO (75). The most promising results were observed on chromosome 16. A Zlr score of 3.41 was observed at position 62.3 cM ($p = 0.0003$). The strongest evidence for linkage was found on chromosome 16, with lod score 2.47 and hlod 2.66 (simple parametric dominant/narrow), lod score 2.22 (recessive/broad), and lod score 2.06 (recessive/narrow), together with Zlr score 3.41 (at marker D16S415, $p = 0.0003$) observed within a span of about 20 cM. This Zlr score is included in a region that spans from position 40.6 to 93.9 where the Zlr score > 1, a region of 53.3 cM. These results may be considered suggestive of linkage to this region (76). The most obvious candidate gene mapped in this region is SLC6A2 ("solute carrier family 6 member 2"), the NE transporter protein locus (protein product, NET1), which maps close to D16S3136 (within the region of interest but not at the linkage peak). These encouraging preliminary observations indicate the need for larger, better-powered studies to replicate and extend this work and for fine-mapping and association studies to confirm the identity of susceptibility gene(s).

An interstitial duplication on chromosome 15, designated by the investigators as DUP25, was found to be linked and associated to a range of anxiety disorders (including social phobia) (77). The linkage described was observed between the DUP25 phenotype and various diagnostic constructs, all involving joint laxity as part of the phenotype. Although this finding generated considerable excitement in the field (78), it has not yet been replicated and, in fact, the validity of the method for identifying DUP25 has been called into question (79,80). It consequently seems unlikely that other investigative groups will replicate this initially intriguing finding.

Although not a linkage study of social phobia per se, recent findings from deCode Genetics of a genomewide scan provide strong support for a susceptibility locus for panic disorder in Icelandic families, a result that may inform the search for social phobia susceptibility genes (81). Linkage analysis of 25 extended families, in each of which at least one affected individual had panic disorder (PD), resulted in a LOD score of 4.18 at D9S271 on chromosome 9q31. The linkage results may be relevant not only to PD but also to anxiety in general, since this linkage study included patients with other forms of anxiety, including social phobia. In fact, when a broader anxiety disorder phenotype (including social phobia, among other anxiety disorders) was tested, the LOD score dropped somewhat but remained highly suggestive of linkage; this finding suggests that at least in the pedigree series studied, social phobia may lie outside the genetic diagnostic spectrum that includes panic disorder. As noted later in this chapter, NMDA (N-methyl-D-aspartate) receptors have been implicated in animal models of anxiety, and this linked region includes at least one candidate susceptibility gene, the gene for the NMDA receptor 3A receptor (*GRIN3A*).

Future linkage studies in social phobia will have to contend with the present uncertainty about precisely what is inherited in families believed to have social phobia. Studies from Columbia and Harvard Universities also tell us that children at high risk for depressive disorders by virtue of parental major depression are also at high risk for social phobia (82,83). These findings underscore the probable etiological link between SP and at least some forms of major depression. It will be necessary in future studies to consider the possibility that a broader array of disorders is inherited and that this might extend to other anxiety disorders (84), or perhaps even more broadly to other anxiety and mood disorders (85). Moreover, the exact diagnostic spectra influenced by each risk locus are likely to differ. A valuable by-product of future, larger linkage studies in social phobia will, in fact, be the information that these studies provide about the range of disorders and traits that run in these families.

B. Linkage and Association Studies in Traits of Potential Relevance to Social Anxiety Disorder

1. Shyness

A polymorphism of the serotonin transporter promoter region polymorphism (a 44-base-pair insertion deletion, referred to as 5-HTTLPR) has recently been related to shyness in a sample of 98 Israeli children attending second grade (86). This polymorphism has been the focus of considerable prior scrutiny, much of it focused on neuroticism, where numerous associations (and nonreplications) have been reported over the past 8 years (87–92). This finding of an association with shyness (86), a trait that is closely tied to social phobia (93,94), strengthens the promise that it will be possible to detect susceptibility genes for social anxiety–related traits and specifically implicates the serotonin transporter gene (*SCL6A4*) among a number of biologically compelling candidates.

2. Neuroticism

Neuroticism is an underlying feature of mood and anxiety disorders, including social phobia (95–99). As such, clarifying the genetic architecture of neuroticism is likely to contribute to our understanding of genetic susceptibility to these disorders (19). In this regard, an important step along the road comes in the form of a recent study of neuroticism (100). In this study, the investigators conducted analyses of a linkage scan in extremely discordant and concordant sibling pairs selected from 34,580 British sibling pairs who completed a personality questionnaire. They performed a genome-wide scan for quantitative-trait loci (QTLs) that influence variation in neuroticism. The maximum LOD scores were found on chromosomes 1q (3.95), 4q (3.84), 7p (3.90), 12q (4.74), and 13q (3.81). The authors note that the locus on 1q is of particular interest because it is syntenic with that reported from QTL mapping of rodent emotionality, an animal model of neuroticism. Further scrutiny of genes in this region (e.g., *GPR88:* G protein–coupled receptor expressed in brain) may be relevant to social phobia.

3. Extraversion

Another personality trait that is of equal (or greater) relevance to social phobia is extraversion (19). Bienvenu and colleagues found that persons in the general population with social phobia or agoraphobia tended to be very low in extraversion (almost 1 standard deviation below average) (101). Studies in clinical and nonclinical (e.g., college-age student) samples similarly find that persons with anxiety disorders are low in extraversion or high on a conceptually and psychometrically related construct that combines aspects of neuroticism and introversion: harm avoidance (102,103). Relatives of probands with certain anxiety disorders (e.g., social phobia) show increased levels of harm avoidance compared to relatives of comparison subjects (10). Taken together, these observations suggest that the study of extraversion, as a complement to the study of neuroticism, is likely to be of considerable importance in our understanding of the genetics of social phobia and other phobic disorders.

Little work has been done looking at genetic aspects of extraversion. Most work in this area has been limited to investigating the relationship between the dopamine D4 receptor gene and harm avoidance (which, as mentioned above, combines aspects of neuroticism and intraversion) (104), or novelty-seeking [which itself shares variance with extraversion (105–108)]. Further genetic investigation of extraversion is, in our opinion, likely to be of considerable value for the understanding of susceptibility for social phobia and other anxiety disorders.

4. Behavioral Inhibition

It has been suggested that BI may represent an "intermediate phenotype" for panic and phobic anxiety disorders that may be more amenable to genetic dissection than the DSM diagnoses (24). Smoller and colleagues have been studying the genetic basis of BI, focusing on candidate loci implicated in murine models of BI-like behavior. In an initial study, they conducted family-based association analyses of BI using four genes derived from genetic studies of mouse models of BI (24). The sample included families of 72 children classified as inhibited by structured behavioral assessments. The investigators observed modest evidence of association ($p = 0.05$) between BI and the glutamic acid decarboxylase gene (65-kDA isoform) that encodes an enzyme involved in GABA synthesis.

More recently, these investigators examined a polymorphism at the corticotropin-releasing hormone (CRH) locus (109). They genotyped a marker tightly linked to the CRH locus in 85 families of children who underwent laboratory-based behavioral assessments of BI. Using family-based association analyses, they observed an inverse association between an allele of the CRH-linked locus and BI ($p = 0.015$). Among offspring of parents with panic disorder, this association was particularly marked ($p = 0.0009$). This work suggests that the CRH locus should be further scrutinized as a potential risk factor for GSP. Moreover, it further illustrates the potential utility of studying anxiety-related traits as an approach to identifying loci involved in GSP and related anxiety disorders.

III. CONCLUSIONS

Although still in its early stages as a subject of scientific scrutiny, the study of the genetics of social anxiety disorder has the potential to improve methods for early intervention, treatment, and/or prevention. Many strong functional candidate genes exist and should be further tested, and several exciting positional candidates have recently emerged from linkage studies that require finer localization and replication. The identification and confirmation of susceptibility genes for social phobia will benefit from techniques that scrutinize quantitative traits (e.g., shyness, low extraversion) that are part of the social phobia spectrum, and examine alternative categorical phenotypes that are seen as either narrow (e.g., selective mutism) or broad (e.g., phobic disorders) manifestations of the true underlying genotype. Such work will not only lead us closer to understanding the genetic underpinnings of social phobia but also give us a better appreciation of the sources of genes influence on complex traits that underlie many of the anxiety and phobic disorders.

REFERENCES

1. Mendlowicz MV, Stein MB. Quality of life in individuals with anxiety disorders. Am J Psychiatry 2000;157:669–682.
2. Chavira DA, Stein MB. Recent developments in child and adolescent social phobia. Curr Psychiatr Rep 2000;2:347–352.
3. Stein MB, Kean Y. Disability and quality of life in social phobia. Am J Psychiatry 2000;157:1606–1613.
4. Stein MB, McQuaid JR, Laffaye C, McCahill ME. Social phobia in the primary care medical setting. J Fam Pract 1999;48:514–519.
5. Katzelnick DJ, Kobak KA, DeLeire T, Henk HJ, Greist JH, Davidson JR, Schneier FR, Stein MB, Helstad CP. Impact of generalized social anxiety disorder in managed care. Am J Psychiatry 2001;158:1999–2007.
6. Hettema JM, Neale MC, Kendler KS. A review and meta-analysis of the genetic epidemiology of anxiety disorders. Am J Psychiatry 2001;158:1568–1578.
7. Stein MB, Jang KL, Livesley WJ. Heritability of social-anxiety related concerns and personality characteristics: a twin study. J Nerv Ment Dis 2002; 190:219–224.
8. Stein MB, Chartier MJ, Hazen AL, Kozak MV, Tancer ME, Lander S, Chubaty D, Furer P, Walker JR. A direct-interview family study of generalized social phobia. Am J Psychiatry 1998;155:90–97.
9. Wittchen H-U, Stein MB, Kessler RC. Social fears and social phobia in a community sample of adolescents and young adults: prevalence, risk factors and co-morbidity. Psychol Med 1999;29:309–323.
10. Stein MB, Chartier MJ, Lizak MV, Jang KL. Familial aggregation of anxiety-related quantitative traits in generalized social phobia: clues to understanding "disorder" heritability? Am J Med Genet (Neuropsychiatr Genet) 2001; 105:79–83.
11. Stein MB, Chavira DA, Jang KL. Bringing up bashful baby: developmental pathways to social phobia. Psychiatr Clin North Am 2001;24:661–675.
12. Daniels D, Plomin R. Origins of individual differences in infant shyness. Dev Psychol 1985;21:118–121.
13. Rowe DC, Plomin R. Temperament in early childhood. J Personality Assess 1977;41:150–156.
14. Warren SL, Schmitz S, Emde RN. Behavioral genetic analyses of self-reported anxiety at 7 years of age. J Am Acad Child Adolesc Psychiatry 1999;38:1403–1408.
15. Leary MR. A brief version of the Fear of Negative Evaluation Scale. Personality Soc Psychol Bull 1983;9:371–376.
16. Livesley WJ, Jang KL, Vernon PA. Phenotypic and genetic structure of traits delineating personality disorder. Arch Gen Psychiatry 1998;55:941–948.

17. Livesley WJ, Jackson D, Schroeder ML. Factorial structure of traits delineating personality disorders in clinical and general population samples. J Abnorm Psychol 1992;101:432–440

18. Samuels J, Eaton WW, Bienvenu OJ III, Brown CH, Costa PT Jr, Nestadt G. Prevalence and correlates of personality disorders in a community sample. Br J Psychiatry 2002;180:536–542.

19. Bienvenu OJ, Stein MB. Personality and anxiety disorders: a review. J Personality Disord 2003;17:139–151.

20. Kagan J, Arcus D, Snidman N, et al. Reactivity in Infants: a cross-national comparison. Dev Psychol 1994; 30:342–345.

21. Kagan J. Temperament and the reactions to unfamiliarity. Child Dev 1997; 68:139–143.

22. Robinson JL, Kagan J, Reznick JS, Corley RP. The heritability of inhibited and uninhibited behavior: a twin study. Dev Psychol 1992;28:1030–1037.

23. Fisher L, Kagan J, Reznick JS. Genetic etiology of behavioral inhibition among 2-year-old children. Infant Behav Dev 1994;17:405–412.

24. Smoller JW, Rosenbaum JF, Biederman J, et al. Genetic association analysis of behavioral inhibition using candidate loci from mouse models. Am J Med Genet (Neuropsychiatr Genet) 2001;105:226–235.

25. Schwartz CE, Wright CI, Shin LM, Kagan J, Rauch SL. Inhibited and uninhibited infants "grown up": adult amygdalar response to novelty. Science 2003;300:1952–1953.

26. Schwartz CE, Wright CI, Shin LM, Kagan J, Whalen PJ, McMullin KG, Rauch SL. Differential amygdalar response to novel versus newly familiar neutral faces: a functional MRI probe developed for studying inhibited temperament. Biol Psychiatry 2003;53:854–862.

27. Torgersen S. Genetic factors in anxiety disorders. Arch Gen Psychiatry 1983; 40:1085–1089.

28. Kendler KS, Neale MC, Kessler RC, Heath AC, Eaves LJ. The genetic epidemiology of phobias in women: the interrelationship of agoraphobia, social phobia, situational phobia, and simple phobia. Arch Gen Psychiatry 1992; 49:273–281.

29. Skre I, Onstad S, Torgesen S, Lygren S, Kringlen E. A twin study of DSM-III-R anxiety disorders. Acta Psychiatr Scand 1993;88:85–92.

30. Kendler KS, Karkowski LM, Prescott CA. Fears and phobias: reliability and heritability. Psychol Med 1999;29:539–553.

31. Kendler KS, Myers J, Prescott CA, Neale MC. The genetic epidemiology of irrational fears and phobias in men. Arch Gen Psychiatry 2001;58:257–265.

32. Nelson EC, Grant JD, Bucholz KK, Glowinski A, Madden PAF, Reich W, Heath AC. Social phobia in a population-based female adolescent twin sample: co-morbidity and associated suicide-related symptoms. Psychol Med 2000;30:797–804.

33. Cooper PJ, Eke M. Childhood shyness and maternal social phobia: a community study. Br J Psychiatry 1999;174:439–443.

34. Biederman J, Hirshfeld-Becker DR, Rosenbaum JF, Hérot C, Friedman D, Snidman N, Kagan J, Faraone SV. Further evidence of association between behavioral inhibition and social anxiety in children. Am J Psychiatry 2001; 158:1673–1679.

35. Hayward C, Killen JD, Kraemer HC, Taylor CB. Linking self-reported childhood behavioral inhibition to adolescent social phobia. Acad Child Adolesc Psychiatry 1998;37:1308–1316.

36. Van Ameringen M, Mancini C, Oakman JM. The relationship of behavioral inhibition and shyness to anxiety disorder. J Nerv Ment Dis 1998;186:425–431.

37. Schwartz CE, Snidman N, Kagan J. Adolescent social anxiety as an outcome of inhibited temperament in childhood. J Am Acad Child Adolesc Psychiatry 1999;38:1008–1015.

38. Rosenbaum JF, Biederman J, Bolduc EA, Hirshfeld DR, Faraone SV, Kagan J. Comorbidity of parental anxiety disorders as risk for childhood-onset anxiety in inhibited children. Am J Psychiatry 1992;149:475–481.

39. Hirshfeld DR, Rosenbaum JF, Biederman J, Bolduc EA, Faraone SV, Snidman N, Reznick JS, Kagan J. Stable behavioral inhibition and its association with anxiety disorder. J Am Acad Child Adolesc Psychiatry 1992; 31:103–111.

40. Martin C, Cabrol S, Bouvard MP, Lepine JP, Mouren-Siméoni MC. Anxiety and depressive disorders in fathers and mothers of anxious school-refusing children. J Am Acad Child Adolesc Psychiatry 1999;38:916–922.

41. Mannuzza S, Schneier FR, Chapman TF, Liebowitz MR, Klein DF, Fyer AJ. Generalized social phobia. reliability and validity. Arch Gen Psychiatry 1995; 52:230–237.

42. Mancini C, Van Ameringen M, Szatmari M, Fugere P, Boyle M. A high-risk pilot study of the children of adults with social phobia. J Am Acad Child Adolesc Psychiatry 1996;35:1511–1517.

43. Fyer AJ, Mannuzza S, Chapman TF, Martin LY, Klein DF. Specificity in familial aggregation of phobic disorders. Arch Gen Psychiatry 1995;52:564–573.

44. Krueger RF. The structure of common mental disorders. Arch Gen Psychiatry 1999;56:921–926.

45. Vollebergh WAM, Iedema J, Bijl RV, de Graaf R, Smit F, Ormel J. The structure and stability of common mental disorders: The NEMESIS study. Arch Gen Psychiatry 2001;58:597–603.

46. Bailey A, Phillips W, Rutter M. Autism: towards an integration of clinical, genetic, neuropsychological and neurobiological perspectives. J Child Psychol Psychiatry 1996;37:89–126.

47. Rapin I, Katzman R. Neurobiology of autism. Ann Neurol 1998;43:7–14.

48. Smalley SL, McCracken J, Tanguay P. Autism, affective disorders, and social phobia. Am J Med Genet 1995;60:19–26.

49. Piven J, Palmer P. Psychiatric disorder and the broad autism phenotype: Evidence from a family study of multiple-incidence autism families. Am J Psychiatry 1999;156:557–563.

50. Autism Consortium. A full genome screen for autism with evidence for linkage to a region on chromosome 7q. Hum Mol Genet 1998;7:571–578.

51. Smith M, Filipek PA, Wu C, Bocian M, Hakim S, Modahl C, Spence MA. Analysis of a 1-Megabase deletion in 15q22-q23 in an autistic patient: identification of candidate genes for autism and of homologous DNA segments in 15q22-q23 and 15q11-q13. Am J Med Genet 2000;96:765–770.

52. Alarcon M, Cantor RM, Liu J, Gilliam TC, Geschwind DH. Evidence for a language quantitative trait locus on chromosome 7q in multiplex autism families. Am J Hum Genet 2002;70:60–71.

53. Jamain S, Quach H, Betancur C, Rastam M, Colineaux C, Gillberg IC, Soderstrom H, Giros B, Leboyer M, Gillberg C, Bourgeron T. Mutations of the X-linked genes encoding neuroligins NLGN3 and NLGN4 are associated with autism. Nat Genet 2003;34:27–29.

54. Buxbaum JD, Silverman JM, Smith CJ, Greenberg DA, Kilifarski M, Reichert J, Cook EH Jr, Fang Y, Song CY, Vitale R. Association between a GABRB3 polymorphism and autism. Mol Psychiatry 2002;7:311–316.

55. Kim SJ, Young LJ, Gonen D, Veenstra-VanderWeele J, Courchesne R, Courchesne E, Lord C, Leventhal BL, Cook EH Jr, Insel TR. Transmission disequilibrium testing of arginine vasopressin receptor 1A (AVPR1A) polymorphisms in autism. Mol Psychiatry 2002;7:503–507.

56. Constantino JN, Todd RD. Genetic structure of reciprocal social behavior. Am J Psychiatry 2000;157:2043–2045.

57. Constantino JN, Todd RD. Autistic traits in the general population: a twin study. Arch Gen Psychiatry 2003;60:524–530.

58. Bergman RL, Piacentini J, McCracken JT. Prevalence and description of selective mutism in a school-based sample. J Am Acad Child Adolesc Psychiatry 2002;41:938–946.

59. Kopp S, Gillberg C. Selective mutism: a population-based study: a research note. J Child Psychol Psychiatry 1997;38:257–262.

60. Dow SP, Sonies BC, Scheib D, Moss SE, Leonard HL. Practical guidelines for the assessment and treatment of selective mutism. J Am Acad Child Adolesc Psychiatry 1995;34:836–846.

61. Dummit ESI, Klein RG, Tancer NK, Asche B, Martin J, Fairbank JA. Systematic assessment of 50 children with selective mutism. J Am Acad Child Adolesc Psychiatry 1997;36:653–660.

62. Anstendig KD. Is selective mutism an anxiety disorder? Rethinking its DSM-IV classification. J Anxiety Disord 1999;13:417–434.

63. Black B, Uhde TW. Elective mutism as a variant of social phobia. J Am Acad Child Adolesc Psychiatry 1990;31:1090–1094.

64. Kristensen H, Torgersen S. MCMI-II personality traits and symptom traits in parents of children with selective mutism: a case-control study. J Abnorm Psychol 2001;110:648–652.

65. Gray RM, Jordan CM, Ziegler RS, Livingston RB. Two sets of twins with selective mutism: Neuropsychological findings. Child Neuropsychol 2002; 8:41–51.

66. Hagerman RJ, Hills J, Scharfenaker S, Lewis H. Fragile X syndrome and selective mutism. Am J Med Genet 1999;83:313–317.
67. Astendig KD. Is selective mutism an anxiety disorder? Rethinking its DSM-IV classification. J Anxiety Disord 1999;13:417–434.
68. Stein MB, Chartier MJ, Kozak MV, Hazen AL, King N, Kennedy JL. Genetic linkage to the serotonin transporter and 5HT2A receptor excluded in generalized social phobia. Psychiatr Res 1998;81:283–291.
69. Kennedy JL, Neves-Pereira M, King N, Lizak MV, Basile VS, Chartier MJ, Stein MB. Dopamine system genes not linked to social phobia. Psychiatr Genet 2001;11:213–217.
70. Colhoun HM, McKeigue PM, Smith GD. Problems of reporting genetic associations with complex outcomes. Lancet 2003;361:865–872.
71. Risch NJ. Searching for genetic determinants in the new millenium. Nature 2000;405:847–856.
72. Gelernter J, Bonvicini KA, Page G, Woods SW, Goddard AW, Kruger S, Pauls DL, Goodson S. Linkage genome scan for loci predisposing to panic disorder or agoraphobia. Am J Med Genet (Neuropsychiatr Genet) 2001; 105:548–557.
73. Gelernter J, Page GP, Bonvicini K, Woods SW, Pauls DL, Kruger S. A chromosome 14 risk locus for simple phobia: results from a genomewide linkage scan. Mol Psychiatry 2003;8:71–82.
74. Gelernter J, Page GP, Stein MB, Woods SW. Genomewide linkage scan for loci predisposing to social phobia: Evidence for a chromosome 16 risk locus. Am J Psychiatry 2004;161:59–66.
75. Gudbjartsson DF, Jonasson K, Frigge ML, Kong A. Allegro, a new computer program for multipoint linkage analysis. Nat Genet 2000;25:12–13.
76. Lander E, Kruglyak L. Genetic dissection of complex traits: guidelines for interpreting and reporting linkage results. Nat Genet 1995;11:241–247.
77. Gratacòs M, Nadal M, Martín-Santos R, Pujana MA, Gago J, Peral B, Armengol L, Ponsa I, Miró R, Bulbena A, Estivill X. A polymorphic genomic duplication on human chromosome 15 is a susceptibility factor for panic and phobic disorders. Cell 2001;106:367–379.
78. Collier DA. FISH, flexible joints and panic: are anxiety disorders really expressions of instability in the human genome? Br J Psychiatry 2002;181:457–459.
79. Tabiner M, Youings S, Dennis N, Baldwin D, Buis C, Mayers A, Jacobs PA, Crolla JA. Failure to find DUP25 in patients with anxiety disorders, in control individuals, or in previously reported positive control cell lines. Am J Hum Genet 2003;72:535–538.
80. Weiland Y, Kraus J, Speicher MR. A multicolor FISH assay does not detect DUP25 in control individuals or in reported positive control cells. Am J Hum Genet 2003;72:1349–1352.
81. Thorgeirsson TE, Oskarsson H, Desnica N, Kostic JP, Stefansson JG, Kolbeinsson H, Lindal E, Gagunashvili N, Frigge ML, Kong A, Stefansson K,

Gulcher JR. Anxiety with panic disorder linked to chromosome 9q in Iceland. Am J Hum Genet 2003;72:1221–1230.

82. Rende R, Warner V, Wickramaratne P, Weissman MM. Sibling aggregation for psychiatric disorders in offspring at high and low risk for depression: 10-year follow-up. Psychol Med 1999;29:1291–1298.

83. Biederman J, Faraone SV, Hirshfeld-Becker DR, Friedman D, Robin JA, Rosenbaum JF. Patterns of psychopathology and dysfunction in high-risk children of parents with panic disorder and major depression. Am J Psychiatry 2001;158:49–57.

84. Klein DN, Lewinsohn PM, Rohde P, Seeley JR, Shankman SA. Family study of co-morbidity between major depressive disorder and anxiety disorders. Psychol Med 2003;33:703–714.

85. Hudson JI, Mangweth B, Pope HG Jr, De Col C, Hausmann A, Gutweniger S, Laird NM, Biebl W, Tsuang MT. Family study of affective spectrum disorder. Arch Gen Psychiatry 2003;60:170–177.

86. Arbelle S, Benjamin J, Golin M, Kremer I, Belmaker RH, Ebstein RP. Relation of shyness in grade school children to the genotype for the long form of the serotonin transporter promoter region polymorphism. Am J Psychiatry 2003;160:671–676.

87. Lesch K-P, Bengel D, Heils A, Sabol SA, Greenberg BD, Petri S, Benjamin J, Müller CR, Hamer DH, Murphy DL. Association of anxiety-related traits with a polymorphism in the serotonin transporter gene regulatory region. Science 1996;274:1527–1531.

88. Mazzanti CM, Lappalainen J, Long JC, Bengel D, Naukkarinen H, Eggert M, Virkkunen M, Linnoila M, Goldman D. Role of the serotonin transporter promoter polymorphism in anxiety-related traits. Arch Gen Psychiatry 1998; 55:936–940.

89. Katsuragi S, Kunugi H, Sano A, Tsutsumi T, Isogawa K, Nanko S, Akiyoshi J. Association between serotonin transporter gene polymorphism and anxiety-related traits. Biol Psychiatry 1999;45:368–370.

90. Greenberg BD, Li Q, Lucas FR, Hu S, Sirota LA, Benjamin J, Lesch K-P, Hamer DH, Murphy DL. Association between the serotonin transporter promoter polymorphism and personality traits in a primarily female population sample. Am J Med Genet (Neuropsychiatr Genet) 2000;96:202–216.

91. Jorm AF, Prior M, Sanson A, Smart D, Zhang Y, Easteal S. Association of a functional polymorphism of the serotonin transporter gene with anxiety-related temperament and behavior problems in children: a longitudinal study from infancy to the mid-teens. Mol Psychiatry 2000;5:542–547.

92. Osher Y, Hamer DH, Benjamin J. Association and linkage of anxiety-related traits with a functional polymorphism of the serotonin transporter gene regulatory region in Israeli sibling pairs. Mol Psychiatry 2000;5:216–219.

93. Chavira DA, Stein MB, Malcarne VL. Scrutinizing the relationship between shyness and social phobia. J Anxiety Disord 2002;16:585–598.

94. Heiser NA, Turner SM, Beidel DC. Shyness: relationship to social phobia and other psychiatric disorders. Behav Res Ther 2003;41:209–221.

95. Hirschfeld RM, Klerman GL, Lavori P, Keller MB, Griffith P, Coryell W. Premorbid personality assesssments of first onset of major depression. Arch Gen Psychiatry 1989;46:345–350.

96. Andrews G. Comorbidity and the general neurotic syndrome. Br J Psychiatry 1996;30:76–84.

97. Bienvenu OJ, Brown C, Samuels JF, et al. Normal personality traits and comorbidity among phobic, panic, and major depressive disorders. Psychiatry Res 2001;102:73–85.

98. Ormel J, Oldehinkel AJ, Brilman E. The interplay and etiological continuity of neuroticism, difficulties, and life events in the etiology of major and sub-syndromal, first and recurrent depressive episodes in later life. Am J Psychiatry 2001;158:885–891.

99. Andrews G, Slade T, Issakidis C. Deconstructing current comorbidity: data from the Australian National Survey of Mental Health and Well-Being. Br J Psychiatry 2002;181:306–314.

100. Fullerton J, Cubin M, Tiwari H, Wang C, Bomhra A, Davidson S, Miller S, Fairburn C, Goodwin G, Neale MC, Fiddy S, Mott R, Allison DB, Flint J. Linkage analysis of extremely discordant and concordant sibling pairs identifies quantitative-trait loci that influence variation in the human personality trait neuroticism. Am J Hum Genet 2003;72:879–890.

101. Bienvenu OJ, Nestadt G, Samuels JF, Howard WT, Costa PT Jr, Eaton WW. Phobic, panic, and major depressive disorders and the five-factor model of personality. J Nerv Ment Dis 2001;189:154–161.

102. Trull TJ, Sher KJ. Relationship between the five-factor model of personality and axis I disorders in a non-clinical sample. J Abnorm Psychol 1994;103:350–360.

103. Samuels J, Nestadt G, Bienvenu OJ, Costa PT Jr, Riddle MA, Liang K-Y, Hoehn-Saric R, Grados M, Cullen BA. Personality disorders and normal personality dimensions in obsessive-compulsive disorder. Br J Psychiatry 2000; 177:457–462.

104. Zohar AH, Dina C, Rosolio N, Osher Y, Gritsenko I, Bachner-Melman R, Benjamin J, Belmaker RH, Ebstein RP. Tridimensional personality questionnaire trait of harm avoidance (anxiety proneness) is linked to a locus on chromosome 8p21. Am J Med Genet 2003;117B:66–69.

105. Livesley WJ, Jang KL. Toward an empirically based classification of personality disorder. J Personality Disord 1998;14:137–151.

106. Costa PT, Jr., McCrae RR. NEO PI-R Professional Manual. Odessa, FL: Psychological Assessment Resources, 1992.

107. Ebstein RP, Novick O, Umansky R, Priel B, Osher Y, Blaine D, Bennett ER, Nemanov L, Katz M, Belmaker RH. Dopamine D4 receptor (DRD4) exon III polymorphism associated with the human personality trait of novelty seeking. Nat Genet 1996;12:78–80.

108. Jonsson EG, Ivo R, Gustavsson JP, Geijer T, Forslund K, Mattila-Evenden M, Rylander G, Cichon S, Propping P, Bergman H, Asberg M, Nothen MM. No association between dopamine D4 receptor gene variants and novelty seeking. Mol Psychiatry 2002;7:18–20.

109. Smoller JW, Rosenbaum JF, Biederman J, Kennedy J, Dai D, Racette S, Laird N, Kagan J, Snidman N, Hirshfeld-Becker DR, Tsuang MT, Sklar PB, Slaugenhaupt SA. Association of a genetic marker at the corticotropin re-leasing hormone locus with behavioral inhibition. Biol Psychiatry 2003;54: 1376–1381.

14

Brain Imaging Studies in Social Anxiety Disorder

Mats Fredrikson and Tomas Furmark
Uppsala University,
Uppsala, Sweden

It is possible and perhaps even likely that most psychiatric conditions are disorders of the brain. Although psychiatric illness often involves negative affect and emotional dysregulation, this is particularly true for anxiety disorders such as social phobia, also known as social anxiety disorder (SAD). In recent years there have been great advances in our understanding of the neurobiological underpinnings of human fear and anxiety. Brain imaging techniques, in particular, have provided unique tools with which to explore neuronal activity in the living human brain during emotionally activated states. In this chapter, we review neuroimaging research pertaining to SAD, focusing mainly on functional imaging studies. The review is preceded by a brief description of the functional neuroanatomy of anxiety as well as common neuroimaging techniques and paradigms used in this field.

I. THE NEURAL BASIS OF FEAR AND ANXIETY

The neurocircuitry of emotion has been described as involving multiple subcortical and cortical areas (1). New leads for understanding this neuro-circuitry have come from cognitive, basic, and affective neuroscience. The

215

brain areas known to correlate with negative emotional behavior in normal healthy individuals may serve as a basis for theoretical predictions of areas involved in social anxiety. Data from animals and human patients with brain lesions as well as functional neuroimaging studies suggest that the amygdala has a central role in mediating and coordinating fearful behaviors. It appears to act as a detector of threat, particularly engaged in attention and vigilance in aversive or ambiguous circumstances (2). The amygdala is also thought to have an important role in the neurocircuitry of social perception and judgment (3), which may be particularly relevant for SAD (4). Further, the amygdala has been consistently implicated in studies of fear conditioning— i.e., the formation of associative fear memories (5). Conditioning paradigms may, in turn, be relevant for understanding the etiology of SAD and other phobic disorders.

Emotional processes also tax other structures in the medial temporal lobe (MTL). For instance, the hippocampus probably assists the amygdala in alerting the individual to threatening stimulation, possibly specializing in contextual or cognitive evaluation of the aversive situation. Also, the surrounding entorhinal, perirhinal, and parahippocampal cortices form an important transit area for sensory and/or memory information into the subcortical MTL structures (6). Besides the MTL, the dorsolateral, ventromedial, and orbitofrontal cortices along with the anterior and posterior (retrosplenial) cingulate, insula, and visual areas have been implicated as involved in emotion and emotional regulation (1,7,8).

Based on the extensive neurobiological corpus of data, the MTL region, particularly the amygdala, would be a prime locus of interest in neuroimaging activation studies of individuals with SAD. With regard to neurotransmitter functioning, it is well documented that treatment regimens that target monoaminergic functions have beneficial effects on mood and anxiety (9). Serotonin in particular has been implicated in animal and human models of fear and anxiety (10). Hence, empirical and theoretical predictions would suggest that SAD is characterized by dysfunction in the serotonergic, dopaminergic, or noradrenergic transmitter systems.

II. BRAIN IMAGING TECHNIQUES AND PARADIGMS

Brain imaging studies use powerful techniques to visualize and quantify brain function and structure. In positron emission tomography (PET), radioactive tracers are utilized to measure regional cerebral blood flow (rCBF) (by means of oxygen 15–labeled water), glucose metabolism [with fluorine-18–labeled fluorodeoxyglucose (FDG)], and also neuroreceptor and transmitter characteristics in the brain. Examples of such PET tracers are [11C]-WAY 100635 to characterize serotonin-1A receptor density and affinity,

[11C]-alpha-methyl-L-tryptophan, and [11C]-5-hydroxy-L-tryptophan to characterize presynaptic serotonin synthesis, and [11C]-DASB to monitor reuptake functions within the serotonergic system. Comparable tracers for other neurotransmitter systems exist. Single-photon-emission tomography (SPECT) is technically different but conceptually similar to PET, also employing tracers that can measure cerebral blood flow [e.g., 99m-technetium-hexamethylpropylene amine oxime (TcHMPAO)] and glucose metabolism [(18F)-FDG]. Functional magnetic resonance imaging (fMRI) measures blood oxygenation level–dependent (BOLD) signal changes in the brain and is perhaps the most commonly used imaging technique in emotional activation studies today.

PET, SPECT, and fMRI can all be used to generate maps that reflect regional brain activity during rest and in response to challenges. They provide measures of subcortical as well as cortical alterations. Other imaging techniques can also generate functional brain maps, although they are more limited to cortical than subcortical areas. These techniques include xenon-133 inhalation, quantitative electroencephalography (EEG), and magneto-encephalography (MEG). Other than functional neuroimaging, there are methods that permit the measurement of structural and neurochemical characteristics of the brain. These include, for example, computed tomography (CT) and structural MRI, which enables volume calculations. Functional magnetic spectroscopy (MRS) can be used to measure compounds like N-acetylaspartate (NAA), held to be a marker of neuronal density or unspecific functional neural activity (11). In sum, imaging tools may reveal both structure and function and provide measures of electrical, magnetic, and metabolic changes, neuroreceptors and neurotransmitters and brain blood flow. Even though most imaging methods yield maps of brain activity, they vary markedly (e.g., with regard to spatial and temporal resolution). Each method has its own set of benefits and drawbacks, which may affect the quality of data obtained by the investigator.

Functional imaging can be used to study brain activity—e.g., during cognitive activation, emotional experiences, and perception (12). Particularly, PET- and fMRI-based measurements of blood flow alterations, expressed as rCBF or BOLD signal changes, in response to task activation have been used to reveal distributed neural representations of emotional processes (13) and social cognition (3). Activation studies frequently use subtractive designs in which a baseline condition (or reference task) is subtracted from the experimental condition of interest (the target task), resulting in regionally specific differences in brain activity corresponding to functionally specialized areas. For example, in studies of anxiety disorders, induction of symptomatic anxiety states could be contrasted with a control condition, presumably revealing brain regions that are specifically engaged in the emotional response. In SAD and other anxiety disorders, such symptom provocation studies have been complemented by studies of various cognitive or perceptual processes and by simple neutral state paradigms where subjects are studied in a nominal resting state only (12). Surprisingly, only a small number of imaging studies have evaluated how anxiolytic treatments affect the manipulated states. In addition to subtractive analyses, event-related approaches as well as various forms of correlative and connectivity analyses exist, allowing more complex research designs to be used in neuroimaging (13).

III. BRAIN IMAGING IN SOCIAL ANXIETY DISORDER

The first wave of imaging studies in anxiety disorders emerged in the early 1980s, starting with pioneering PET studies of panic disorder conducted by Reiman and colleagues (14). The first imaging reports on social phobia appeared about a decade later. To date, we have located a total of 16 published, peer-reviewed imaging reports on SAD, with one reporting on brain structure (MRI), two on unspecific markers of neural activity (MRS), three on receptor and transmitter characteristics (PET), while 10 functional imaging studies report on measures of rCBF (5), BOLD (4), and EEG (1) during rest or in response to challenges and treatments. The vast majority of these reports have been published within the last 5 years.

A. Structural Neuroimaging in Social Anxiety Disorder

In the first published brain imaging study in SAD, Potts and co-workers (15) used structural MRI to evaluate differences in basal ganglia volumes between 22 patients with SAD and an equal number of healthy control subjects. The caudate and putamen were selected specifically for volume calculations, on the basis of previous studies implicating dopamine and the basal ganglia in the pathophysiology of SAD. No statistically significant differences between phobics and controls were obtained. The authors did note a greater age-related reduction in putamen volumes in patients with SAD relative to controls, but that did not correlate with symptom severity (15).

B. Magnetic Resonance Spectroscopy in Social Anxiety Disorder

Magnetic resonance spectroscopy was used by Davidson and colleagues (16) to evaluate CNS metabolic activity in a group of 20 individuals with SAD and an equally large healthy control group. Results showed that choline, creatine and N-acetylaspartate (NAA) signal-to-noise ratios were lower in SAD patients than controls in the thalamus and caudate nucleus, and in addition NAA ratios were lower also in white matter. Results were attributed to altered metabolic activity and possibly a lower number of neurons or neural activity in SAD. In a follow-up study, the investigators sought to replicate and extend their original findings using enhanced methodology (17). Results pointed to differences between social phobics and healthy controls in cortical and subcortical gray matter, while between-group differences were minimal for white matter. The authors concede, however, that the significance and specificity of the findings to SAD remain unclear.

C. Imaging Neurotransmitter Systems in Social Anxiety Disorder

There have been a few attempts to image neurotransmitter systems in SAD. Because neurobiological research indicates that the dopamine and serotonin systems could be compromised in SAD (10), these two systems have been of prime interest.

1. The Dopaminergic System

Tiihonen and co-workers reported data from a SPECT study in which it was found that the density of the striatal dopamine reuptake site was markedly lower in patients with SAD than in age- and gender-matched comparison subjects (18). Significant correlations between severity of illness or duration of symptoms and dopamine reuptake density were not observed. The authors argued that their findings of lower dopamine reuptake site density probably reflect a smaller number of dopaminergic synapses and neurons in the basal ganglia of patients with SAD. This in agreement with observation in Parkinson's disease, which is associated with an increased rate of SAD (10).

In another SPECT study focusing on dopaminergic functioning in SAD, Schneier and co-workers reported that dopamine D_2 receptor binding was significantly lower in subjects with social phobia than in comparison subjects (19). The authors also noted a trend toward a negative correlation of binding potential with Liebowitz social anxiety (LSAS) scores within the SAD group. Thus, two independent imaging studies point to an altered dopamine system activity in SAD.

2. The Serotonergic System

The imaging of serotonergic functions in SAD has only recently begun. In a PET study based on the radiotracer [11C](+)-McN 5652, Kent and colleagues (20) studied the occupancy of the serotonin reuptake transporter resulting from treatment with the selective serotonin reuptake inhibitor (SSRI) paroxetine in 5 patients with SAD. After 3 to 6 months of continuous treatment, occupancy of the serotonin reuptake transporter was high in all patients and in all regions measured. There have also been initial attempts to image presynaptic serotonin processes in SAD by means of PET and the [11C]-5-hydroxy-L-tryptophan tracer (21). Preliminary evaluations indicate a lower uptake of the tracer mainly in temporal lobe regions in patients versus controls, which could correspond to a regionally specific suppressed serotonin synthesis in SAD.

Future studies of this kind might help to unravel the mechanisms whereby serotonin modulates anxiety and how serotonergic drugs act. It would be interesting to learn whether serotonin synthesis rate, serotonergic receptor density or affinity, or serotonin reuptake processes are affected by treatments—e.g., with SSRIs or even cognitive-behavioral therapy. It would also be interesting to find out if individuals with SAD differ from normal, healthy controls with regard to serotonin neurotransmitter, receptor, and reuptake mechanisms.

D. Functional Neuroimaging in Social Anxiety Disorder: Activation Studies

1. Face Perception Studies

Face perception paradigms may be used to assess brain responsivity to threat-relevant social stimuli. Several imaging studies have demonstrated that the amygdala is activated when normal, healthy volunteers passively view slides of faces with fearful expressions as compared with neutral or happy facial expression (12). The question arises whether patients with SAD differ from nonanxious controls with regard to amygdalar responsivity to facial stimuli.

In the first published activation study in SAD, Birbaumer and co-workers (22) used fMRI to determine activation of the amygdala in 7 male social phobics and 5 male healthy controls while they were exposed to slides of neutral faces. The authors used a region-of-interest approach focusing on the amygdala. Enhanced bilateral amygdalar activation in response to faces as compared to a fixation cross was observed in social phobics when compared to the normal, healthy controls. This finding was conceptually replicated by Veit et al. (23), who reported activation of the right amygdala in patients with SAD in response to neutral faces as compared to a fixation point. This was observed during the habituation phase in a fear conditioning paradigm. In addition, neural activity increased bilaterally in the orbito-frontal, dorsomedial prefrontal, and left inferior frontal cortices. These data suggest that amygdalar activity is exaggerated in SAD patients even when presumably neutral social cues are evaluated.

Recently, Stein and co-workers (24) performed an elegant fMRI-study of brain responsivity to disorder salient and nonsalient stimuli in individuals with generalized SAD. Subjects were exposed to harsh (angry, fearful, and contemptuous) as well as accepting (happy) facial emotional expressions while BOLD signal changes were measured. Collectively, harsh faces induced relatively increased neural activity in SAD patients compared to controls in the left amygdala, the rhinal and parahippocampal cortical regions, and also in frontal cortical territories bilaterally. This effect was mainly driven by robust BOLD signal changes when comparing contemptuous with happy faces and angry with happy faces, whereas the fearful versus happy comparison remained insignificant. Stein and colleagues (24) suggested that an enhanced amygdala responding to danger signals could be a feature shared by a number of anxiety disorders, while the selectivity of response to particular danger stimuli could be what differentiates them. One obvious hypothesis is that nature/nurture interactions determine what is salient for the amygdala, and that an easily triggered amygdala could be a vulnerability factor perhaps associated with comorbidity with other anxiety disorders.

2. Fear Conditioning Studies

In experimental fear conditioning, the emotional impact of a stimulus is altered—i.e., it is transformed into a conditioned stimulus capable of eliciting fear reactions after pairings with aversive unconditioned stimuli such as electric shocks. Fear conditioning is one possible etiological mechanism through which SAD could evolve. For instance, making a mistake or an unfavorable impression in a social situation, as when talking in class (situation becoming the conditioned stimuli), might result in the individual being ridiculed, laughed at, or exposed to hostility from others (the unconditioned stimuli). A social situation could thereby acquire the potential to elicit fear or anxiety reactions (a conditioned response) in the future. As previously outlined, numerous animal studies support a crucial role for the amygdala in the expression and acquisition of such associative fear memories (5,6). Lesion and neuroimaging studies have supported the theory that the amygdala is involved in fear conditioning processes in humans as well (2,25,26).

In view of this, it is interesting that Schneider and co-workers (27) noted that patients with SAD had an increased activation, and a healthy comparison group decreased activation, in the amygdala and the hippocampus when presented with neutral faces that had been previously paired with an aversive odor stimulus. This raises the possibility that patients with SAD have an altered threshold for amygdalar responses to affective stimuli and possibly for fear conditionability. A subsequent report could not demonstrate evidence for an enhanced fear conditionability in generalized social phobics as compared to controls (28). However, enhanced unconditioned stimulus expectancy and a delayed extinction of conditioned autonomic responses were observed in the SAD group. The authors concluded that subjects with generalized SAD may be more prone to associate neutral social cues with aversive outcomes and also that delayed extinction may be related to the maintenance of social anxiety (28). An easily aroused subcortical emotional network, a specifically enhanced capability for fear conditioning, or both may characterize SAD. However, a recent fMRI study failed to demonstrate increased amygdalar activation during the acquisition of conditioned aversive reactions in subjects with SAD, although altered neural responding in widespread cortical areas was observed (23).

3. Anxiety Provocation Studies

a.   Public Speaking Situational Anxiety.   Even though studies of face perception and experimental fear conditioning have yielded interesting results in SAD, the ecological validity of such studies could be questioned. For instance, it could be argued that facial stimuli are not truly phobogenic in SAD, or at least not anxiety-provoking in the way snakes or spiders are in individuals with animal phobias. Also, laboratory fear conditioning studies do not resemble naturalistic situations in which associative fear memories can be formed and recalled. The cardinal symptom in social phobia is anxiety in situations in which scrutiny by others is likely and in which embarrassment and humiliation are possible outcomes. Thus, symptom provocation studies in which the dreaded and avoided emotion is produced would be likely to reveal neural underpinnings of the core symptomatic emotional experience.

In the first published imaging study of symptom provocation in SAD, Tillfors and co-workers (29) used PET and oxygen 15–labeled water to measure rCBF in 18 subjects with DSM-IV–defined social phobia and a nonfearful comparison group while they were speaking in presence of an audience and in private. Heart rate and subjective anxiety ratings confirmed a more profound public speaking distress reaction in SAD patients than in healthy controls. This was associated with an enhanced rCBF in the right amygdaloid complex in the social phobics relative to the comparison subjects (Fig. 1). There was a seemingly linear relationship between ratings of fear and increased activity in the right but not in the left amygdala in individuals with SAD.

Brain responsivity in going from private to public speaking differed between SAD patients and controls also in widespread cortical areas. In the orbitofrontal and insular cortices as well as in the temporal pole, rCBF diminished somewhat in the social phobics while it increased in the comparison subjects. In the parietal and secondary visual cortices, neural activity increased less in SAD than in comparison subjects. Furthermore, rCBF increased in the comparison but not the SAD group in the perirhinal and retrosplenial cortices. It is conceivable that pathways involving the amygdala

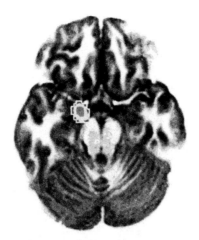

FIGURE 1 Increased normalized relative rCBF in the amygdaloid complex in 18 social phobics as compared to 6 controls during public versus private speaking.

or limbic structures, activated in SAD subjects during anxiety provocation, may elicit rapid emotional responses. Simultaneously, the failure to activate cortical areas of importance for emotional appraisal could indicate that cognitive evaluative or self-regulatory processes may be compromised in patients with SAD when they are in an anxious state (3,29). Thus, during symptom provocation, there seems to be a fear-related shift from cortical to subcortical processing in subjects with SAD, suggesting that a phylogenetically old danger recognition system dominates the influence on behavior.

    b. Anticipatory Social Anxiety. In a follow-up report, Tillfors and co-workers (30) also studied the effect of anticipatory social anxiety on neural activity. This was performed by evaluating rCBF during the private-speaking control condition in social phobics who performed their private speech before their public performance, compared with those who did the reverse. Presumably, worry or anticipatory anxiety is higher in the former group because of the forthcoming public speech. Statistical techniques were used to exclude the possibility of changes in outcome measures being related to time effects. The statistical evaluation confirmed that subjective anxiety ratings and heart rate were increased in the anticipation group relative to the comparison group. This was accompanied by enhanced cerebral blood flow in the left temporal lobe, including the amygdaloid-hippocampal region and also the right dorsolateral prefrontal cortex (Fig. 2).

    Generally, the anxiety related rCBF alterations in the amygdala and MTL structures are consistent with studies identifying the amygdala as

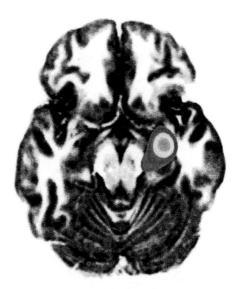

FIGURE 2 Enhanced normalized relative rCBF in the left amygdaloid-hippocampal region in social phobics speaking alone before (i.e., the anticipation group) compared to after (i.e., the comparison group) speaking in public.

important for perception and production of negative affect (2,26,31), including social anxiety (30) and dispositional pessimism (32). The prefrontal cortex has been suggested to participate in the conscious experience of emotions (33). Because anticipatory anxiety is characterized by worry but also activates memories of the past, it was speculated that the enhanced perfusion in the right dorsolateral prefrontal cortex could reflect affective working memory. This finding is similar to an increased right-sided prefrontal activation found at rest in patients with generalized anxiety disorder, a syndrome that is also characterized by worry and anticipatory anxiety (34).

Combining the results from the two studies on anxiety induction with right amygdalar activation resulting from situationally induced anxiety symptoms (29) and left amygdalar activation resulting from worry induction (30) points to a functional segregation of the left and right amygdala. Some previous lesion and imaging studies suggest that cognitive processes are more left-lateralized, whereas right-lateralized activity is associated with pure emotive functions (35). Thus, the pattern of amygdalar activation may distinguish different types of anxiety. This notion is generally consistent with neuroimaging studies reporting that noncognitive processes, like implicit emotional memory recall, activate the right amygdala (36) whereas more cognitive processes, like explicit emotional memory recall, activate the left amygdala (35). Also, right amygdalar responses have been found to habituate faster than the responses in the left amygdala, and it has been suggested that the right amygdala is part of a dynamic emotional stimulus-detection system while the left one is involved in sustained stimulus evaluation (37).

In another imaging study of anticipatory social anxiety, Davidson and coworkers studied a group of patients with SAD and a healthy control group while they anticipated making a public speech. They recorded electroencephalograms (EEGs) from scalp locations as well as heart rate and blood pressure (38). As in the data presented by Tillfors et al. (30), anticipatory anxiety in social phobics was associated with a marked right-sided activation in the lateral prefrontal regions and also in the anterior temporal cortex. This pattern of activation is generally consistent with what Rauch and coworkers (39) found when they analyzed findings across three different anxiety disorders (obsessive compulsive disorder, simple phobia, and posttraumatic stress disorder). They reported right-sided activation in various territories of the prefrontal cortex when anxiety symptoms were provoked (39). The right-sided cortical activation is also consistent with theories of emotion and emotionality as being relatively right lateralized (40).

c. Treatment Effects on Social Anxiety. Very few neuroimaging activation studies have investigated the effects of treatment on brain activity. This is especially the case for psychological treatments such as cognitive-behavioral therapy. However, in a recent report, Furmark and co-workers (41) studied the effect of the SSRI citalopram and cognitive-behavioral group therapy on rCBF during symptom provocation in SAD. Subjects were scanned during an anxiety-provoking public speaking task before and after treatment. It was noted that both types of treatment were successful in alleviating social anxiety. Two-thirds of the patients were classified as responders after 9 weeks of either pharmacological or behavioral therapy. Results were compared with a waiting-list control group that remained unimproved after the 9-week period. The evaluation of rCBF changes showed that symptom improvement, regardless of treatment approach, was accompanied by a decreased neural response to public speaking in the MTL including the amygdala, hippocampus, and the surrounding cortical areas—i.e., the perirhinal, entorhinal, and parahippocampal cortices (Fig. 3). Interestingly, patients who exhibited the greatest decrease of activity in the amygdala and other subcortical regions were the most improved at follow-up a year later.

Thus, the SSRI and cognitive-behavioral therapy produced a similar pattern of change on rCBF. This could mean that effective pharmacological and psychological treatment acts by reducing neuronal activity in the MTL. Attenuation of neurons in the amygdala, in particular, may be crucial to

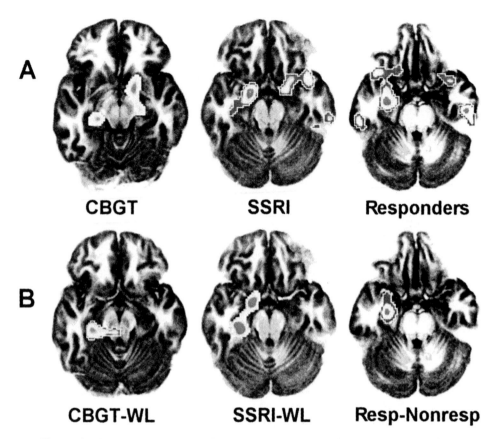

FIGURE 3 A. Lower normalized rCBF in response to an axiogenic public speaking task after as compared to before treatment. Images display decreases in rCBF for social phobics treated with cognitive-behavioral group therapy (CBGT; left), the selective serotonin reuptake inhibitor citalopram (SSRI; middle) and for responders regardless of treatment approach (right). Points of neural convergence were observed in the amygdala, hippocampus, and surrounding temporal cortical regions. B. Corresponding between-group differences in the amount of rCBF change with treatment. Images show a greater reduction in the neural response to public speaking in CBGT relative to waiting list (WL) subjects (left), SSRI relative to WL subjects (middle), and in responders relative to nonresponders (right).

obtaining robust and enduring therapeutic effects. It has previously been speculated that anxiolytic medications work "bottom up," perhaps through stabilization of brainstem nuclei (42). Cognitive-behavioral therapy, on the other hand, might work "topdown," through modification of dysfunctional cognitions presumably involving the prefrontal cortex, thereby resembling extinction of fear conditioning (12,42). However, given the lack of cortical activations, the data of Furmark et al. (41) may seem more compatible with a bottom-up mechanism also in psychotherapy. This may be true for exposure-based therapies that could permit systematic habituation of limbic neurons. It is also possible that top-down modulation, or a cognitive treatment mechanism, is more prominent when a treated patient anticipates phobic exposure rather than during the actual exposure.

4. Resting State Studies

Resting or neutral-state paradigms are most often used to evaluate between-group differences in brain activity without focusing on the specific state of the subject at the time of scanning (12). There are two studies reporting on rCBF in the resting state in SAD. In an early SPECT study, Stein and Leslie (43) reported that brain perfusion in a group of patients with generalized SAD and healthy controls did not differ. Neither were significant correlations observed between brain activity in various regions of interest and anxiety or mood ratings. This indicates that neural activity, as measured by brain blood flow, does not distinguish social phobics from nonphobics during resting conditions. Other data—for example, those demonstrating an increased comorbidity with depression and other amygdala-related disorders in SAD—might indicate that amygdalar hyperactivity constitutes more of a trait than a state-like character. However, the Stein and Leslie (43) study supports that alterations observed in imaging studies of emotional perception, learning, and induction in SAD most likely are state specific, to the state induced reflecting brain responsivity rather than trait characteristics only.

Finally, in another SPECT study, Van der Linden and co-workers (44) reported on resting rCBF before and after pharmacotherapy in individuals with SAD. They observed that 8 weeks of SSRI (citalopram) treatment was associated with reduced activity in the anterior and lateral part of the left temporal cortex but also in the midfrontal, cingulate, and occipital areas. The alterations were mainly left-sided and could either represent a treatment-related response or the effect of repetition testing, because no comparison group was included to control for time effects. In addition, these data suggest that alterations observed by Furmark and co-workers (41) do not simply reflect an altered resting activity but are instead consistent with a reduced neural response to anxiety provocation following treatment.

5. Functional Imaging Studies: Conclusions

Results from functional brain imaging studies of SAD are summarized in Table 1. The MTL region in general and the amygdala in particular has consistently been reported to display an enhanced activity in patients with SAD as compared to healthy controls, both in response to neutral and harsh

TABLE 1 Functional Neuroimaging Studies of Social Phobia (Social Anxiety Disorder): Main Findings

Task	Method	Cortical changes	Subcortical changes	Reference
1. Face perception:				
Neutral faces vs. fixation (Phobics vs. controls)	fMRI		+ amygdala B	Birbaumer et al. (22)
Neutral faces vs. fixation (Phobics vs. controls)	fMRI	+ orbitofrontal B + dosomedial prefrontal R + inferior frontal L	+ amygdala R	Veit et al. (23)
Harsh vs. accepting faces (Phobics vs. controls)	fMRI	+ medial temporal B + inferior frontal L + superior frontal R + dorsomedial prefrontal B	+ amygdala L	Stein et al. (24)
2. Aversive conditioning:				
Face predicting negative odor (Phobics vs. controls)	fMRI		+ amygdala B + hippocampus B	Schneider et al. (27)
Face predicting painful pressure	fMRI	+ insula R + orbitofrontal B + dosolateral prefrontal R + somatosensory B		Veit et al. (23)
3. Anxiety provocation:				
a. Private vs. public speaking (Δ Phobics vs. controls)	PET	− insula B − inferior/anterior temporal B − parietal R − posterior cingulate B − occipital R	+ amygdala R	Tillfors et al. (29)

b. Anticipation of a public speech High vs. low anxiety groups	PET	+ inferior temporal L + dorsolateral prefrontal R − temporal pole L	+ amygdala L + hippocampus L − cerebellum B	Tillfors et al. (30)
Phobics vs. controls	EEG	+ anterior temporal R + lateral prefrontal R		Davidson et al. (38)
c. After treatment CBT or citalopram 9 weeks (Public speaking post vs. pre) Responders vs. nonresponders	PET	− medial temporal B − medial temporal R − anterior cingulate B − dorsolateral prefrontal R	− amygdala B − hippocampus B − amygdala R − hippocampus R	Furmark et al. (41)
4. Resting state a. Phobics vs. controls	SPECT	*no change*	*no change*	Stein and Leslie (43)
b. After treatment Citalopram 8 weeks	SPECT	− anterior/lateral temporal L − mid frontal L − cingulate L − occipital B		van der Linden et al. (44)

Key: + increases, − decreases; B = bilateral, L = left, R = right hemisphere; CBT = Cognitive-behavior therapy; fMRI = functional magnetic resonance imaging, PET = positron emission tomography, EEG = electroencephalography, SPECT = single photon emission tomography; Δ changes in brain blood flow in going from private to public speaking in phobics compared with controls.

faces, during acquisition of aversive memories (fear conditioning) and when anticipating and performing a stressful public speech. In addition, treatment-related changes were associated with reduced activity in the MTL, including the amygdala, and reductions predicted behavioral outcome over a year. This consistency with respect to amygdalar involvement is not observed for other anxiety disorders with the possible exception of posttraumatic stress disorder. It is not possible to determine whether the exaggerated activation of the amygdala and other MTL structures in emotional activation studies precedes or is a consequence of SAD. In the future, imaging techniques could perhaps be used in longitudinal research to address topics of this kind.

Aside from the MTL, other areas of the brain show a more diversified pattern of activation and deactivation. This might reflect qualitative or quantitative differences associated with study designs, imaging methods, and arousal levels with, for example, emotional perception producing low-level arousal, anxiety provocation producing high-level arousal, and anticipation being in an intermediate position. It is noteworthy that the dorsolateral prefrontal cortex is often implicated in the activation studies, at least during low or moderate arousal levels. Neural activity in this region also decreased when comparing treatment responders versus nonresponders in the Furmark et al. (41) study. It is possible that worry-like processes are associated with prefrontal activity, whereas panic and fear are more related to amygdaloid activation.

IV. FUTURE DIRECTIONS

Neuroimaging studies of SAD and other anxiety disorders have only begun. Looking at the future, it is conceivable that imaging studies will be increasingly sophisticated in addressing diagnostic issues, such as distinguishing social phobics from nonphobics and other anxiety disorders, and identifying subgroups of SAD on the basis of brain activity. Moreover, there is clearly a need for more treatment studies evaluating anxiolytic drugs, psychotherapeutic interventions, and their combination. Even though current treatments of SAD are helpful, they often produce only partial improvement. Exploring novel treatment approaches is therefore important. Brain imaging studies could be of great assistance in this process, since they can provide unique information about the pathophysiology of anxiety disorders and the brain mechanisms underlying the therapeutic effect. Imaging data can also be used to fine-tune existent treatments, e.g., with regard to dose optimization in pharmacotherapy or in identifying the beneficial components in psychotherapy. The effects of treatment on brain activity could be studied using several activation paradigms such as anxiety provocation, emotional face processing, fear conditioning, and fear-potentiated startle. Also, how successful treatment affect neurotransmitter and receptor dynamics is largely unexplored. In view of the rapid development of novel PET tracers, it is likely that the near future will see more studies of this kind in SAD.

ACKNOWLEDGMENTS

Supported by grants from the Swedish Research Council, the Bank of Sweden Tercentenary Foundation, and the Swedish Brain Foundation.

REFERENCES

1. Davidson RJ, Jackson DC, Kalin NH. Emotion, plasticity, context, and regulation: perspectives from affective neuroscience. Psychol Bull 2000;126:890–909.
2. Davis M, Whalen PJ. The amygdala: vigilance and emotion. Mol Psychiatry 2001;6:13–34.
3. Adolphs R. Cognitive neuroscience of human social behaviour. Nat Rev Neurosci 2003;4:165–178.
4. Amaral DG. The primate amygdala and the neurobiology of social behavior: implications for understanding social anxiety. Biol Psychiatry 2002;51:11–17.
5. LeDoux JE. Emotion circuits in the brain. Annu Rev Neurosci 2000;23:155–184.
6. LeDoux JE. The Emotional Brain: The Mysterious Underpinnings of Emotional Life. New York: Simon & Schuster, 1996.
7. Davidson RJ, Irwin W. The functional neuroanatomy of emotion and affective style. Trends Cogn Sci 1999;3:11–21.
8. Maddock RJ. The retrosplenial cortex and emotion: new insights from functional neuroimaging of the human brain. Trends Neurosci 1999;22:310–316.
9. Gorman JM, Kent JM. SSRIs and SMRIs: broad spectrum of efficacy beyond major depression. J Clin Psychiatry 1999;60(suppl 4):33–38.
10. Bell CJ, Malizia AL, Nutt DJ. The neurobiology of social phobia. Eur Arch Psychiatry Clin Neurosci 1999;249(suppl 1):S11–S18.
11. Castillo M, Kwock L, Mukherji SK. Clinical applications of proton MR spectroscopy. Am J Neuroradiol 1996;17:1–15.
12. Rauch SL, Shin LM, Wright CI. Neuroimaging studies of amygdala function in anxiety disorders. Ann NY Acad Sci 2003;985:389–410.
13. Illes J, Kirschen MP, Gabrieli JDE. From neuroimaging to neuroethics. Nat Neurosci 2003;3:205.
14. Reiman EM, Raichle ME, Butler FK, Herscovitch P, Robins E. A focal brain abnormality in panic disorder, a severe form of anxiety. Nature 1984;310:683–685.
15. Potts NLS, Davidson JRT, Krishnan KRR, Doraiswamy PM. Magnetic resonance imaging in social phobia. Psychiatr Res 1992;52:35–42.
16. Davidson JRT, Krishnan KRR, Charles HC, Boyko O, Potts NLS, Ford SM, Patterson L. Magnetic resonance spectroscopy in social phobia: preliminary findings. J Clin Psychiatry 1993;54:19–25.

17. Tupler LA, Davidson JR, Smith RD, Lazeyras F, Charles HC, Krishnan KR. A repeat proton magnetic resonance spectroscopy study in social phobia. Biol Psychiatry 1997;42:419–424.
18. Tiihonen J, Kuikka J, Bergström K, Lepola U, Koponen H, Leinonen E. Dopamine reuptake site densities in patients with social phobia. Am J Psychiatry 1997;154:239–242.
19. Schneier FR, Liebowitz MR, Abi-Darham A, Zea-Ponce Y, Lin S-H, Laruelle M. Low dopamine D_2 receptor binding potential in social phobia. Am J Psychiatry 2000;157:457–459.
20. Kent JM, Coplan JD, Lombardo I, Hwang DR, Huang Y, Mawlawi O, Van Heertum RL, Slifstein M, Abi-Dargham A, Gorman JM, Laruelle M. Occupancy of brain serotonin transporters during treatment with paroxetine in patients with social phobia: a positron emission tomography study with 11C. McN 5652. Psychopharmacology 2002;164:341–348.
21. Marteinsdottir I, Furmark T, Tillfors M, Agren H, Hartvig P, Fredrikson M, Långström B, Fischer H, Antoni G, Hagberg G. Presynaptic serotonin imaging in social phobia using [3-11C]-5-hydroxy-L-tryptophan and PET. Neuroimage 2001;13:S1070.
22. Birbaumer N, Grodd W, Diedrich O, Klose U, Erb M, Lotze M, Schneider F, Weiss U, Flor H. fMRI reveals amygdala activation to human faces in social phobics. Neuroreport 1998;9:1223–1226.
23. Veit R, Flor H, Erb M, Hermann C, Lotze M, Grodd W, Birbaumer N. Brain circuits involved in emotional learning in antisocial behavior and social phobia in humans. Neurosci Lett 2002;328:233–236.
24. Stein MB, Goldin PR, Sareen J, Zorrilla LT, Brown GG. Increased amygdala activation to angry and contemptuous faces in generalized social phobia. Arch Gen Psychiatry 2002;59:1027–1034.
25. Whalen PJ. Fear vigilance and ambiguity: initial neuroimaging studies of the human amygdala. Curr Direct Psychol Sci 1998;7:177–188.
26. Furmark T, Fischer H, Wik G, Larsson M, Fredrikson M. The amygdala and individual differences in human fear conditioning. Neuroreport 1997;8:3957–3960.
27. Schneider F, Weiss U, Kessler C, Müller-Gärtner H-W, Posse S, Salloum JB, Grodd W, Himmelmann F, Gaebel W, Birbaumer N. Subcortical correlates of differential classical conditioning of aversive emotional reactions in social phobia. Biol Psychiatry 1999;45:863–871.
28. Hermann C, Ziegler S, Birbaumer N, Flor H. Psychophysiological and subjective indicators of aversive Pavlovian conditioning in generalized social phobia. Biol Psychiatry 2002;52:328–337.
29. Tillfors M, Furmark T, Marteinsdottir I, Fischer H, Pissiota A, Långström B, Fredrikson M. Cerebral blood flow in subjects with social phobia during stressful speaking tasks: a PET study. Am J Psychiatry 2001;158:1220–1226.
30. Tillfors M, Furmark T, Marteinsdottir I, Fredrikson M. Cerebral blood flow during anticipation of public speaking in social phobia: a PET study. Biol Psychiatry 2002;52:1113–1119.

31. Fredrikson M, Furmark T. Amygdaloid regional cerebral blood flow and subjective fear during symptom provocation in anxiety disorders. Ann NY Acad Sci 2003;985:341–347.

32. Fischer H, Tillfors M, Furmark T, Fredrikson M. Dispositional pessimism and amygdala activity: a PET study in healthy volunteers. Neuroreport 2001; 12: 1635–1638.

33. Lane RD, Reiman EM, Axelrod B, Yun LS, Holmes A, Schwartz GE. Neural correlates of levels of emotional awareness. Evidence of an interaction between emotion and attention in the anterior cingulate cortex. J Cogn Neurosci 1998; 10:525–535.

34. Wu JC, Buchsbaum MS, Hershey TG, Hazlett E, Sicotte N, Johnson JC. PET in generalized anxiety disorder. Biol Psychiatry 1991;29:1181–1199.

35. Isenberg N, Silbersweig D, Engelien A, Emmerich S, Malavade K, Beattie B, Leon AC, Stern E. Linguistic threat activates the human amygdala. Proc Natl Acad Sci USA 1999;96:10456–10459.

36. Rauch SL, Whalen PJ, Shin LM, McInerney SC, Macklin ML, Lasko NB, Orr SP, Pitman RK. Exaggerated amygdala response to masked facial stimuli in post traumatic stress disorder: a functional MRI study. Biol Psychiatry 2000; 47:769–776.

37. Wright CI, Fischer H, Whalen PJ, McInerney SC, Shin LM, Rauch SL. Differential prefrontal cortex and amygdala habituation to repeatedly presented emotional stimuli. Neuroreport 2001;12:379–383.

38. Davidson RJ, Marshall JR, Tomarken AJ, Henriques JB. While a phobic waits: regional brain electrical and autonomic activity in social phobics during anticipation of public speaking. Biol Psychiatry 2000;47:85–95.

39. Rauch SL, Savage CR, Alpert NM, Fischman AJ, Jenike MA. The functional neuroanatomy of anxiety: a study of three disorders using positron emission tomography and symptom provocation. Biol Psychiatry 1997;42:446–452.

40. Davidson RJ, Irwin W. The functional style and affective disorders: perspectives from affective neuroscience. Cognition Emotion 1998;12:307–330.

41. Furmark T, Tillfors M, Marteinsdottir I, Fischer H, Pissiota A, Langstrom B, Fredrikson M. Common changes in cerebral blood flow in patients with social phobia treated with citalopram or cognitive-behavioral therapy. Arch Gen Psychiatry 2002;59:425–433.

42. Gorman JM, Kent JM, Sullivan GM, Coplan JD. Neuroanatomical hypothesis of panic disorder, revised. Am J Psychiatry 2000;157:493–505.

43. Stein MB, Leslie WD. A brain single-photon-emission computed tomography (SPECT) study of generalized social phobia. Biol Psychiatry 1996;39:825–828.

44. Van Der Linden G, Van Heerden B, Warwick J, Wessels C, Van Kradenburg J, Zungu-Dirwayi N, Stein DJ. Functional brain imaging and pharmacotherapy in social phobia: single photon emission computed tomography before and after treatment with the selective serotonin reuptake inhibitor citalopram. Progr Neuropsychopharmacol Biol Psychiatry 2000;24:419–438.

15

Cognitive-Behavioral Therapy for Social Anxiety Disorder: A Treatment Review

Robert M. Holaway and
Richard G. Heimberg
Temple University,
Philadelphia, Pennsylvania, U.S.A.

I. INTRODUCTION

Since its inception as a nosological category in the third edition of the *Diagnostic and Statistical Manual of Mental Disorders* (DSM-III) (1), investigations of the efficacy of treatments for social anxiety disorder have greatly increased. Much of this research has focused on those approaches falling under the rubric of cognitive-behavioral therapy (CBT). This chapter provides an overview of the various cognitive-behavioral techniques used in the treatment of social anxiety disorder as well as a review of the current literature on the efficacy of these approaches. (A review of the relative efficacy of CBT and medication approaches is provided by Zaider and Heimberg in another chapter in this volume.) A review of empirical findings regarding the influence of particular factors on treatment outcome is also provided. Finally, practical guidelines for the implementation of CBT and directions for future research are discussed.

II. COGNITIVE-BEHAVIORAL APPROACHES TO SOCIAL ANXIETY DISORDER

Cognitive-behavioral therapy encompasses a number of different strategies for the treatment of psychological disorders (e.g., exposure therapy, progressive muscle relaxation, cognitive restructuring techniques). In general, CBT is a time-limited, present-oriented approach that aims to teach patients the cognitive and behavioral skills that will allow them to adapt adequately and function efficiently in their internal and external environments (2). Central to most CBT approaches is the collaboration between patient and therapist in their journey toward positive change. The therapist serves as a coach as he or she teaches adaptive coping skills and brings to attention maladaptive thinking and behavior patterns that may serve to maintain the patient's distress.

With respect to social anxiety disorder, recent variations of CBT have been informed by theoretical models (3,4) that emphasize the interdependence of the socially anxious person's dysfunctional belief system and tendencies toward behavioral avoidance. The most widely studied cognitive-behavioral approaches to the treatment of social anxiety disorder are cognitive restructuring, exposure therapy, relaxation training, and social skills training. Each of these modalities is described below.

A. Social Skills Training

The use of social skills training for social anxiety disorder is based on the idea that socially anxious patients display behavioral deficiencies in their interpersonal communications (e.g., poor eye contact, poor conversation skills) that elicit negative reactions from others, consequently leading to awkward and uncomfortable social exchanges. The goal of social skills training is to increase patients' social knowledge and behavioral skills and thereby increase the likelihood of favorable social outcomes. Training typically includes therapist modeling, behavioral rehearsal, corrective feedback, social reinforcement, and homework assignments.

Though some socially anxious individuals do have deficits in their abilities to effectively interact with others, it is often unclear whether their behaviors are a function of social skills deficiencies or behavioral inhibition driven by their social anxiety. Research on the behavior of socially anxious individuals has produced mixed results, with some studies suggesting deficits in social behaviors (5,6) and others finding no indication that the performance of individuals with social anxiety is less adequate than the performance of those without the disorder (7,8). It is clear, however, that socially anxious individuals often underestimate the adequacy of their behavioral performance during social exchanges (6,8) and believe they are being perceived much more negatively than the true opinions held by those with whom they interact (9). Therefore, reduction in social anxiety following social skills training may not always be attributable to the remediation of behavioral deficiencies. For example, social skills training may decrease a patient's social anxiety through repeated confrontation with feared stimuli and corrective feedback regarding the adequacy of social behaviors (2). Some researchers have successfully used a combination of social skills training and cognitive restructuring or exposure therapy in their approach to the treatment of social anxiety disorder (10).

B. Exposure to Feared Situations

Exposure to anxiety-evoking situations has long been an integral component of CBT for the anxiety disorders (11). Behavioral models of fear reduction suggest that confrontation with feared situations allows the natural conditioning processes of extinction and habituation to occur, providing patients with opportunities for greater access to positively reinforcing stimuli and consequently decreasing behavioral avoidance. From a cognitive perspective, exposure provides the patient with corrective information that allows for the modification of maladaptive beliefs and information processing biases, which ultimately leads to reevaluation of feared situations as less threatening (3,4). For individuals with social anxiety disorder, this usually occurs when they are repeatedly exposed to feared social situations but do not encounter anticipated negative outcomes.

The first stage in the collaborative development of planned exposures is the generation of a rank-ordered list of social situations that evoke anxiety for the patient (most often referred to as the fear and avoidance hierarchy). Patients then put themselves into these feared situations, starting with those low on this list. To make exposures maximally effective, it is essential that patients fully engage themselves in the situation (i.e., maintain a focus on the situation and all its various aspects rather than attempting to filter the distressing aspects of the situation from awareness or engage in some other form of distraction) and remain in the situation until their anxiety naturally begins to subside (12). Recent research indicates that individuals who are instructed to maintain focus on the feared situation are more likely to benefit from exposure than those who do not receive these specific instructions (13). As a sense of mastery over less anxiety-evoking situations is obtained and lower levels of anxiety are elicited, patients are encouraged to approach increasingly more anxiety-evoking circumstances and gradually work towards their most feared social situations. Exposure to feared situations may be administered via imagery, role-play with the therapist or therapy assistants, confrontation of feared situations in everyday life outside of session, or a combination of these approaches. Exposure procedures may vary with respect to the amount of therapist involvement, length of exposure sessions, and number of exposure sessions. Further, exposure is often implemented in combination with other treatment components, such as applied relaxation or cognitive restructuring.

C. Relaxation Training

Many individuals with social anxiety disorder report troubling physiological arousal (e.g., heart palpitations, trembling) when confronted with feared social situations or in anticipation of them. Several relaxation training techniques have been developed over the years with the primary goal of providing patients with a means of coping with these physiological manifestations of anxiety, which often interfere with their ability to perform optimally in social situations. Most current approaches are derived from the pioneering work of Wolpe (14) and Bernstein and Borkovec (15). These primarily involve exercises aimed at the relaxation of different muscle groups (both in session and as homework assignments), a technique known as progressive muscle relaxation (see also the recent work of Bernstein and colleagues, Ref. 16). This approach focuses on the induction of tension and relaxation in particular muscle groups with the specific goal of learning the difference between sensations accompanying tension and those accompanying relaxation (e.g., warmth, heaviness). An additional component often used with progressive muscle relaxation is cue-controlled relaxation, which involves the repeated pairing of a word (e.g., *relax*) with a relaxed physical state. Later, the paired word can be used as a cue to achieve a relaxed state during everyday activities.

Relaxation training for social anxiety disorder has been found to be effective only when applied in feared situations. Therefore *applied relaxation* has typically entailed a combination of relaxation strategies and exposure techniques to help individuals effectively cope with anxiety-evoking situations (17). Applied relaxation training consists of three main skills to be acquired in treatment: recognition of the early sensations of anxiety and physiological arousal, proficiency in achieving a relaxed state quickly while engaging in daily activities, and use of relaxation strategies in actual anxiety-evoking situations. Interestingly, recent research suggests that socially anxious individuals do not exhibit higher levels of autonomic arousal during stressful tasks than those with low levels of social anxiety even though they report the subjective experience of greater anxiety (18). This finding suggests that individual differences in social anxiety are more the result of cognitive mechanisms than autonomic activation and may be directly related to the negative interpretation of arousal. However, there are also differences in activity of areas such as the amygdala in social anxiety disorder and healthy controls (this volume, chapter by Fredrikson and Furmark). Nevertheless, applied relaxation may functionally be (at least partially) a cognitive technique.

D. Cognitive Restructuring

A core feature of social anxiety disorder is the intense fear that others may judge one negatively. Central to cognitive-behavioral models of social anxiety disorder is the idea that patients exhibit maladaptive patterns of thinking, including overestimation of the dangers inherent in social situations, negative predictions concerning the outcomes of these situations, and information-processing biases that increase the apparent danger in social situations. The goal of cognitive restructuring is to teach patients to assess their thoughts and beliefs regarding social situations more objectively. First, patients are taught to identify the negative thoughts that occur prior to, during, and following exposure to feared situations. The patient and therapist then examine the validity of the patient's belief system in light of facts derived from Socratic dialogue (19). As a result of these efforts, patients accumulate evidence supportive of less catastrophic interpretations of social situations. By utilizing these more rational thoughts during exposures to anxiety-evoking situations, patients are ultimately able to modify their habitual negative beliefs about social situations.

Most cognitive approaches to the treatment of social anxiety disorder rely heavily on systematic exposures to feared stimuli. For example, exposure to anxiety-provoking situations allows patients to access their negative thoughts regarding a particular situation and to obtain evidence to evaluate the accuracy of these cognitions. Behavioral experiments are designed to provide patients with opportunities to treat their thoughts as hypotheses and test whether their beliefs (e.g., "everyone will laugh at me" or "I will be unable to speak") are realistic or exaggerated appraisals of the situation. Behavioral experiments may require patients to enter feared situations without engaging in or relying on their safety behaviors (20,21). Patients commonly hold erroneous beliefs that engaging in certain behaviors will allow them to manage their anxiety successfully and prevent the occurrence of feared outcomes. For example, patients with fears of blushing may attempt to hide their faces by walking with their heads down, allowing their hair to shield their faces, or wearing excessive amounts of makeup. Individuals who fear other types of social situations may remain reserved and avoid contributing to conversations or other activities, or they may carefully rehearse every line to be spoken for fear of saying or doing the wrong thing and consequently being criticized by others. As a result, they may think they survived the feared situation only because they engaged in these behaviors.

However, these behaviors actually prevent them from learning that they could have managed the situation adequately and may actually disrupt their efforts to perform well. Instructing patients to resist safety behaviors during exposures as well as in their everyday lives is essential for achieving a favorable treatment outcome (21).

III. EFFICACY OF CBT FOR SOCIAL ANXIETY DISORDER: A METAANALYTIC REVIEW

Over the past 20 years, a number of studies have examined the efficacy of CBT for social anxiety disorder. Many of these studies have evaluated the overall utility of CBT interventions as well as the relative importance of particular components of the cognitive-behavioral approach (e.g., exposure, cognitive restructuring). Because the treatment outcome literature for social anxiety disorder has grown rather large, metaanalyses have been increasingly used to evaluate treatment efficacy, as they allow one to examine the outcomes of several studies simultaneously. This is made possible by reducing the results of each study to a common quantitative metric, the effect size. The within-group effect size (also referred to as "uncontrolled") denotes the number of standard deviation units of improvement for patients within a particular treatment group and is most often measured using the formula for Cohen's d $[(M_{pre} - M_{post})/SD_{pooled}]$ (22). An average within-group effect size of 1.0 for a specific treatment indicates that, on average, the patients in all the studies who received that particular treatment improved by one standard deviation. Between-group, or controlled, effect sizes, on the other hand, provide an index of the degree of improvement of patients in a treatment condition compared to those in a control condition. A between-group effect size of one standard deviation indicates that the treatment group improved one standard deviation unit more than the control group $[(M_{treatment} - M_{control})/SD_{control}]$ (23). Guidelines for the interpretation of the magnitude of effect sizes have been provided by Cohen (22), who states that 0.20, 0.50, and 0.80 correspond to small, medium, and large effects, respectively.

To date, five metaanalytic studies have examined the efficacy of CBT for social anxiety disorder (24–28). Overall, the various cognitive-behavioral approaches to treatment (e.g., exposure, cognitive restructuring, social skills training) appear to be rather efficacious, with a number of studies reporting significant improvements in social anxiety. Chambless and Hope (24) meta-analyzed eight controlled studies in which group CBT, applied relaxation training, and exposure with anxiety management were examined. The average within-group effect size for group CBT was 0.94, a large effect, suggesting that individuals receiving CBT had significant reductions in their social anxiety following treatment. Gould and Johnson (29) more recently reviewed the results of three metaanalytic investigations examining the efficacy of CBT for social anxiety disorder (26–28). Overall, CBT treatments were superior to control conditions and appeared to be effective interventions at posttreatment (8 to 12 weeks). Patients were improved on measures of social anxiety, cognitive change, and depression, with moderate to large between-group effect sizes in all three metaanalyses (0.74 to 1.06). Similarly, Fedoroff and Taylor (25) found CBT to be efficacious, further supporting its effectiveness as a short-term treatment for social anxiety disorder.

CBT for social anxiety disorder has also shown to be effective over the long term, maintaining treatment gains through 6-month follow-up (29), with some evidence for additional improvement 3 months after termination (28). Uncontrolled effect sizes for pretreatment to follow-up periods have generally ranged from 0.78 to 1.31, strongly supporting the effectiveness of CBT as a longer-term treatment option (24–26,28). The uncontrolled effect size for change between posttreatment and follow-up in one metaanalysis was 0.23, providing empirical support for the enduring and potentially growing effects of CBT following active therapy (27).

Across both short- and long-term investigations, CBT appears to be an efficacious approach to the treatment of social anxiety disorder. However, due to the heterogeneous nature of cognitive-behavioral treatments, it is important to examine the relative efficacy of its individual components (e.g., cognitive restructuring, exposure), and several metaanalyses have attempted to do so. Studies employing exposure alone appear to yield more favorable outcomes than studies using cognitive restructuring alone (29). Fedoroff and Taylor (25) examined the relative efficacy of social skills training, applied relaxation, cognitive restructuring, cognitive restructuring plus exposure therapy, and exposure alone. All treatment variations demonstrated moderate to large effects, with average within-group effect sizes of 0.64, 0.51, 0.72, 0.84, and 1.08, respectively. However, there was a great deal of variability among studies using exposure alone, leading the confidence interval around the effect size of 1.08 to overlap with zero, suggesting a nonsignificant effect. Another metaanalysis found the largest within-group effect sizes to be associated with approaches combining cognitive restructuring and exposure (1.06) (28). In this investigation, the effect size for exposure alone was also large (0.82). However, the only treatment with effects significantly greater than placebo at posttreatment was the combination of cognitive restructuring and exposure. In the metaanalysis by Fedoroff and Taylor (25), there were no differences between exposure, cognitive restructuring, combined exposure and cognitive restructuring, and social skills training at follow-up.

CBT appears to be a rather efficacious approach to treating social anxiety disorder. A number of empirical investigations have supported its utility as a viable and powerful treatment option for ameliorating the effects of social anxiety both in the short-term and over the long-term. Exposure alone and exposure combined with cognitive restructuring have generally been shown to be the most effective variations of CBT. However, it remains unclear whether the addition of a cognitive component augments the benefits achieved by exposure alone. Although cognitive change is an important or even necessary part of reduction in social anxiety, it is not clear whether changes in maladaptive thinking require the use of cognitive techniques or if these results can be achieved solely with the use of exposure treatments. Further research will likely resolve this question; however, it is important to discuss potential explanations for the lack of differences observed when comparing exposure to combined treatments. First, there are very few exposure-based treatments, if any, that strictly adhere to a behavioral regimen that is void of some type of cognitive component. For example, exposure treatments often include therapist feedback about the patient's performance, providing corrective information that may bring about cognitive change (30). Though such methods may not be considered "cognitive," there is a great deal of overlap among approaches, suggesting that exposure-alone methods may be very similar to combination treatments. Second, exposure-only treatments may be sufficient to bring about significant improvements in some patients, whereas others may require the addition of cognitive restructuring to achieve optimal outcomes. Whether or not cognitive techniques are shown to be necessary in the treatment of social anxiety disorder, it appears that individuals who demonstrate more cognitive change (as assessed with measures of rational thinking, positive and negative self-statements, or through listing procedures after behavior tests) show greater improvements in social anxiety (31,32). Future research that adheres to more consistent boundaries between treatment components is essential to better understanding this phenomenon and will likely provide improved methods of treatment.

IV. FACTORS INFLUENCING TREATMENT OUTCOME

Though CBT has generally been found to be efficacious in the treatment of social anxiety disorder, a percentage of patients do not achieve clinically significant improvement by the end of therapy. A number of studies have examined the role of particular variables in predicting response to treatment and their influence on overall therapeutic outcome.

A. Homework Compliance

An integral ingredient of CBT for social anxiety disorder has been the completion of between-session homework assignments. These assignments most often consist of exposures to anxiety-evoking situations as well as self-administered cognitive-restructuring activities. To date, three studies have examined the relationship between homework compliance and outcome of CBT for social anxiety disorder. For the most part, patients labeled as homework compliant did not achieve better outcome scores at posttreatment than those who were classified as less compliant (33,34). However, in one study, compliant patients reported greater decreases in avoidant behaviors and less anxiety while giving a speech at 6-month follow-up (33). The contribution of homework compliance to treatment outcome during each phase of therapy has also been examined, with differential effects evident as the focus and content of homework assignments systematically changes over the course of treatment (i.e., psychoeducation and self-monitoring, cognitive-restructuring, and in vivo exposure) (35). The completion of assignments during the first phase of treatment was minimally related to treatment outcome, whereas compliance during the last phase of treatment showed a strong relationship to outcome. Interestingly, compliance with homework assignments during the middle phase of treatment was *positively* correlated with social anxiety. Further investigations on this topic are warranted.

B. Subtype of Social Anxiety Disorder and Avoidant Personality Disorder

A number of studies have examined the influence of subtype of social anxiety disorder (i.e., generalized versus nongeneralized) and avoidant personality disorder (APD) on CBT outcome. Most studies assessing the impact of subtype on response to treatment have found few differences with respect to degree of improvement; however, individuals with the generalized subtype of social anxiety disorder have consistently been found to be more impaired prior to and following treatment. For example, individuals with generalized social anxiety disorder and those with nongeneralized social anxiety disorder have shown equivalent improvement at posttreatment; however, individuals with the generalized subtype were more impaired prior to and following treatment and were less likely to make clinically significant gains as a result of therapy (36). Two other studies reported similar findings (37,38), with one study finding individuals with nongeneralized social anxiety disorder more likely to achieve moderate or high end-state functioning at the end of treatment (38). Thus, CBT appears to be effective for patients with both types of social anxiety disorder. Differences are evident, however, when examining posttreatment outcome, likely an artifact of differences in pretreatment severity.

Individuals with social anxiety disorder and comorbid APD have consistently demonstrated more severe symptomatology before and after treatment than those without APD, a finding very similar to that observed in individuals with the generalized subtype. Nevertheless, most studies have found both groups to improve at the same rate, suggesting that a comorbid diagnosis of APD has little effect on outcome and may be more an indicator of greater severity of social anxiety disorder than a separate diagnostic category (36,37,39,40). Two studies have examined the effect of APD on treatment outcome among persons with generalized social anxiety disorder. Brown and colleagues (36) found similar rates of response to group CBT among individuals with generalized social anxiety disorder with and without APD. However, Feske and colleagues (41) found patients with comorbid generalized social anxiety disorder and APD to improve at a poorer rate than those with generalized social anxiety disorder alone. Studies that did not consider subtype of social anxiety disorder have found patients with comorbid APD to benefit much more slowly from treatment than patients without APD (40). The undesirable effect of APD, or more severe types of social anxiety disorder, on outcome in some studies may be due to the reluctance of individuals with these characteristics to fully engage in treatment, particularly those components involving interaction with others (e.g., in-session exposures).

C. Axis I Comorbidity

Social anxiety disorder has commonly been found to be highly comorbid with other axis I disorders, such other anxiety disorders, depression, and substance use disorders (42,43). Therefore it is important to understand how comorbidity affects the course of treatment, and several studies have examined the influence of comorbidity on the outcome of CBT. In an examination of the effect of axis I comorbidity on response to group CBT at both posttreatment and 12-month follow-up, patients with a comorbid anxiety disorder responded similarly to those with uncomplicated social anxiety disorder (44). However, individuals with a comorbid mood disorder were found to have more severe social anxiety, both before and after treatment. However, they did not differ in their response to treatment. Therapeutic gains were maintained by individuals in all three groups through 12-month follow-up. Chambless and colleagues (45) found pretreatment levels of self-reported depression to be the single most significant predictor of treatment outcome. More depressed individuals were less likely to improve on measures of anxious apprehension and anxiety than less depressed individuals. Other studies examining the influence of comorbid axis I disorders (i.e., dysthymia, generalized anxiety disorder, or simple phobia) on treatment outcome have found similar results, with some suggesting the presence of additional axis I disorders to have little to no influence on the rate of overall improvement or the level of end-state functioning (38,40,46).

D. Expectancy for Improvement

Expectancy for change at pretreatment has been shown to be significantly related to outcome among individuals receiving group CBT. In one study, individuals who reported higher expectancy for benefit and had stronger beliefs regarding the efficacy of the treatment were more likely to improve and maintain their gains on anxious apprehension and self-ratings of conversation role-play anxiety and performance (45). In another study (47), patients' expectancy ratings prior to treatment significantly predicted clinicians' ratings of the severity of social anxiety disorder at posttreatment above and beyond patients' pretreatment scores. Expectancy for change was also strongly related to posttreatment scores on self-report measures of social anxiety and depression. Interestingly, patients' expectancy ratings were strongly related to pretreatment severity, duration of illness, and subtype of social anxiety disorder, suggesting that individuals with more severe and enduring forms of social anxiety are less likely to expect to make gains as a result of treatment. Low expectancy for improvement may affect treatment outcome in a number of ways, such as the degree to which patients are willing to engage in challenging exposures or homework assignments. Early detection of low expectancy for improvement among patients seeking treatment for social anxiety disorder may allow clinicians to improve the likelihood of treatment response by addressing these beliefs prior to focusing on presenting concerns.

E. Anger

Though some evidence exists to suggest that individuals with social anxiety may be more likely to experience difficulties with anger than those without an anxiety disorder (48,49), only one study has examined the influence of anger on response to treatment in individuals receiving CBT for social anxiety disorder (50). Individuals with higher levels of trait anger were more likely to terminate treatment prematurely. Among those who completed treatment, elevations in state anger, trait anger, and the tendency to suppress the expression of angry feelings at pretreatment were significantly associated with greater posttreatment social anxiety and depressive symptoms. Further research should examine whether anger exerts an effect on outcome by increasing attributions for one's anxiety to others' behavior rather than one's own, which may undermine motivation for self-change. It will also be important to examine whether intervening with problematic anger and anger suppression helps the patient become more available to the treatment experience.

V. PRACTICAL GUIDELINES

Though research over the years has shed much light on what constitutes effective treatment for social anxiety disorder, clinical experience and anecdotal reports have provided additional guidelines on how to maximize therapeutic effectiveness.

As suggested by a number of metaanalytic investigations, treatments employing exposure alone or in combination with cognitive techniques have consistently yielded the largest improvements. However, the rate of success of such approaches may be contingent on a number of factors. For example, patients who are encouraged to abandon their safety behaviors and maintain their focus on the feared situation during exposures are likely to experience greater gains than those who do not. Patients often attempt to filter the distressing aspects of a feared situation from awareness or engage in some other form of distraction. However, individuals who remain engaged in and focused on the situation until their anxiety naturally begins to subside allow the natural conditioning processes of extinction and habituation to occur, making future confrontation with such stimuli less aversive (12). Patients must be willing to tolerate the anxiety brought on by exposure assignments and be encouraged to do so in order to obtain the greatest benefit (29).

In metaanalytic studies, cognitive-behavioral approaches have been shown to yield long-term benefits up to 6 months, with one study suggesting continued improvement at 3-month follow-up. One follow-up study suggests that gains may be maintained for as long as 5 years (51). Anecdotal evidence suggests that these enduring benefits are likely due to the continued practice of exposure to feared situations after the termination of formal treatment (29). Patients should be encouraged to view their treatment as the beginning of a long journey toward positive change. Though most will experience a significant reduction in their anxiety as a result of treatment, those who continue to use the skills obtained during therapy (e.g., cognitive restructuring, exposure to feared situations) will likely see further benefits.

Though patients are likely to improve after receiving CBT for social anxiety disorder, the course of treatment can be difficult for some to endure. Many patients do not experience improvement until the later stages of treatment. Thus, it is essential to set intermediate goals that can be achieved along the way. It is preferable for these goals to be couched in terms of behavioral accomplishment rather than anxiety reduction, as changes in anxiety often follow changes in behavior and are less under the control of the patient. As patients begin to build their confidence by conquering less anxiety-evoking circumstances, they will likely be more willing to put themselves into increasingly more difficult situations. As setbacks are likely to occur along the way, patients should be encouraged to accept success and avoid negative postevent processing (3).

VI. CONCLUSIONS

As evident by a number of randomized controlled studies and metaanalytic investigations, CBT approaches appear to treat social anxiety disorder effectively. These treatments have produced reliable and robust improvements in many patients and have demonstrated efficacy in modifying the behavioral, cognitive, and affective components of social anxiety, with improvements above and beyond wait-list and placebo control conditions.

One specific most effective variant of CBT has yet to emerge; however, most investigations suggest that individuals receiving exposure or exposure combined with cognitive treatments experience the greatest improvement. Further, a number of investigations have evaluated the influence of particular variables (e.g., homework compliance, axis I comorbidity, APD) on treatment outcome. Homework compliance, treatment expectancy, and anger-related variables have been found to be related to outcome. Other factors, such as subtype of social anxiety disorder and comorbid depression, are related to greater pretreatment severity of social anxiety disorder and greater posttreatment severity as well. However, the slope of improvement during treatment does not appear to differ as a function of depression or generalized social anxiety disorder. This complex pattern suggests that more depressed patients or patients with generalized social anxiety disorder may require a longer course of cognitive-behavioral treatment.

In sum, CBT is an efficacious treatment strategy for social anxiety disorder. Nevertheless, some patients show only partial response to therapy and some do not benefit at all. Further research will likely provide valuable evidence regarding the most effective variations of these treatments. Additionally, identifying predictors of response to treatment should be a priority for future investigations.

REFERENCES

1. American Psychiatric Association. Diagnostic and Statistical Manual of Mental Disorders. 2d ed. Washington, DC: American Psychiatric Press, 1980.
2. Heimberg RG. Cognitive-behavioral therapy for social anxiety disorder: current status and future directions. Biol Psychiatry 2002; 51:101–108.
3. Clark DM, Wells A. A cognitive model of social phobia. In: Heimberg RG, Liebowitz MR, Hope DA, Schneier FR, eds. Social Phobia: Diagnosis, Assessment, and Treatment. New York: Guilford Press, 1995:69–93.

4. Rapee RM, Heimberg RG. A cognitive-behavioral model of anxiety in social phobia. Behav Res Ther 1997; 35:741–756.

5. Halford K, Foddy M. Cognitive and social skills correlates of social anxiety. Br J Clin Psychol 1982; 21:7–28.

6. Stopa L, Clark DM. Cognitive processes in social phobia. Behav Res Ther 1993; 31:255–267.

7. Glasgow RE, Arkowitz H. The behavioral assessment of male and female social competence in dyadic heterosexual interactions. Behav Ther 1975; 6:488–498.

8. Rapee RM, Lim L. Discrepancy between self- and observer ratings of performance in social phobics. J Abnorm Psychol 1992; 101:728–731.

9. Christensen PN, Stein MB, Means-Christensen A. Social anxiety and interpersonal perception: a social relations model analysis. Behav Res Ther 2003; 41:1355–1371.

10. Turner SM, Beidel DC, Cooley MR, Woody SR, Messer SC. A multicomponent behavioral therapy for social phobia. Behav Res Ther 1994; 32:381–390.

11. Barlow DH, Wolfe BE. Behavioral approaches to anxiety disorders: a report on the NIMH-SUNY, Albany research conference. J Consult Clin Psychol 1981; 49:448–454.

12. Foa EB, Kozak MJ. Emotional processing of fear: exposure to corrective information. Psychol Bull 1986; 99:20–35.

13. Wells A, Papageorgiou C. Social phobia: effects of external attention of anxiety, negative beliefs, and perspective taking. Behav Ther 1998; 29:357–370.

14. Wolpe J. Psychotherapy by Reciprocal Inhibition. Stanford: Stanford University Press, 1958.

15. Bernstein DA, Borkovec TD. Progressive Relaxation Training: A Manual for the Helping Professions. Champaign, IL: Research Press, 1973.

16. Bernstein DA, Borkovec TD, Hazlett-Stevens H. New Directions in Progressive Relaxation Training: A Guidebook for Helping Professionals. Westport, CT: Praeger/Greenwood, 2000.

17. Öst LG. Applied relaxation: description of a coping technique and review of controlled studies. Behav Res Ther 1987; 25:397–409.

18. Mauss IB, Wilhelm FH, Gross JJ. Autonomic recovery and habituation in social anxiety. Psychophysiology 2003; 40:648–653.

19. Beck AT, Rush J, Shaw BF, Emery G. Cognitive Therapy of Depression. New York: Guilford Press, 1979.

20. Morgan H, Raffle C. Does reducing safety behaviours improve treatment response in patients with social phobia? Aust NZ J Psychiatry 1999; 33:503–510.

21. Wells A, Clark DM, Salkovskis P, Ludgate J, Hackman A, Gelder M. Social phobia: the role of in-situation safety behaviors in maintaining anxiety and negative beliefs. Behav Ther 1995; 26:153–161.

22. Cohen J. Statistical Power Analysis for the Behavioral Sciences. 2d ed. New York: Academic Press, 1988.

23. Glass GV, McGraw B, Smith ML. Meta-analysis in social research. Beverly Hills, CA: Sage, 1981.

24. Chambless DL, Hope DA. Cognitive approaches to the psychopathology and treatment of social phobia. In: Salkovskis PM, ed. Frontiers of Cognitive Therapy. New York: Guilford Press, 1996:345–382.

25. Fedoroff IC, Taylor S. Psychological and pharmacological treatments of social phobia: a meta-analysis. J Clin Psychopharmacol 2001; 3:311–324.

26. Feske U, Chambless DL. Cognitive behavioral versus exposure only treatment for social phobia: a meta-analysis. Behav Ther 1995; 26:695–720.

27. Gould RA, Buckminster S, Pollack MH, Otto MW, Yap L. Cognitive-behavioral and pharmacological treatment for social phobia: a meta-analysis. Clin Psychol Sci Prac 1997; 4:291–306.

28. Taylor S. Meta-analysis of cognitive-behavioral treatments for social phobia. J Behav Ther Exp Psychiatry 1996; 27, 1–9.

29. Gould RA, Johnson MW. Comparative effectiveness of cognitive-behavioral treatment and pharmacotherapy for social phobia: meta-analytic outcome. In: Hofmann SG, DiBartolo PM, eds. From Social Anxiety to Social Phobia: Multiple Perspectives. Needham Heights, MA: Allyn & Bacon, 2001:379–390.

30. Newman MG, Hofman SG, Trabert W, Roth WT, Taylor S. Does behavioral treatment of social phobia lead to cognitive changes? Behav Ther 1994; 25:503–517.

31. Mattick RP, Peters L. Treatment of severe social phobia: effects of guided exposure with and without cognitive restructuring. J Consult Clin Psychol 1988; 56:251–260.

32. Mattick RP, Peters L, Clark JC. Exposure and cognitive restructuring for social phobia: a controlled study. Behav Ther 1989; 20:3–23.

33. Edelman RE, Chambless DL. Adherence during session and homework in cognitive-behavioral group treatment of social phobia. Behav Res Ther 1995; 33:573–577.

34. Woody SR, Adessky RS. Therapeutic alliance, group cohesion, and homework compliance during cognitive-behavioral group treatment of social phobia. Behav Ther 2002; 33:5–27.

35. Leung AW, Heimberg RG. Homework compliance, perceptions of control, and outcome of cognitive-behavioral treatment for social phobia. Behav Res Ther 1996; 34:423–432.

36. Brown EJ, Heimberg RG, Juster HR. Social phobia subtype and avoidant personality disorder: effect on severity of social phobia, impairment, and outcome of cognitive-behavioral treatment. Behav Ther 1995; 26:467–486.

37. Hope DA, Herbert JD, White C. Diagnostic subtype, avoidant personality disorder, and efficacy of cognitive-behavioral group therapy for social phobia. Cogn Ther Res 1995; 19:399–417.

38. Turner SM, Beidel DC, Wolff PL, Spaulding S, Jacob RG. Clinical features affecting treatment outcome of social phobia. Behav Res Ther 1996; 34:795–804.

39. Hofmann SG, Newman MG, Becker E, Taylor CB, Roth WT. Social phobia with and without avoidant personality disorder: preliminary behavior therapy outcome findings. J Anxiety Disord 1995; 9:427–438.

40. van Velzen CJM, Emmelkamp PMG, Scholing A. The impact of personality disorders on behavioral treatment outcome for social phobia. Behav Res Ther 1997; 35:889–900.

41. Feske U, Perry KJ, Chambless DL, Renneberg B, Goldstein A. Avoidant personality disorder as a predictor for treatment outcome among generalized social phobics. J Personality Disord 1996; 10:174–184.

42. Kessler RC, McGonagle KA, Zhao S, Nelson CB, Hughes M, Eshleman S, Wittchen HU, Kendler KS. Lifetime and 12-month prevalence of DSM-III-R psychiatric disorders in the United States: results from the National Co-morbidity Survey. Arch Gen Psychiatry 1994; 51:8–19.

43. Schneier FR, Johnson J, Hornig CD, Liebowitz MR, Weissman MM. Social phobia: comorbidity and morbidity in an epidemiologic sample. Arch Gen Psychiatry 1992; 49:282–288.

44. Erwin BA, Heimberg RG, Juster H, Mindlin M. Comorbid anxiety and mood disorders among persons with social anxiety disorder. Behav Res Ther 2002; 40:19–35.

45. Chambless DL, Tran GQ, Glass CR. Predictors of response to cognitive-behavioral group therapy for social phobia. J Anxiety Disord 1997; 11:221–240.

46. Mennin DS, Heimberg RG, Jack MS. Comorbid generalized anxiety disorder in primary social phobia: symptom severity, functional impairment, and treatment response. J Anxiety Disord 2000; 14:325–343.

47. Safren SA, Heimberg RG, Juster HR. Clients' expectancies and their relation-ship to pretreatment symptomatology and outcome of cognitive-behavioral group treatment for social phobia. J Consult Clin Psychol 1997; 65:694–698.

48. Fitzgibbons L, Franklin ME, Watlington C, Foa EB. Assessment of anger in generalized social phobia. 31st Annual Convention of the Association for Advancement of Behavior Therapy, Miami, FL, November 1997.

49. Meier VJ, Hope DA, Weilage M, Elting D, Laguna L. Anger and social phobia: its expression and relation to treatment outcome. 29th Annual Convention of the Association for Advancement of Behavior Therapy, Washington DC, November 1995.

50. Erwin BA, Heimberg RG, Schneier FR, Liebowitz MR. Anger experience and expression in social anxiety disorder: pretreatment profile and predictors of attrition and response to cognitive-behavioral treatment. Behav Ther 2003; 34:331–350.

51. Heimberg RG, Salzman D, Holt CS, Blendell K. Cognitive behavioral group treatment of social phobia: effectiveness at 5-year follow-up. Cogn Ther Res 1993; 17:325–339.

16

Psychodynamic Theory and Treatment of Social Anxiety Disorder

Fredric N. Busch

Weill Medical College of Cornell University
and Columbia University Center for
Psychoanalytic Training and Research,
New York, New York, U.S.A.

Barbara L. Milrod

Weill Medical College of Cornell University
and New York Psychoanalytic Institute,
New York, New York, U.S.A.

I. INTRODUCTION

Social anxiety disorder is a severe psychiatric syndrome that results in significant suffering and impairment in psychosocial function (1,2) (this volume, chapter by Baldwin and Buis). Many theoretical models exist to describe the causes of this disorder. Although psychoanalysts have developed several theoretical models of the development of anxiety, they have rarely focused on specific anxiety disorders as described in the *Diagnostic and Statistical Manual of Mental Disorders*, fourth edition, text revision (DSM-IV-TR) (3). More systematic assessment of psychological factors and the development of therapeutic approaches to specific psychiatric syndromes has occurred only in recent years and remains outside mainstream psychoanalysis.

The syndrome of social anxiety disorder has been almost absent from the psychoanalytic literature. In contrast, randomized controlled studies have demonstrated effectiveness for both cognitive-behavioral therapy (this volume, chapter by Holaway and Heimberg) and medication (this volume, chapter by Bandelow and Stein). Nevertheless, we believe that psychoanalysis has the potential to make a valuable contribution to the understanding and treatment of social anxiety disorder. Psychoanalytic theory encompasses a broad array of psychological constructs, including unconscious conflicts and fantasies and defense mechanisms that are not addressed by other modes of treatment. In addition, psychodynamic psychotherapy focuses on the meanings and unconscious significance of symptoms, as well as developmental factors, and makes use of the transference that arises between the patient and therapist to further understanding.

Use of these therapeutic approaches in the treatment of panic disorder has appeared promising in two studies (4–6). Panic disorder overlaps with social anxiety disorder in phenomenology. Symptoms shared by the two disorders include anticipatory anxiety, panic attacks in social anxiety disorder in feared situations, and phobic avoidance (3). It is not surprising, then, that from a psychodynamic perspective, social anxiety disorder and panic disorder also overlap in specific dynamic constellations, including core unconscious conflicts with separation, ambivalent attachments, and difficulties with the experience of anger.

Review of clinical theory and cases from the psychoanalytic literature indicates, however, that additional dynamisms are present in patients with social anxiety disorder, in particular conflicted fantasies of inadequacy, grandiosity, and exhibitionism (7–12). Clarification and delineation of these dynamics can aid in the development of a psychodynamic treatment approach specific to social anxiety disorder and provide useful information for clinicians using treatment approaches other than psychodynamic psychotherapy. In order to elaborate on these ideas, core dynamic concepts, research and clinical data, treatment approaches, and clinical material are discussed.

II. PSYCHODYNAMIC THEORY OF SOCIAL ANXIETY DISORDER

A. Relevant Core Dynamic Concepts

Employing a psychodynamic approach to social anxiety disorder begins with a working knowledge of certain core psychodynamic concepts. These concepts derive from Sigmund Freud's work and were expanded upon by subsequent psychoanalytic clinicians and theorists.

1. *The Unconscious.* Psychoanalytic theory posits that mental life functions on both conscious and unconscious (out of awareness) levels (13). Wishes, fantasies, and impulses that may be considered dangerous to the self, or the ego, are often unconscious; commonly, their potential emergence into consciousness is experienced as threatening.

2. *Traumatic Anxiety versus Signal Anxiety.* Freud (14) described traumatic anxiety, in which anxiety overwhelms the ego, in contrast to signal anxiety, in which a small dose of anxiety alerts the ego to the potential emergence of wishes, impulses, or feelings that are considered to be dangerous to the self.

3. *Defenses.* Defenses, or unconscious psychological mechanisms that ward off or disguise dangerous wishes and impulses to render them safer, are often triggered by signal anxiety. If defenses are ineffective at diminishing the danger experienced from internal wishes and unconscious fantasies (15), traumatic anxiety, or panic, results. In the unconscious process of avoiding the experience of traumatic anxiety, the patient may also develop symptoms that bind anxiety, or magically control or symbolize it, such as phobic avoidance, including the avoidance symptoms seen in social anxiety disorder.

4. *Compromise Formation.* Using another unconscious mechanism to diminish the danger experienced from unconscious fantasies and wishes, the ego may synthesize a "compromise formation," often a psychological symptom, which symbolically represents a compromise between the wish and the defenses that are being employed to neutralize the threat from the wish (13). Symptoms of social anxiety disorder represent compromise formations.

5. *The Pleasure Principle.* Individuals consciously or unconsciously attempt to behave, think, or feel in ways that will bring about the least amount of unpleasure (16). Paradoxical as it may seem to patients who are suffering from severe anxiety, anxiety symptoms represent the least unpleasurable solution available to the person as he or she faces threatening fantasies and ideas. In other words, from a psychodynamic perspective, the perceived danger of acknowledging or experiencing warded off feelings or fantasies would be more disruptive than the discomfort experienced from the anxiety symptoms themselves. For example, in social anxiety disorder, a preoccupation with fears of rejection by others can prevent the patient from becoming aware of aggressive urges or fantasies that may be experienced as overwhelmingly disorganizing or threatening to the integrity of the self or to key dependent relationships.

6. *Self and Object Representations.* Over the course of psychological development, people internalize mental representations of themselves and others and of the self in relation to others. Patients with anxiety disorders often have representations of others as being demanding, controlling, threatening, and anxiety-inducing. These object representations add to the idea

that fantasies and feelings can be dangerous or disorganizing and that attachments are insecure and easily disrupted.

B. Neurophysiological Vulnerability and Psychodynamic Factors in Social Anxiety Disorder

Evidence (17–20) (this volume, chapter by Van Ameringen and Mancini) indicates that neurophysiological vulnerabilities may increase the likelihood that an individual will develop social anxiety disorder. An individual's sense of self and others, as well as the danger of certain feelings and fantasies, are affected by a fearful temperament. Kagan and colleagues (17–19) identified a cohort of children, described as "behaviorally inhibited," who developed fear responses when exposed to novelty. Children determined to have behavioral inhibition at age 21 months were found to have an increased risk of anxiety disorders at age 8, including phobic disorders (19). Parents of children with behavioral inhibition were found to have higher rates of anxiety disorders, particularly social anxiety disorder (20). Thus there may be a genetic backdrop for this fearfulness that interacts with particular environmental factors to trigger social anxiety disorder.

Environmental stressors can include critical and/or humiliating parents or siblings, family conflicts, and loss of or separation from a parent (21). Indeed, systematic assessments of patients' perceptions indicate that people with social phobia viewed parents as less caring and more rejecting and overprotective compared to normal controls (22,23). Based on the interaction of neurophysiological underpinnings and developmental stressors, individuals who develop social anxiety disorder internalize views of themselves as inadequate, shameful, and easily rejected and perceive others as ridiculing and abandoning. They become acutely socially sensitive, intensely vulnerable to pecking orders and social slights. Others are avoided due to these fears and sensitivities, and the avoidance interferes further with the development of effective coping strategies. Persistent feelings of ineffectiveness add to a view of themselves as incompetent, childlike, and inadequate, particularly as compared to their view of their parents as powerful.

These perceptions also lead to a set of unconscious constellations, the understanding of which can aid further in understanding the dangers perceived internally and between themselves and others.

1. Due to anxiety about being rejected and abandoned, disdainful and critical feelings toward others are often experienced as threatening and damaging. Patients with social anxiety disorder are often plagued by anger at those whom they have experienced as rejecting, creating a conflict between wishes to maintain the attachment, and hostile feelings and fantasies. As Fenichel (7) noted: "Anyone who needs the opinion of others to maintain

his own mental equilibrium has good reason to fear this opinion, especially if he feels that he actually hates the person whose opinion is about to become decisive" (p. 519). In order to avert anger, several unconscious situations commonly occur.

- Anger can be denied and projected onto others, who are seen as disdainful and critical of the person with social phobia, which can lead to increasing levels of anger and anxiety in a vicious cycle.
- Seeing oneself as humiliated and anxious rather than as hostile and aggressive can reduce the risk of viewing oneself as being dangerous and threatening.
- The patient can employ the defense mechanism of reaction formation, in which angry feelings are avoided by being overly polite or accommodating.

2.   Socially anxious individuals may harbor an underlying grandiosity, which is often associated with conflicted wishes to exhibit oneself sexually (7). These wishes may derive from an attempt to compensate for a sense of personal inadequacy. Alternatively, this grandiosity may be primary. Grandiose fantasies intensify the disappointment experienced in normal social situations and increase the vulnerability patients feel to social slights. Because exhibitionistic and grandiose fantasies trigger embarrassment, guilt, and fears of punishment, the patient often needs to deny them. Social anxiety represents both a means of avoidance of these wishes and a punishment for them, and avoidance of social situations aids in avoidance of these fantasies.

3.   Patients with social anxiety disorder commonly experience a form of separation anxiety: they fear that their efforts to become autonomous and connected to others will result in their losing the love of parents or caregivers. The threat of such loss is heightened by the contrasting views of themselves as being incapable and of their parents as being powerful. Autonomy comes to represent not only abandonment but also contains within it the threat of disorganization and fragmentation. Other people are therefore avoided to prevent catastrophic cutoffs, and relationships with parents can remain close and conflicted.

Summarizing the concepts described above, people with social phobia may harbor grandiose fantasies with a sense they should be treated in a special way; they therefore experience intense disappointment in contacts with others. Grandiose and accompanying sexually exhibitionistic fantasies create emotional conflict and are denied via the symptoms of social anxiety, in which these fantasies are turned into their opposite with avoidance and self-contempt. Additionally, people with social phobia struggle with unconscious fantasies that their intense anger and disparagement of others will damage needed relationships. The threat to relationships is intensified by the sense that powerful others are required for love, organization, and coherence. Assertive fantasies or behaviors trigger increased fears of loss of these needed relationships. Finally, social anxiety and avoidance can serve as a specific punishment for grandiose, sexual, angry, and competitive feelings and fantasies.

The defense mechanisms commonly employed by people with social phobia include the denial of grandiose and sexual wishes by turning them to their opposite, self-contempt, and by socially phobic behavior itself. In addition, patients deny their angry feelings and project these feelings onto others, who are experienced as critical and rejecting. They may demonstrate reaction formation, in which anger is turned into positive, helping feelings and behaviors in a further attempt to disguise their own aggressive fantasies from themselves. Efforts at idealization of self or others in an attempt to ward off painful feelings of inadequacy add to the potential for disappointment.

Avoidance of others commonly expresses a particularly painful self-punishment for fantasies of grandiosity and may also represent an unconscious expression of contempt. Social avoidance may also preserve an underlying sense of specialness by not directly testing these beliefs with others. Feelings of guilt about aggressive wishes can be eased via the distress of social anxiety symptoms per se as well as with loss of social contacts. In short, from a psychodynamic perspective, these patients find it less difficult to experience literally "painful" shyness than the threat seen from loss of dependency or specialness.

III. PSYCHODYNAMIC TREATMENT OF SOCIAL ANXIETY DISORDER

A. Introduction

In psychodynamic psychotherapy, unconscious and warded-off fantasies and conflicts that underlie social phobic symptoms are brought into consciousness and explored. The interrelationships of the various fantasies, conflicts, compromise formations, and defense mechanisms with social phobic symptoms are identified. In this process, the imagined catastrophic threat and magical ideas that patients experience from certain fantasies and conflicts are diminished. Symptoms are reduced as patients become more aware of their wishes and more able to express them effectively. As a result of this process, social situations become less threatening.

In addition, patients' intense self-criticism can be modified by the internalization of more soothing attitudes. From the perspective of the self psychological model (24), one branch of psychoanalytic theory, patients with anxiety disorders lack a capacity for self-soothing, and their internal perceptions of self and others are often tinged with hostility and rejection. The lack of the capacity to soothe oneself is believed to develop from parenting that is traumatically unempathic to children's emotional needs. From the self-psychological viewpoint, patients' perceptions of parents as humiliating, rejecting, and abandoning represent actual empathic failures of parents. The experience of therapy, with the nonjudgmental and empathic support of the therapist, can aid in the development of self-soothing capacities and allow patients to internalize more benign or supportive representations of themselves and others, thereby diminishing the perceived danger of social interactions.

In order to elicit fantasies and conflicts, therapists must maintain an open-ended and exploratory stance. The therapist does not directly instruct the patient to confront feared situations, as this may disrupt a clear view of the development of the transference. *Transference* refers to the phenomenon in which emotional reactions, fantasies, and conflicts that originated with childhood relationships are unconsciously focused on current relationships (25). Transference articulation by the therapist is crucial in elucidating the underlying significance of the specific fantasy nature of the social phobic threat. As this psychodynamic exploration leads to a reduction in fears, the patient ultimately becomes more curious about confronting previously avoided situations.

B. Exploring Unconscious Fantasies and Conflicts

The unconscious fantasies and conflicts underlying social anxiety disorder can be brought to the surface by exploring the emotional meanings of specific symptoms, the stressors surrounding symptom onset or exacerbation, the patient's developmental history, and fantasies and feelings that develop with and about the therapist.

1. Emotional Meanings of Symptoms

Although patients with social anxiety disorder meet the phenomenological set of standardized criteria outlined in the DSM IV-R (3), the symptoms of any given individual patient have unique aspects. Thus, the therapist explores specific symptoms in detail to aid in determining emotional meanings, fantasies, and conflicts that the symptom represents.

2. Stressors Surrounding Symptom Onset

In addition, stressors surrounding symptom onset are identified for their relationship to underlying psychological meanings and conflicts.

For example, one socially anxious patient began to experience near panic levels of anxiety as he took on a leadership role at his office and had to make more presentations to colleagues. Initially it emerged that the patient felt he would be attacked or humiliated by others for expressing power and competence in his new role. Subsequently, therapist and patient discovered that the presentations represented the realization of his conflicted exhibitionistic wishes to be admired and to be the center of attention. The intense anxiety signaled the catastrophic alarm these exhibitionistic fantasies triggered and also punished him for the expression of these wishes.

3. Developmental Factors

Developmental factors are explored to ascertain a sense of the milieu in which precursor conflicts or early symptoms, if present, originated. The patient's perceptions of early caretakers' behavior and attitudes and family interrelationships are highly relevant in this regard.

The patient mentioned above described his mother as overprotective and threatened by any assertive behavior he evinced. He began to see any demonstrations of aggression or capability as dangerous. This formed a component of his fear that his promotion and speaking opportunities were somehow too dangerous to himself and others.

4. Exploring the Transference

Working with patients' experience of the therapist reveals significant aspects of the conflicts and fantasies underlying the symptoms. For example, people with social phobia often fear that they will be criticized or rejected by the therapist in a similar way to what they perceived in childhood or they anticipate will occur in other social situations (8). Fears of humiliation or ridicule may cause patients to miss sessions or even to leave treatment. Addressing expectations of criticism and feelings of inadequacy experienced in the transference, therapists can point out that patients' views of how others see them may be misperceptions and may not correspond to the actual attitudes of others.

C. Addressing Conflicted Feelings and Fantasies

An important component of therapy is helping patients to become aware of their anger and angry fantasies more tolerant of them, and more able to express them. Because of the inherent danger these patients experience about self-assertion of any kind, rage is often experienced as disorganizing and threatening, and patients often deny these feelings. However, such anger frequently emerges as treatment progresses. Kaplan (9) noted that "the shy patient has lively impulses of derogation and disdain which arise toward others with intense self-righteousness" (p. 442). In psychotherapy, these feelings invariably occur in relation to the therapist, providing an opportunity for exploration in an atmosphere of greater safety.

Grandiose fantasies are often important phenomenological components in people with social phobia. Patients may be aware of having fantasies of grand power and being the center of attention but often do not connect the fantasies to their social anxiety or tend to minimize the importance of the fantasies, given their manifest feelings of inadequacy. The therapist can identify these fantasies as they emerge in the treatment and note their potential importance. The patient can be informed that grandiose fantasies form a guilty backdrop of high expectations that trigger recurrent disappointments.

For instance, one patient recurrently compared his fantasy of becoming a rock star, surrounded by acolytes, with the tepid reactions he usually received from others.

D. Countertransference

Psychodynamic psychotherapy emphasizes the importance of therapists becoming aware of their reactions to patients (26). Countertransference is sometimes defined more narrowly as therapists' often unconscious reactions to patients' transferences and, at other points, as the full range of therapists' reactions to patients. Being alert to countertransference helps therapists to avoid attitudes or behaviors that may be disruptive to the treatment. Awareness of emotional reactions and fantasies about patients can also provide information about patients' conflicts.

Therapists must be alert to feelings of criticism or frustration that may arise in working with social phobia patients. Frustration can be triggered by these patients' level of dependency and by their difficulty taking more autonomous steps to change their lives. Covert expression of critical feelings can lead to an enactment that can intensify patients' feelings of inadequacy. Patients may attempt to induce contempt in the therapist so as to confirm an expectation that they will be rejected, as they have felt in so many other situations, in response to central transference pressures to reenact core relationships. The experience of a nonjudgmental, helpful therapist is critical in modification of negative, tormenting self and object representations.

E. Combining Psychodynamic Psychotherapy with Other Treatment Approaches

Psychodynamic therapy can be employed in combination with cognitive-behavioral therapy and/or medication. Many psychodynamic psychotherapeutic interventions can be viewed as cognitive in that they highlight and comment upon the irrational nature of the patient's self-critical beliefs.

However, rather than being the central focus of treatment, these observations are used as tools toward understanding the origins and meanings of these beliefs. Behavioral interventions, such as encouraging a patient to enter a frightening social situation, can aid in exploring the unconscious fantasies that are triggered in that setting. Nonetheless, a purer form of dynamic treatment may be preferable for many patients, in which the therapist comments on the patient's reluctance to expose himself or herself to feared situations, thereby addressing the topic of the roots of the patient's avoidance rather than merely circumventing it with instructions from the therapist. Dangers of direct behavioral interventions include continuing passivity on the patient's part as well as passive negativism as an expression of transference rage. Medication can play an important adjunctive role in psychodynamic treatment of social anxiety disorder, particularly in more severe cases, where symptoms can overwhelm the patient's capacity for psychodynamic exploration and self-observation. As with other interventions, psychodynamic psychotherapists often explore the meaning of medications to the patient.

IV. CASE EXAMPLES

A. Ms. A

Ms. A, a 30-year-old nurse, was fearful of criticism by others in many situations. She felt that she was inadequate, that her shyness was evident to others, and that others would invariably be highly critical of her. In particular, she felt that others would reject her for her small stature, which she felt made her appear child-like. Due to her shyness and what she saw as physical flaws, she was certain that men would reject her. She frequently avoided parties and dates, assuming that she would be ignored or rejected.

Ms. A described her parents as pleasant but passive figures, not actively engaging in their children's lives or activities. Of foremost significance in Ms. A's experience of shyness is the fact that she was tormented over many years during childhood by an older sister, Sarah, who seemed to feel that it was necessary to "whip" the patient and her siblings "into shape." In the sister's view, she had to take over the role of the parents, who were ineffective. Sarah was harshly critical of the patient's capabilities, including both her social and academic skills. Ms. A saw no other possibility but to submit to her attacks. Attacks by her siblings and father on her mother, who was viewed as "spacey," intensified Ms. A's internal struggles. She felt sorry for her mother while at the same time furious with her for not defending herself.

Only over time did it emerge that Ms. A was highly critical of others. For example, Ms. A, who was strongly committed to her job, felt disdain for other nurses who she felt did not really care about their patients and could not wait until the workday was over. Ms. A had done very well academically, in part in response to her sister's constant pressure, and she was critical of others who were less well read and not intellectual. As her negative views emerged, Ms. A was surprised about their extent. The therapist noted that Ms. A wrote off most people with whom she could be involved in a relationship.

Additionally, it emerged that Ms. A felt very threatened by the idea of having power. This blocked her from viewing herself as successful, as she equated success with a damaging power. This included success in relationships and on the job, where Ms. A avoided promotion in subtle, self-destructive ways that kept her from moving into nursing management despite her hard work. In Ms. A's perception, power, as employed by her sister, could only be used in hurtful and damaging ways. Indeed, she was preoccupied by revenge fantasies toward Sarah and others whom she psychologically identified with her. In conjunction with these fantasies, she unconsciously identified with her sister, viewing herself as potentially abusive and sadistic toward others. In a compensatory effort to undo these fantasies, Ms. A found it safer to experience herself as inadequate and downtrodden and a protector of the downtrodden than as someone with power.

Conflicted exhibitionistic fantasies of controlling men through sexuality were also revealed. These fantasies, in which men would be tortured with longing for her while she was unresponsive, were conflated with Ms. A's feared sadistic wishes. Out of a fear of acting on these fantasies, she avoided meeting men and viewed herself as unattractive as a compensatory fantasy of inadequacy to protect against these dangerous and disorganizing fantasies of power and control.

An additional reduction in her self-contempt and social anxiety developed by further understanding of the history of problems with Sarah. It was important for the patient to be able to vent her anger and hurt at her sister and at her parents for not intervening. Ms. A identified herself with her mother, vulnerable to attacks by others in the family due to her inadequacy. She was particularly conflicted about this issue, since she was also disdainful of her mother, critical of the family's attitudes toward the mother, yet strongly influenced by them. Untangling of these mixed loyalties allowed for more assertive social behavior and reduction in social anxiety.

B. Mr. B

Mr. B, a 28-year-old physical therapist, presented with severe social anxiety disorder. He regularly avoided social situations, which left him somewhat alone and isolated. However, he was capable of being witty and charming when not anxious. He was frustrated with his profession, which he had pursued after giving up an acting career. Mr. B had had dreams of being a movie star and still felt disappointed and bereft that this did not work out.

As Mr. B's anxiety was explored, it emerged that he was as fearful about making inappropriate hostile remarks because he was worried about others rejecting him. For instance, Mr. B felt the urge to make a nasty remark about another person's clothes being "dorky" or to tell a pregnant woman "I hope the child doesn't look like you." He experienced a disruption in his conversation when these thoughts came to mind and was concerned that others might be aware of his hostile feelings.

Mr. B's mother had moved to another town with him when he was 12 years old, leaving his father behind. He was ridiculed in his new environment, where his accent and style were quite different from those of others. He also missed the support of his father, whom he rarely saw. Ultimately, his mother married a man whom he experienced as highly critical and humiliating. In Mr. B's view, his stepfather attacked every assertive effort the patient made, viewing them as reflecting poor judgment. When Mr. B pursued acting, his stepfather gave him constant lectures about how acting was not a practical choice.

Mr. B's mother ignored the stepfather's attacks. She also appeared to have mixed feelings about Mr. B's growing up, as she focused on his having enough to eat and supported him financially without considering that he should learn to handle his own financial affairs. Mr. B's fantasies of movie stardom in part related to feelings of specialness and entitlement he experienced with his mother. He was frequently disappointed when he did not receive the attention he hoped for from others, and anxiety was triggered by anticipation of these disappointments. Helping Mr. B to moderate his expectations in social situations and to become more aware of the impact of his grandiose fantasies helped to reduce his disappointment.

In addition, exhibitionistic wishes became conflicted because Mr. B anticipated punishment, such as that which he had received from his stepfather. Fears of humiliation also related to the teasing he underwent when he moved at age 12 and functioned as guilty self-punishment for his gratifying, forbidden fantasies. Thus Mr. B struggled between wishes to exhibit his talents alongside intense fears of "standing out," which would lead invariably to a panic attack. At the same time, he feared his own criticisms of others, which were found to be related to retaliatory wishes to humiliate others in ways that he had been humiliated. Exploring these wishes helped to diminish the anxiety he experienced from being assertive.

Exploration of the transference proved particularly valuable in relieving Mr. B's anxiety. Critical feelings toward the therapist—including the therapist's posture, office furniture, and clothing—were accepted and explored for their meaning in relation to the patient's experience of attack. Over time, Mr. B felt safer in revealing other talents, which were numerous, including building furniture, skiing, and surfing. He had viewed the revelation of these talents as "bragging" or potentially disturbing to the therapist. This included fears that the therapist would feel threatened by his abilities and attack or undermine him, as his stepfather had done. The ability to safely reveal his criticisms and his talents helped to diminish his social anxiety in other spheres.

V. CONCLUSION

Despite the lack of specific attention and systematic research in psychodynamic approaches to social anxiety disorder, psychodynamic treatment potentially has much to offer in treatment of this disorder. Unconscious, conflicted, angry, grandiose, and exhibitionistic fantasies, which are typically not explored in other treatments, are often important contributors to social anxiety. Understanding the relevance of developmental factors can give patients a greater sense of comprehension and control over their symptoms. Exploration of various aspects of the transference provides a valuable opportunity for relief of anxiety in the therapist-patient dyad, which frequently generalizes to other social settings. Given the significant impact of social anxiety disorder on psychosocial function, it is of value to continue to refine and assess psychodynamic approaches to this disorder.

REFERENCES

1. Wittchen HU, Fehm L. Epidemiology, patterns of comorbidity, and associated disabilities of social phobia. Psychiatr Clin North Am 2001; 24 (4): 617–641.
2. Wittchen HU, Beloch E. The impact of social phobia on quality of life. Int Clin Psychopharmacol 1996; 11 (suppl 3): 15–23.
3. American Psychiatric Association. Diagnostic and Statistical Manual of Mental Diseases, 4th ed. text revision. Washington, DC: American Psychiatric Association, 2000.
4. Milrod B, Busch F, Leon AC, Shapiro T, Aronson A, Roiphe J, Rudden M, Singer M, Goldman H, Richter D, Shear MK. Open trial of psychodynamic psychotherapy for panic disorder: a pilot study. Am J Psychiatry 2000; 157: 1878–1880.
5. Milrod BL, Busch FN, Leon AC, Aronson A, Roiphe J, Rudden M, Singer M, Shapiro T, Goldman H, Richter D, Shear MK. A pilot open trial of brief psychodynamic psychotherapy for panic disorder. J Psychother Pract Res 2001; 10: 239–245.
6. Wiborg IM, Dahl AA. Does brief psychodynamic psychotherapy reduce the relapse rate of panic disorder? Arch Gen Psychiatry 1996; 53: 689–694.

7. Fenichel O. The Psychoanalytic Theory of Neurosis. New York: Norton, 1945.
8. Gabbard GO. Psychodynamic Psychiatry in Clinical Practice, 3d ed. Washington, DC: American Psychiatric Press, 2000.
9. Kaplan DM. On shyness. Int J Psychoanal 1972; 53: 439–454.
10. Gabbard GO. Psychodynamics of panic disorder and social phobia. Bull Menninger Clin 1992; 56(2, suppl A): A3–A13.
11. Zerbe KJ. Uncharted waters: Psychodynamic considerations in the diagnosis and treatment of social phobia. Bull Menninger Clin 1994; 58(2, suppl A): A3–20.
12. Lipsitz JD, Marshall RD. Alternative psychotherapy approaches for social anxiety disorder. Psychiatr Clin North Am; 24: 817–829.
13. Breuer J, Freud S. Studies on hysteria (1895). In: Strachey J, trans and ed. Standard Edition of the Complete Psychological Works of Sigmund Freud. Vol. 2. London: Hogarth Press, 1955: 1–181.
14. Freud S. Inhibitions, symptoms and anxiety (1926). In: Strachey J, trans and ed. Standard Edition of the Complete Psychological Works of Sigmund Freud. Vol. 20. London: Hogarth Press, 1959: 77–174.
15. Shapiro T. The concept of unconscious fantasy. J Clin Psychoanal 1992; 1: 517–524.
16. Freud S. Formulations on the two principles of mental functioning (1911). In: Strachey J, trans and ed. Standard Edition of the Complete Psychological Works of Sigmund Freud, Vol 12. London: Hogarth Press, 1958: 213–226.
17. Kagan J, Reznick JS, Snidman N, Johnson MO, Gibbons J, Gersten M, Biederman J, Rosenbaum JF. Origins of panic disorder. In: Ballenger J, ed. Neurobiology of Panic Disorder. New York: Wiley, 1990: 71–87.
18. Rosenbaum JF, Biederman J, Hirshfeld DR, Bolduc EA, Chaloff J. Behavioral inhibition in children: a possible precursor to panic disorder or social phobia. J Clin Psychiatry 1991; 52(11 suppl): 5–9.
19. Biederman J, Rosenbaum JF, Hirshfeld DR, Faraone SV, Bolduc EA, Gersten M, Meminger SR, Kagan J, Snidman N, Reznick JS. Psychiatric correlates of behavioral inhibition in young children of parents with and without psychiatric disorders. Arch Gen Psychiatry 1990; 47: 21–26.
20. Rosenbaum JF, Biederman J, Hirshfeld DR, Bolduc EA, Faraone SJ, Kagan J, Snidman N, Reznick JS. Further evidence of an association between behavioral inhibition and anxiety disorders: results from a family study of children from a non-clinical sample. J Psychiatr Res 1991; 25: 49–65.
21. Kagan J, Reznick JS, Snidman N. Biological bases of childhood shyness. Science 1988; 240: 167–171.
22. Arrindell WA, Emmelkamp PMG, Monsma A, Brilman E. The role of perceived parental rearing practices in the aetiology of phobic disorder: A controlled study. Br J Psychiatry 1983; 143: 183–187.
23. Parker G. Reported parental characteristics of agoraphobics and social phobics. Br J Psychiatry 1979; 135: 555–560.
24. Kohut H. The Analysis of the Self. New York: International Universities Press, 1971.

25. Freud S. Fragment of an analysis of a case of hysteria (1905). In: Strachey J, trans and ed. Standard Edition of the Complete Psychological Works of Sigmund Freud. Vol. 7. London: Hogarth Press, 1953: 3–122.
26. Gabbard GO. Countertransference: the emerging common ground. Int J Psychoanal 1995; 76: 475–485.

17

Pharmacotherapy of Social Anxiety Disorder

Borwin Bandelow

University of Göttingen,
Göttingen, Germany

Dan J. Stein

University of Stellenbosch,
Cape Town, South Africa
and University of Florida,
Gainesville, Florida, U.S.A.

I. INTRODUCTION

It is only recently that medication has become viewed as an acceptable treatment for social anxiety disorder (SAD). At the time of the first drug trials for SAD in the 1980s, many clinicians believed that this condition was best conceptualized as a personality disorder and that pharmacological intervention was therefore inappropriate. Similarly, in a survey of laypersons, only 4% of respondents stated that psychopharmalogical drugs were a therapeutic option for SAD (Tables 1 and 2), while 68% believed that psychological interventions were helpful (1).

A range of findings have led to the current view that medication is useful in SAD. As detailed elsewhere in this volume, there is a growing awareness that SAD is a chronic and disabling disorder. Furthermore,

TABLE 1   Categories of Evidence[a]

↑	**A. Positive evidence** is based on: Two or more randomized double-blind studies showing superiority to placebo *and* One or more positive double-blind studies showing superiority to or equal efficacy as established comparator drug. In the case of existing negative studies (studies showing nonsuperiority to placebo or inferiority to comparator drug), these must be outweighed by at least two more positive studies. Studies must fulfill established methodological standards (e.g., standard diagnostic criteria, optimal sample sizes, adequate psychometric scales, adequate statistical methods, adequate comparator drug etc.).
(↑)	**B. Preliminary positive evidence** is based on: **B1.** one or more randomized double-blind study showing superiority to placebo *or* **B2.** one or more positive naturalistic open studies *or* **B3.** one or more positive case reports *and* No negative studies exist
↔	**C. Inconsistent results** Controlled positive studies are outweighed by an approximately equal number of negative studies
↓	**D. Negative evidence** The majority of controlled studies show nonsuperiority to placebo or inferiority to comparator drug
?	**E. Lack of evidence** Adequate studies proving efficacy or nonefficacy are lacking

[a]In Table 2, the categories of evidence for all recommended drugs are given. These recommendations are based on randomized, double-blind clinical studies published in peer-reviewed journals. Not all of the recommended drugs are licensed for these indications in every country.

comorbid disorders such as depression are common in SAD and are known to respond to medication (alcohol is commonly used as self-medication of SAD, but with obvious adverse consequences) (2). Clinical experience has demonstrated that the concern that pharmacological therapy would impact negatively on cognitive behavioral therapy (CBT) is not warranted (3). Most persuasively, however, a growing database of rigorous trials has demonstrated that specific pharmacological agents are effective and safe in the treatment of SAD. This review considers the pharmacotherapy of SAD from an evidence-based perspective, emphasizing data from randomized controlled trials but also considering open-label data (Tables 3 and 4). Data were extracted from the MEDLINE database and the Science Citation Index at Web of Science (ISI). A range of medications have now been studied, and additional considerations, such as side-effect profiles and drug interactions can be considered in choosing the optimal pharmacological agent for any particular patient. It should be noted that not all agents proven effective for SAD have been licensed in all countries, as local marketing factors often influence this process. Now that a number of agents are available for the treatment of SAD, one can expect that comparator trials

TABLE 2 Evidence for Pharmacological Treatment of Social Anxiety Disorder[a]

Treatment	Examples	Category of Evidence	Recommended Daily Dose for Adults
SSRI	Fluvoxamine	A	100–300 mg
	Paroxetine	A	20–50 mg
	Sertraline	A	50–150 mg
	Escitalopram	A	10–20 mg
SNRI	Venlafaxine	A	75–225 mg
RIMA	Moclobemide	A	300–600 mg
MAOI	Phenelzine	A	45–90 mg
Alpha$_2$-calcium channel modulator	Pregabalin	B1	150–600 mg
When other treatment strategies are not effective or not tolerated:			
Benzodiazepines	Clonazepam	B1	1.5–8 mg
Anticonvulsant	Gabapentin	B1	600–3600 mg
SSRI	Citalopram	B2	20–60 mg
Antipsychotic	Olanzapine	B2	5–10 mg
Anticonvulsant	Valproic acid	B2	500–2500 mg
Negative evidence			
SSRI	Fluoxetine	D	
Tricyclic antidepressant	Imipramine	D	
Beta blocker	Atenolol	D	
5-HT$_{1A}$ agonist	Buspirone	D	
5-HT$_{2A}$ blocker	Nefazodone	D	

[a] Categories of evidence are based only on efficacy without regard to other properties (e.g., side effects). See text for abbreviations; see Table 1 for categories of evidence.

TABLE 3 Randomized Controlled Studies in SAD, Sorted by Drug[a]

Authors	Ref.	Treatment, N Patients	Efficacy	Daily Dose
Turner et al., 1994	64	Exposure 26/21, Atenolol 24/21, placebo 21/20	Exposure > Atenolol = placebo	Atenolol 25–100 mg
Clark and Agras, 1991	58	Cognitive therapy + placebo 9/7, Cognitive therapy + Buspirone 8/8, Buspirone 9/7, placebo 8/7	Cognitive therapy > Buspirone = placebo	Buspirone 15–50 mg
van Vliet et al., 1992	40	Brofaromine[b] 15/15, placebo 15/14	Brofaromine > placebo	Brofaromine 50–150 mg
Fahlen et al., 1995	41	Brofaromine 37/29, placebo 40/35	Brofaromine > placebo	Brofaromine 150 mg
Lott et al., 1997	42	Brofaromine 52/38, placebo 50/33	Brofaromine > placebo	Brofaromine 50–150 mg
van Vliet et al., 1997	55	Buspirone 15/15 placebo15/12	Buspirone = placebo	Buspirone 30 mg
Davidson et al., 1993	47	Clonazepam 39/29, placebo 36/27	Clonazepam > placebo	Clonazepam 0,5–3 mg
Munjack et al., 1990	46	Clonazepam 12/10, Waiting list 11/10	Clonazepam > waiting list	Clonazepam 1–6 mg
Kasper et al., 2002	5	Escitalopram 181/145 placebo 177/145	Escitalopram > placebo	Escitalopram 10–20 mg
Montgomery et al., 2003	7	Escitalopram 190/126, placebo 181/80	Escitalopram > placebo	Escitalopram 10–20 mg
Lader et al., 2003	6	Escitalopram 504/365, paroxetine 169/123, placebo 166/116	Escitalopram = paroxetine > placebo	Escitalopram 5–20 mg, paroxetine 20 mg

Study		Sample sizes	Result	Drug/dose
van Vliet et al., 1994	8	Fluvoxamine 15/14, placebo 15/14	Fluvoxamine > placebo	Fluvoxamine 150 mg
Stein et al., 1999	95	Fluvoxamine 48/43, placebo 44/43	Fluvoxamine > placebo	Fluvoxamine 202 mg
Westenberg et al., 2003	10	Fluvoxamine 149/146, placebo 151/148	Fluvoxamine > placebo	Fluvoxamine 100–300 mg
Kobak et al., 2002	96	Fluoxetine 30, placebo 30	Fluoxetine = placebo	Fluoxetine 20–60 mg
Pande et al., 1999	69	Gabapentin 34/21, placebo 34/18	Gabapentin > placebo	Gabapentin 900–3600 mg
Versiani et al., 1992	35	Moclobemide 26/17, Phenelzine 26/20, placebo 26/7	Phenelzine = Moclobemide > placebo	Phenelzine 30–90 mg, Moclobemide 200–600 mg
IMCTGMSP, 1997	33	Moclobemide 384/?, placebo 194/?	Moclobemide > placebo	Moclobemide 300–600 mg
Noyes et al., 1997	37	Moclobemide 521, placebo 85	Moclobemide = placebo	Moclobemide 75–900 mg
Schneier et al., 1998	36	Moclobemide 40/33, placebo 37/32	Moclobemide = /> placebo	Moclobemide 300–600 mg
Stein et al., 2002	34	Moclobemide 191/188, placebo 193/189	Moclobemide > placebo	Moclobemide 300–600 mg
Van Ameringen, 2003	66	Nefazodone 52/36, placebo 52/46	Nefazodone = placebo	Nefazodone 300–600 mg
Barnett et al., 2002	65	Olanzapine 7/4, placebo 5/3	Olanzapine > placebo	Olanzapine 5–20 mg
Baldwin et al., 1999	12	Paroxetine 139/104, placebo 151/109	Paroxetine > placebo	Paroxetine 20–50 mg

(continued)

TABLE 3 (cont.)

Authors	Ref.	Treatment, N Patients	Efficacy	Daily Dose
Allgulander, 1999	13	Paroxetine 44/36, placebo 48/29	Paroxetine > placebo	Paroxetine 20–50 mg
Stein et al., 1998	11	Paroxetine 92/72, placebo 91/62	Paroxetine > placebo	Paroxetine 20–50 mg
Liebowitz et al., 2002	14	Paroxetine 289/175, placebo 95/67	Paroxetine > placebo	Paroxetine 20–60 mg
Liebowitz et al., 1988, 1992	63	Phenelzine 25/21, Atenolol 23/15, placebo 26/24	Phenelzine > Atenolol = placebo	Phenelzine 15–90 mg, Atenolol 50–100 mg
Heimberg et al., 1998	97	Phenelzine 31/26, placebo 33/27, Cognitive therapy 36/28, psychological placebo 33/26	Phenelzine > placebo Cognitive therapy > psychological placebo; phenelzine > cognitive therapy	Phenelzine 15–90 mg
Gelernter et al., 1991	50	Cognitive therapy + self-exposure 20/17, Phenelzine + self-exposure 15/13, Alprazolam + self-exposure 15/14, placebo + self-exposure 15/15	Cognitive therapy + self-exposure = phenelzine + self-exposure = alprazolam + self-exposure = placebo + self-exposure	Phenelzine 30–90 mg, Alprazolam 2,1–6,3 mg
Feltner et al., 2000	53	Pregabalin 89, placebo 46	Pregabalin > placebo	Pregabalin 150–600 mg
Falloon et al., 1981	98	Exposure + Propranolol 8/6, Exposure + placebo 8/6	Exposure + propranolol = Exposure + placebo	Propranolol 160–320 mg
Katzelnick et al., 1995	15	Sertraline, placebo crossover 12/11	Sertraline > placebo	Sertraline 50–200 mg

Blomhoff et al., 2001	17	Sertraline 96/87, Sertraline + Exposure 98/88, Exposure + placebo 98/91, placebo 95/88	Sertraline + exposure = Sertraline > placebo; Exposure + placebo = placebo	Sertraline 50–150 mg
Van Ameringen et al., 2001	16	Sertraline 135/104, placebo 69/54	Sertraline > placebo	Sertraline 50–200 mg
Liebowitz et al., 2003	18	Sertraline 205/152, placebo 196/141	Sertraline > placebo	Sertraline 50–200 mg
Liebowitz and Mangano, 2002	99	Venlafaxine 133/88, placebo 138/85	Venlafaxine > placebo	Venlafaxine 75–225 mg
Stein and Mangano, 2003	30	Venlafaxine 277/124, placebo 129/44	Venlafaxine > placebo	Venlafaxine 75–225 mg
Liebowitz et al., 2003	100	Venlafaxine 144/122, paroxetine 144/122 placebo 146/119	Venlafaxine = paroxetine > placebo	Venlafaxine 75–225 mg, paroxetine 20–50 mg
Liebowitz et al., 2003	100	Venlafaxine 141/103, paroxetine 142/102 placebo 146/113	Venlafaxine = paroxetine placebo	Venlafaxine 75–225 mg, paroxetine 20–50 mg

[a]Explanation: "Clonazepam 39/29": 39 patients were included and 29 were evaluable. "clonazepam > placebo": clonazepam was significantly more effective than placebo.
[b]Brofaromine has been withdrawn from development.

will be undertaken and will further contribute to optimal decision making in this area.

II. INDICATION FOR TREATMENT

Treatment is indicated for most patients who fulfill the criteria for SAD of the tenth edition of the *International Classification of Diseases* (ICD-10) or the fourth edition of the *Diagnostic and Statistical Manual of Mental*

TABLE 4   Open Studies in SAD[a]

Authors	Ref.	Treatment, N Patients	At Least Very Much or Much Improved	Daily Dose
Reich and Yates, 1988	101	Alprazolam 16/14	88%	1–7 mg
Gorman et al., 1985	62	Atenolol 10/10	81%	50–100 mg
Emmanuel et al., 2000	67	Bupropion 15/10	50%	200–400 mg
Munjack et al., 1991	56	Buspirone 16/11	81%	10–60 mg
Schneier et al., 1993	57	Buspirone 21/17	47%	15–60 mg
Bouwer and Stein, 1998	19	Citalopram 22/22	86%	40 mg
Atmaca et al., 2002	20	Citalopram 36/36, moclobemide 35/35	Citalopram 75% Moclobemide 74%	Citalopram 20–60 Moclobemide 300–900
Reiter et al., 1990	102	Clonazepam 11/11	81%	0.75–3 mg
Black et al., 1992	21	Fluoxetine 14/14	71%	20–80 mg
Van Ameringen et al., 1993	22	Fluoxetine 16/13	63%	20–60 mg
DeVane et al., 1999	103	Fluvoxamine 15/10	52% reduction of BFBS[b] in completers	50–150 mg
Simpson et al., 1998	54	Imipramine 15/9	42%	50–300 mg
Bisserbe and Lépine, 1994	38	Moclobemide 35/18	45%	300–600 mg
Liebowitz et al., 1986	104	Phenelzine 11/11	100%	30–90 mg
Simpson et al., 1998	68	Selegiline 10/10	33%	
Kinrys et al., 2003	70	Valproic acid	41%	500–2500 mg
Kelsey, 1995	32	Venlafaxine 9/9	81%	75–300 mg
Versiani et al., 1988	44	Tranylcypromine 32/29	79%	40–60

[a]Explanation: "Alprazolam 16/14": 16 patients were included and 14 were evaluable.
[b]Brief Social Phobia Rating Scale.

Diseases (DSM-IV). The treatment plan should be based on the patient's preference, severity of illness, psychiatric comorbidity, concomitant medical illnesses, complications like suicide risk, and the history of previous treatments. In most health systems, costs of treatment also need to be considered. The goals of drug treatment are to target relevant symptom domains, including socially mediated anxiety symptoms and panic attacks, anticipatory anxiety, cognitive misperceptions, avoidance behavior, and comorbid conditions such as depression. There is growing awareness of the importance of obtaining symptom remission rather than merely response.

Before drug treatment is initiated, the mechanisms underlying psychic and somatic anxiety should be explained to the patient. Cooperation with drug treatment can be improved when the advantages and disadvantages of the drug, such as the delayed onset of effect or common side effects, are explained carefully to the patient before treatment. Patients with SAD are particularly sensitive to some side effects—such as initial jitteriness, nervousness, or insomnia—or they may sometimes express groundless or exaggerated fears of the side effects of psychopharmacological drugs (e.g., addiction), even if the drugs are known not to have any potential for addiction.

III. AVAILABLE AGENTS

This section reviews controlled studies (Table 3) and open studies (Table 4), before considering the advantages and disadvantages of the different classes of drugs (Table 5). Specific details of particular agents are not provided here but are readily obtainable from the relevant literature (4).

A. Selective Serotonin Reuptake Inhibitors (SSRIs)

The efficacy of the SSRIs in SAD has been demonstrated in a number of controlled studies. The anxiolytic effect may start with a latency of 2 to 6 weeks (although in some cases efficacy is seen only between weeks 8 and 12). To avoid overstimulation and insomnia, doses should be given in the morning and at midday.

1. Mechanism of Action

Although the exact mechanism by which selective serotonin reuptake inhibitors exhibit their anxiolytic properties is unknown, it is believed that, because they inhibit serotonin reuptake transport into the presynaptic cell, more serotonin is available in the synaptic cleft, thus enhancing serotonergic neurotransmission. Serotonergic neurons from the raphe nuclei can be assumed to inhibit pathological arousal in specific areas of the brain responsible for anxiety symptoms.

TABLE 5 Advantages and Disadvantages of Psychopharmacological Drugs in SAD

Substance	Advantages	Disadvantages

SSRI	No dependency
	Sufficient evidence from
	  clinical studies
	Relatively safe in overdose
		Latency of effect 2–6 weeks
		  or longer; initial jitteriness,
		  nausea, restlessness, sexual
		  dysfunctions and other
		  side effects

SSNRI
  venlafaxine
	No dependency
	Sufficient evidence from
	  clinical studies
	Relatively safe in overdose
		Latency of effect 2–6 weeks
		  or longer; nausea and other
		  side effects

Moclobemide	No dependency
	Benign side effect profile;
	  relatively safe in overdose
		Latency of effect 2–6 weeks
		  or longer; inconsistent study
		  results in SAD, no efficacy
		  proofs for other anxiety
		  disorders

Phenelzine	No dependency
	Sufficient evidence from
	  clinical studies
		Latency of effect 2–6 weeks
		  or longer; serious side effects
		  and interactions possible

Benzodiazepines	Fast onset of action
	Few clinical studies available
	Relatively safe in overdose
		Dependency possible;
		  sedation, slow reaction time
		  and other side effects

Pregabalin (only
  preliminary
  data)
	Fast onset of action
	No dependency
		Side effects: dizziness,
		  somnolence and others

Key: SSRI, selective serotonin reuptake inhibitor; SSNRI, selective serotonin noradrenaline reuptake inhibitor.

2. Clinical Studies

Escitalopram (5–7), fluvoxamine (8–10), paroxetine (11–14), and sertraline (15–18) have all been shown to be effective in double-blind, placebo-controlled studies of SAD. Citalopram showed positive results in two open studies (19,20). Although small open-label trials of fluoxetine have suggested potential efficacy in social anxiety disorder (21,22), fluoxetine failed to separate from placebo in a controlled trial with 60 patients (23).

3. Dosing

Recommended dosages are given in Table 2. SSRIs have a relatively flat response curve—i.e., approximately 75% of patients respond to the initial (low) dose. In some patients, treatment may be started with half the recommended dose in order to reduce side effects. There are relatively few fixed-dose studies of SSRIs in SAD. In a study of paroxetine 20, 40, or 60 mg versus placebo, a linear dose-response curve was not seen, with efficacy of the different dosage groups depending in part on the rating scale used (14).

4. Side Effects

Restlessness, jitteriness, an increase in anxiety symptoms, and insomnia in the first days or weeks of treatment may hamper compliance with treatment. In particular, patients with anxiety disorders can be sensitive to the side effects of antidepressants and may discontinue treatment because of initial discomfort. Lowering the starting dose of an SSRI may reduce this over-stimulation. Other side effects that occur predominantly in the first 2 to 3 weeks of treatment include headache, nausea, diarrhea, and sweating. Later on, both weight loss and weight gain (perhaps particularly with par-oxetine) can be seen (24,25). Sexual dysfunction may also be a problem during long-term treatment with SSRIs. Finally, discontinuation syndromes have been observed during tapering of medication (26,27). In general, however, the side-effect profiles of SSRIs are relatively benign.

5. Contraindications

SSRIs must be used with caution in patients with epilepsy, although these drugs have less propensity to lower the seizure threshold than other anti-depressants (28). Patients with severe liver impairment, diabetes, heart failure, and respiratory depression should also be treated with caution.

6. Interactions

Most SSRI interactions are due to competition in the cytochrome P450 system. Fluvoxamine and fluoxetine are more likely than other SSRIs to produce interactions in this system. The combination of SSRIs and irre-versible monoamine oxidase inhibitors may result in a serotonin syndrome, and should be avoided.

B. Selective Serotonin Noradrenaline Reuptake Inhibitor (SSNRI) Venlafaxine

The efficacy of the antidepressant venlafaxine, a selective serotonin noadrenaline reuptake inhibitor, in SAD has been shown in a number of controlled studies. The antianxiety effect may occur with a latency of 2 to 4 weeks or longer.

1. Clinical Studies

A short-term and a long-term study with venlafaxine showed superiority over placebo. One was a 12-week study (29); the other was a long-term study over 28 weeks (30).

Two other studies compared venlafaxine with paroxetine and placebo (31). Venlafaxine was superior to placebo, and the average reduction of the Liebowitz Social Anxiety Scale (LSAS) scores was similar in the venlafaxine and paroxetine group. These findings confirm early promising open studies of venlafaxine (32,33).

2. Dosing

Recommended dosages are given in Table 2.

3. Side Effects

The side-effect profile of venlafaxine is similar to that of the SSRIs. At the beginning of treatment, side effects like nausea, dry mouth, sweating, restlessness, or insomnia may occur and hamper compliance with treatment. In general, the extended-release formulation of the drug is recommended in order to reduce side effects.

Other adverse events include loss of appetite, fatigue, headache, gastrointestinal complaints, sweating, constipation, hypertension, hypotension, dizziness, tachycardia, palpitations, and withdrawal symptoms similar to those seen with the SSRIs.

4. Contraindications and Precautions

Patients with severe liver or kidney dysfunction, epilepsy, diabetes, cardiac or respiratory insufficiency, myocardial infarction, and hypertension should be treated with caution.

5. Interactions

Venlafaxine should not be combined with irreversible monoamine oxidase inhibitors (MAOIs). Coadministration with the selective MAOIs moclobemide or selegiline may increase noradrenergic or serotonergic effects.

C. Reversible Inhibitor of Monoamine Oxidase A (RIMA) Moclobemide

Moclobemide is not available in the United States but is obtainable in Canada and many other countries. It is a reversible inhibitor of monoamine oxidase A. Brofaromine is a RIMA and serotonin reuptake inhibitor that, despite early promising data, was not brought to market.

1. Mechanism of Action

The enzyme monoamine oxidase (MAO) metabolizes serotonin to 5-hydroxy-indoleacetic acid (5-HIAA). Drugs that inhibit this enzyme reduce the metabolization of neurotransmitter, thus increasing the amount of serotonin in the synaptic cleft. There are two forms of MAO, A and B. Moclobemide is a selective inhibitor of MAO_A. Thus there is still enough MAO_B left to metabolize tyramine. Unlike the nonselective MAOIs, moclobemide does not cause the potentially dangerous "cheese effect" when taken together with tyramine, which is found in various food products (such as certain cheeses).

2. Clinical Studies

Although the majority of studies of moclobemide have been positive, the data have been somewhat inconsistent. The compound was superior to placebo in two studies (33,34) and also more effective than placebo and as effective as phenelzine on most measures in a third study (35). In a fourth study, the size of its clinical effect was small (36), and in a fifth study (37), no superiority against placebo could be demonstrated. Open studies have similarly shown mixed results (20,38).

Frequently, SAD is comorbid with other anxiety disorders. In one study (34), patients with SAD with or without comorbid other anxiety disorders were investigated. Superiority of medication over placebo was similar in patients with and without comorbid anxiety disorders as well as in patients with different subtypes of SAD. Nevertheless, given the inconsistent data on moclobemide, it is not surpising that effect sizes for efficacy of this agent are smaller than those seen with SSRIs (39).

Three trials with brofaromine in social phobia showed superiority over placebo (40–42).

3. Dosing

Moclobemide is prescribed at a dose of 300 to 600 mg/day or higher. Higher doses should be used as these are not associated with substantially more side effects, and improvement is seen more often than at lower doses. To avoid overstimulation and insomnia, doses should be given in the morning and at midday.

4. Side Effects

The side-effect profile of moclobemide is benign and includes agitation, insomnia, dry mouth, headache, dizziness, gastroinstestinal complaints, and nausea.

5. Contraindications

Moclobemide should be used with caution in patients with severe liver dysfunction. The strict precautions that have to be followed when using irreversible nonselective MAOIs do not apply to moclobemide. However, in unusually high doses, MAO inhibition may be less selective.

6. Interactions

Moclobemide should not be used together with selegeline, a selective MAO_B inhibitor. In combination with L-tryptophan, a serotonin syndrome may occur. The combination with opioids should also be avoided. Increased serotonergic effects may occur when moclobemide is combined with other antidepressants or triptans. Antiarhythmics may increase moclobemide plasma levels. Combination with sympathomimetics may lead to hypertensive crises.

Treatment with moclobemide does not require a special diet.

D. Irreversible Monoamine Oxidase Inhibitors

The efficacy of the irreversible, nonselective MAOI phenelzine in SAD has been shown in a number of controlled studies. Phenelzine is not available in some countries, but controlled data with other MAOIs, such as tranylcypromine, are lacking.

1. Mechanism of Action

The MAOIs phenelzine and tranylcypromine are nonselective—i.e., they affect both MAO_A and MAO_B. Also, the inhibition of MAO is "irreversible"— i.e., the effect lasts for 1 or 2 weeks. Therefore these drugs have a high liability for producing unwanted side effects and interactions. Phenelzine may also increase brain levels of GABA (43).

2. Clinical Studies

Early work suggested that phenelzine was associated with a high response rate (35). Controlled studies comparing phenelzine to placebo and to moclobemide (27) and atenolol (33,34) confirmed its efficacy. However, phenelzine was less well tolerated than moclobemide (35). In an open study over one year, tranylcypromine was associated with continued improvement of SAD; however, side effects were frequent (44).

3. Dosing

Recommended dosages are provided in Table 2.

4. Side Effects

Irreversible MAOIs are generally less well tolerated than modern antidepressants. Side effects may include dizziness, headache, agitation, anxiety, tremor, sweating, sleep disorders, orthostatic hypotension, and hypertensive crises with agitation, hypertension, or intracerebral hemorrhage. Because of the possibility of severe side effects and interactions with other drugs or food components, phenelzine and tranylcypromine are not considered first-line drugs and should be used only by experienced psychiatrists when other treatment modalities have been unsuccessful or have not been tolerated. To avoid overstimulation and insomnia, doses should be given in the morning and at midday.

5. Contraindications and Precautions

Patients with diabetes, epilepsy, hypertension, or hyperthyroidism should be treated with caution.

6. Interactions

Due to their possibly dangerous interactions with a number of drugs, irreversible MAOIs are considered only as third line drugs in SAD. During treatment with MAOIs, patients must avoid tyramine-containing food products.

E. Benzodiazepines

The efficacy of benzodiazepines in SAD has been shown in only a few studies. Given that patents have expired for the available benzodiazepines, this may partly reflect a lack of industry interest in sponsoring relevant trials.

One advantage of the benzodiazepines is the immediate onset of anxiolytic effect after oral or parenteral administration. In contrast to antidepressants, they do not lead to initially increased nervousness.

In general, the benzodiazepines have a good record of safety. Due to the possibility of addiction, treatment with benzodiazepines requires a careful weighing of risks and benefits. In particular, in patients in whom other treatment modalities were not effective or were not tolerated due to side effects, treatment with benzodiazepines may be justified. Patients with a history of benzodiazepine abuse should be excluded from treatment. Benzodiazepines may also be used in combination with antidepressants during the first weeks before the onset of efficacy of the antidepressants (45).

Benzodiazepines may be used in the "as needed" treatment of short-term distress (e.g., exams). When treating comorbid anxiety disorders, one should be aware that benzodiazepines do not treat some comorbid conditions, such as depression or obsessive-compulsive disorder.

1. Clinical Studies

Controlled studies have demonstrated that the benzodiazepine clonazepam was superior to placebo or a waiting list condition, respectively (46,47). After a 6-month open trial, a 5-month extension study with placebo controlled tapering suggested maintained efficacy and declining dosage during long-term clonazepam treatment, increased relapse during switch to placebo, and a lack of significant problems during slow taper (48,49). A study by Gelernter et al. (50) did not detect a significant difference between alprazolam and placebo, but this may have reflected the fact that all subjects also received exposure instructions.

2. Dosing

Benzodiazepine doses should be as low as possible to avoid side effects but as high as necessary to achieve a complete treatment result.

3. Side Effects

Benzodiazepine treatment may be associated with sedation, dizziness, prolonged reaction time and other side effects. Cognitive functions and driving skills may be affected. After long-term treatment with benzodiazepines (e.g., over 4 to 8 months), dependency may occur in some patients, especially in predisposed patients. Withdrawal reactions have their peak severity at 2 days for short-half-life and 4 to 7 days for long-half-life benzodiazepines (51). It is claimed that prolonged withdrawal reactions may occasionally occur. Tolerance seems to be rare (52).

F. Pregabalin

The anticonvulsant pregabalin has no activity at the GABA receptor. It appears to bind at the $alpha_2$ subunit of the voltage-dependent calcium channels. In recent years, this drug has been investigated in a number of indications.

1. Clinical Studies

In a double-blind, placebo-controlled study, patients in the pregabalin group had a significant reduction in SAD symptoms as compared to the placebo group (53). Data from additional studies have not yet been reported.

2. Side Effects

The most frequent adverse events reported for pregabalin are somnolence and dizziness. Other side effects include weight gain, asthenia, headache, nausea, ataxia, confusion, and amblyopia.

G. Tricyclic Antidepressants (TCAs)

TCAs have not been studied in controlled trials in patients with SAD. The only existing open trial with imipramine was disappointing. However, it would be premature to conclude from this single study that tricyclics are not effective in SAD. Given the proven efficacy of tricyclic antidepressants, particularly the serotonergic tricyclic clomipramine, in other anxiety disorders, such agents may be a treatment option for otherwise treatment-refractory cases.

The dosage should be titrated up slowly until dosage levels as high as in the treatment of depression are reached. Patients should be informed that the onset of the anxiolytic effect of the drug may have a latency of at least 2 to 4 weeks.

1. Clinical Studies

There is only one open study using TCAs in SAD. In this 8-week open trial, 15 patients received imipramine. Of these, 9 patients completed the trial; 6 dropped out early because of adverse effects. The overall response rate [based on the Clinical Global Impression Scale of Improvement (CGI-I) of "very much" or "much improved"] was 20 and 22%, respectively. The reductions in the Liebowitz Social Anxiety Scale (LSAS) were only modest (54).

2. Side Effects

Especially at the beginning of treatment, compliance may be hampered by adverse effects such as initially increased anxiety, dry mouth, postural hypotension, tachycardia, sedation, and impaired psychomotor function. Weight gain and sexual dysfunction may be a problem during long-term treatment. In general, the frequency of adverse events is higher for TCAs than for newer antidepressants, such as the selective serotonin reuptake inhibitors (SSRIs) or selective serotonin noradrenaline reuptake inhibitors (SSNRIs).

G. 5-HT$_{1A}$ Agonist Buspirone

The 5-HT$_{1A}$ agonist buspirone is effective in generalized anxiety, but the results of a double-blind study do not support the efficacy of buspirone in SAD (55). Open studies had mixed results (56,57).

According to a placebo-controlled study by Clark and Agras (58), buspirone was not effective in treating performance anxiety in musicians.

H. Beta Blockers

Because beta blockers may influence autonomic anxiety symptoms such as palpitations, tremor, etc., they have been used in the treatment of anxiety disorders.

Beta blockers have been shown to improve peripheral symptoms in musicians with performance anxiety. Oxprenolol (59), pindolol (60), and nadolol (61) showed beneficial effects on peripheral but not central anxiety symptoms. Although the available studies did not demonstrate clear effects on performance anxiety, beta blockers have become widely used for this purpose. The findings obtained with musicians with performance anxiety should not be generalized to SAD.

Although an open study suggested benefits of atenolol (62), available double-blind studies were not able to show efficacy of this beta blocker in SAD (63,64).

I. Neuroleptics

In a number of European countries, neuroleptics have been widely used to treat anxiety disorders. High- or low-potency neuroleptics have been prescribed in lower doses than are used in the treatment of schizophrenia. Nevertheless, studies conducted with neuroleptics in the 1970s and 1980s in patients suffering from "anxiety neuroses" had methodological flaws, and there is little evidence for their value from more recent studies. Indeed, there are reports of increased social anxiety secondary to administration of antipsychotic agents. Moreover, the risk of irreversible tardive dyskinesia is an important concern when these agents are prescribed for nonpsychotic disorders.

Newer-generation antipsychotics, however, have a lower liability for extrapyramidal symptoms and tardive dyskinesia. Therefore, investigation of the role of these compounds in anxiety disorders may be warranted. Newer neurobiological findings have associated SAD with a dysfunction of dopamine systems (this volume, chapter by van Ameringen and Mancini). It would be interesting to determine whether new-generation antipsychotics are effective in SAD. In a first small pilot study with 12 patients, olanzapine was shown to be superior to placebo (65).

J. Homeopathic and Herbal Preparations

In some countries, herbal preparations such as St. John's wort, kava-kava* (*Piper methysticum*), or valerian are being used widely in the treatment of anxiety disorders. Sufficient proof of efficacy is not available for these preparations.

In addition, there is no proof of efficacy for the treatment of SAD with any homeopathic preparations.

Initial improvement with these compounds may be due to placebo effects, spontaneous remission, or the tendency of regression to the mean. Herbal and homeopathic preparations are sometimes used in the hope that

---

*Kava-kava products have been associated with hepatotoxicity; therefore, the license for their sale has been withdrawn in some countries.

advantage can be taken of these nonspecific effects and that adverse events can be minimized. However, placebo effects are usually not long-lasting, and a recurrence or deterioration of the symptomatology may result in loss of confidence in the physician. Also, these preparations often have not undergone a safety evaluation similar to the one required for other drugs. Indeed, the prescription of these compounds may result in considerable costs for the health system.

K. Other Compounds

Nefazodone, a blocker of postsynaptic serotonin 5-HT_{2A} receptors and an inhibitor of serotonin and noradrenaline reuptake, was studied in a placebo-controlled trial with 104 patients (66). There was no statistical difference between the groups regarding the CGI-I or LSAS scores. In an open-label trial with bupropion, a noradrenaline-dopamine reuptake inhibitor, 5 of 10 patients improved (67).

In an open trial of selegiline, a selective inhibitor of MAO_B in a small group of patients with social phobia, there was only a 33% response rate (68). This does not, however, rule out the possibility that this agent might be effective at higher, nonselective doses.

The anticonvulsant gabapentin acts to increase central gamma-aminobutyric acid (GABA), the principal inhibitory neurotransmitter in the brain. It also has activity at voltage-sensitive sodium and calcium channels. In a double-blind, placebo-controlled, 14-week study in patients with SAD, gabapentin was superior to placebo. Gabapentin was dosed flexibly between 900 and 3600 mg daily in three divided doses. Adverse events were consistent with the known side-effect profile of gabapentin. Dizziness, dry mouth, somnolence, nausea, flatulence, and decreased libido occurred at a higher frequency among patients receiving gabapentin than among those receiving placebo (69). In a small open study, the anticonvulsant valproic acid showed a moderate response rate in patients with SAD (70). Clonidine was successful according to a single-case report (71).

IV. ADVANTAGES AND DISADVANTAGES
OF ANTIANXIETY DRUGS

None of the available drug treatments for SAD can be seen as ideal for every patient. In Table 5, risks and benefits of the available compounds are reviewed. Treatments should be chosen individually for each patient. Medication costs may also have to be taken into account. Usually, the prices of newer drugs are relatively high.

V. LONG-TERM TREATMENT

A number of controlled long-term studies exist for the treatment of SAD. Two relapse-prevention studies have demonstrated the long-term efficacy of SSRIs. Following a 20-week double-blind, placebo-controlled study (16) in which the superiority of sertraline over placebo was demonstrated, 50 patients who were rated much or very much improved on the CGI-I were randomly assigned to either continue double-blind treatment with sertraline or immediately switch to placebo for another 24 weeks (72). A total of 15 responders to placebo also continued to receive double-blind placebo treatment in the continuation study. Only 1 of 25 patients in the sertraline-continuation group, but 9 (36%) of 25 patients in the placebo-switch group had relapsed at study endpoint.

In a 24-week double-blind study that examined the efficacy of sertraline or exposure therapy administered alone or in combination, sertraline was found to be superior to placebo (17).

In the extension of a 12-week single-blind treatment study with paroxetine, responders were randomized to a further 24 weeks of paroxetine or placebo. Relapse rates were significantly lower in the paroxetine group (73).

The efficacy of escitalopram in the relapse prevention of SAD was shown in a 24-week, double-blind comparison and placebo study that followed a 12 week open-label treatment period with escitalopram (7).

In a 24-week study, both phenelzine and moclobemide were superior to placebo (35). In a double-blind study comparing moclobemide and placebo (34), patients had the option of continuing for an additional 6 months of treatment. In the extension phase, response rates remained higher in the moclobemide group, and ratings of tolerability were equally high in both groups.

The efficacy and safety of venlafaxine were demonstrated in a 28-week study (30).

VI. GENERALIZED VERSUS NONGENERALIZED SAD

The DSM-IV includes the specifier *generalized* to refer to SAD patients if the fears include "most social situations." As most patients included in SAD trials belong to the generalized subgroup, it is interesting to know whether these findings can also be applied to the nongeneralized type. To compare response of more generalized and less generalized SAD to pharmacotherapy (74), pooled data from three randomized placebo-controlled double-blind multicenter trials of the SSRI paroxetine in SAD were analyzed. There were no significant differences in response in the patients with more generalized as compared to those with less generalized SAD.

VII. TREATMENT RESISTANCE

There are few data to guide treatments recommendations for nonresponders to a standard pharmacotherapy for SAD. Nevertheless, some general principles can be formulated.

Before considering a patient to be treatment-resistant, it should be ascertained whether the diagnosis is correct, the patient is compliant with therapy, the dosage prescribed is therapeutic, and the trial period has been adequate. Concurrent prescription drugs may interfere with efficacy—e.g., metabolic enhancers or inhibitors. Psychosocial factors may affect response, and comorbid personality disorders may lead to poor outcome. Depression and substance abuse are especially likely to complicate anxiety disorders. Psychological treatments such as cognitive behavioral therapy must be considered.

Before a medication trial is considered as a failure, a treatment period of at least 6 to 8 weeks or longer at adequate doses is required. An analysis of the paroxetine database showed that a number of nonresponders at 8 weeks responded by 12 weeks. The trial period should perhaps be extended in the case of a partial response. Elderly patients may take longer to show a response.

Although "switching studies" are lacking, many treatment-resistant patients are reported to respond when a different class of antidepressants is tried (e.g., switching from an SSRI to moclobemide or vice versa). Open-label work has suggested that venlafaxine may be effective when SSRIs have failed (31).

There are few controlled studies of treatment-refractory SAD patients. In a double-blind, placebo-controlled, crossover design, 14 patients with generalized SAD who were less than "very much improved" on the CGI-I after at least 10 weeks of treatment with a maximally tolerated dose of paroxetine, either 5 mg of pindolol, t.i.d., or placebo was added to a steady paroxetine dose. However, pindolol was no more effective than placebo in augmenting the effects of SSRI treatment for generalized SAD (75). An open-label study has suggested that buspirone augmentation may be a useful clinical strategy in SAD patients who show a partial response to an SSRI (76).

VIII. DURATION OF DRUG TREATMENT

In most cases, SAD is a chronic disorder, albeit with a waxing and waning course. After remission, treatment should continue for at least several months in order to prevent relapses. In general, few studies have examined relapse prevention after a period of more than 1 year. The existing relapse-prevention studies have demonstrated that patients who were switched to placebo after initial improvement with SSRI treatment of 12 to 24 weeks had a higher relapse rate than patients on the active drug (72,73). These results suggest that treatment should be extended for at least 24 weeks after stable remission has occurred. An expert consensus conference recommended a duration of pharmacotherapy of at least 12 months (77). Antidepressants should be tapered off very gradually in order to avoid withdrawal reactions.

IX. TREATMENT UNDER SPECIAL CONDITIONS

A. Pregnancy

According to the majority of reviews, the use of SSRIs and TCAs in pregnancy imposes no increased risk for the infant that is detectable during the newborn period, although minor anomalies, prematurity, and neonatal complications have been reported with the use of these drugs. The use of these medications is not associated with intrauterine death or major fetal malformations (78–84). Case reports describe direct drug effects and withdrawal syndromes in some neonates whose mothers were treated with antidepressants near term (85,86). However, preschool age children exposed to fluoxetine in utero show no significant neurobehavioral changes (87).

An association between the use of benzodiazepines during pregnancy and congenital malformations has been reported (88). However, there has been no consistent proof that benzodiazepines at this time are hazardous, and the available literature suggests that it is safe to take diazepam or chlordiazepoxide during pregnancy. It has been suggested that would be prudent to avoid alprazolam during pregnancy (89). To avoid the potential risk of congenital defects, physicians should use benzodiazepines that have long safety records.

B. Breast Feeding

SSRIs and TCAs are excreted into breast milk, and low levels have been found in infant serum (80–91). In mothers receiving TCAs with the exception of doxepine, it seems unwarranted to recommend that breast feeding should be discontinued. Fluoxetine should probably be avoided during lactation (91). Treatment with other SSRIs (citalopram, fluvoxamine, paroxetine, or sertraline) seems to be compatible with breast feeding, although this view should be considered as preliminary due to the relative lack of data (91).

For venlafaxine, only limited data are available from case reports (92).

Regarding benzodiazepines, adverse drug reactions in infants have been described during maternal treatment with diazepam. During maternal treatment with all benzodiazepines, infants should be observed for signs of sedation, lethargy, poor suckling, and weight loss; if high doses have to be used and long term administration is required, breast feeding should probably be discontinued (89,91).

C. Treating Children and Adolescents

Although SAD is an anxiety disorder with onset in childhood or adolescence, controlled studies in this population are lacking. There is only one small open study. In a combined psychoeducational and pharmacological treatment program for children and adolescents (ages 8 to 17 years) with generalized SAD, 12 participants received 12 weeks of citalopram treatment with a maximum dose of 40 mg/day and eight brief counseling sessions, which included education about social anxiety, skills coaching, and behavioral exercises. Based on clinician global ratings of change, 10 of 12 (83.3%) youths reported much or very much improvement. Significant changes were also found on self-report ratings of social anxiety, depression, and parents' perceptions of the children's social skills during the course of treatment (93).

D. Treatment of the Elderly

Factors that have to be considered in the treatment of the elderly include an increased sensitivity for anticholinergic properties of drugs, an increased risk for orthostatic hypotension and electrocardiographic (ECG) changes, and possible paradoxical reactions to benzodiazepines. Thus, treatment with TCAs or benzodiazepines is considered less favorable, while SSRIs, buspirone, and moclobemide appear to be safe.

However, no studies exist that investigate the treatment of SAD in the elderly, as this population rarely seeks treatment for this condition.

E. Comorbid Alcohol Use

As stated above, alcohol abuse is common in SAD. In a study of adults with co-occurring SAD and alcohol use disorder, Randall et al. (94) assessed the efficacy of the SSRI paroxetine on social phobia symptoms and alcohol-consuming behavior in a small double-blind study. Six patients received paroxetine and nine patients received placebo for 8 weeks using a flexible dosing schedule. Dosing began at 20 mg/day and increased to a target dose of 60 mg/day. Patients treated with paroxetine improved more than those treated with placebo on social phobia measures, including the CGI-I and the LSAS. On alcohol use, there was no significant effect on quantity or frequency measures of drinking, but there was for the CGI ratings for alcohol drinking. A total of 50% of the paroxetine patients but only 11% of placebo patients were responders on drinking. Further study is warranted to investigate the efficacy of SSRIs in helping affected individuals reduce alcohol use.

X. CONCLUSIONS

Not all persons suffering from shyness are candidates for drug therapy. However, SAD is associated with suffering, restrictions in quality of life, depression, suicidality, and substance abuse. The risks of drug therapy with modern antidepressants are relatively insignificant in comparison to the risks of untreated SAD.

The SSRIs may be regarded as first-line drugs in SAD. In addition, the SSNRI venlafaxine was found effective in several controlled studies. Its side effect profile is similar to the SSRIs. Pregabalin, a new drug acting at the alpha$_2$ subunit of the voltage-dependent calcium channels, showed promising results in preliminary work. The MAOI phenelzine shows robust results in terms of efficacy. However, this drug is less well tolerated than alternative treatments. The results with moclobemide are somewhat inconsistent, and effect sizes observed in clinical studies were only moderate. The database for benzodiazepines is small. Benzodiazepines are not recommended as first-line agents in treating SAD because they are associated with abuse and long-term dependence. However, they may play a role as an adjunctive agent or for patients who are refractory to other treatments. They may also be used as an adjunct to antidepressant therapy during the first period of 2 to 3 weeks before the onset of action of these drugs. Tricyclic antidepressants have not been investigated in controlled studies. An open study did not suggest efficacy of imipramine in SAD. SAD patients refractory to treatment with SSRIs may benefit from second-line drugs, such as phenelzine, moclobemide, or clonazepam.

In summary, due to increased efforts in the systematic clinical evaluation of psychopharmacological agents in the treatment of SAD in recent years, there is now a growing database of trials that can be drawn upon when formulating guidelines for the treatment of this condition. In clinical practice, pharmacotherapy is often combined with cognitive behavioral therapy to optimize symptom reduction and quality-of-life enhancement, although additional work on how best to combine and sequence different treatment modalities is still needed.

REFERENCES

1. Graf-Morgenstern M, Benkert O. Urteile und Meinungen zur Pharmako-therapie und Psychotherapie in der Bevölkerung—eine repräsentative Bev-ölkerungsumfrage. ZNS J 2001; 5:22–31.
2. Marshall JR. The diagnosis and treatment of social phobia and alcohol abuse. Bull Menninger Clin 1994; 58:A58–A66.
3. Bandelow B, Zohar J, Hollander E, Kasper S, Möller HJ. World Federation of Societies of Biological Psychiatry (WFSBP) guidelines for the pharmacol-ogical treatment of anxiety, obsessive-compulsive and posttraumatic stress disorders. World J Biol Psychiatry 2002; 3:171–199.
4. Bezchlibnyk-Butler KZ, Jeffries JJ. Clinical Handbook of Psychotropic Drugs, 13th ed. Seattle/Toronto/Goettingen/Bern: Hogrefe & Huber, 2003.
5. Kasper S, Loft H, Smith JR. Escitalopram is efficacious and well tolerated in the treatment of social anxiety disorder. Poster, American Psychiatric Asso-ciation (APA), Philadelphia, PA, 2002.
6. Lader M, Stender K, Bürger V, Nil R. Fixed doses of escitalopram and par-oxetine for the treatment of social anxiety disorder. Poster, European College of Neuropsychopharmacology (ECNP) Congress, Prague, 2003.
7. Montgomery SA, Dürr-Pal N, Loftus EF, Nil R. Relapse prevention by escitalopram treatment of patients with social anxiety disorder (SAD). Poster, European College of Neuropsychopharmacology (ECNP) Congress, Prague 2003.
8. van Vliet I, den Boer JA, Westenberg HGM. Psychopharmacological treatment of social phobia—a double blind placebo controlled study with fluvoxamine. Psychopharmacology 1994; 115:128–134.
9. Stein DJ, Berk M, Els C, Emsley RA, Gittelson L, Wilson D, Oakes R, Hunter B. A double-blind placebo-controlled trial of paroxetine in the man-agement of social phobia (social anxiety disorder) in South Africa. S Afr Med J 1999; 89:402–406.
10. Westenberg HGM, Stein DJ, Yang HM, Li D, Barbato L. A double-blind, placebo-controlled study of controlled release fluvoxamine for the treatment of generalized social anxiety disorder. Poster, European College of Neuro-psychopharmacology (ECNP) Congress, Prague 2003.
11. Stein MB, Liebowitz MR, Lydiard RB, Pitts CD, Bushnell W, Gergel I. Paroxetine treatment of generalized social phobia (social anxiety disorder): a randomized controlled trial. JAMA 1998; 280:708–713.
12. Baldwin D, Bobes J, Stein DJ, Scharwachter I, Faure M. Paroxetine in social phobia/social anxiety disorder. Randomised, double- blind, placebo-controlled study. Paroxetine Study Group. Br J Psychiatry 1999; 175:120–126.
13. Allgulander C. Paroxetine in social anxiety disorder: a randomized placebo-controlled study. Acta Psychiatr Scand 1999; 100:193–198.
14. Liebowitz MR, Stein MB, Tancer M, Carpenter D, Oakes R, Pitts CD. A randomized, double-blind, fixed-dose comparison of paroxetine and placebo

in the treatment of generalized social anxiety disorder. J Clin Psychiatry 2002; 63:66–74.

15. Katzelnick DJ, Kobak KA, Greist JH, Jefferson JW, Mantle JM, Serlin RC. Sertraline for social phobia: placebo-controlled crossover study. Am J Psychiatry 1995; 152:1368–1371.

16. Van Ameringen MA, Lane RM, Walker JR, Bowen RC, Chokka PR, Goldner EM, Johnston DG, Lavallee YJ, Nandy S, Pecknold JC, et al. Sertraline treatment of generalized social phobia: a 20-week, double- blind, placebo-controlled study. Am J Psychiatry 2001; 158:275–281.

17. Blomhoff S, Tangen Haug T, Hellstrom K, Holme I, Humble M, Madsbu HP, Wold JE. Randomised controlled general practice trial of sertraline, exposure therapy and combined treatment in generalised social phobia. Br J Psychiatry 2001; 179:23–30.

18. Liebowitz MR, DeMartinis NA, Weihs K, Londborg PD, Smith WT, Chung H, Fayyad R, Clary CM. Efficacy of sertraline in severe generalized social anxiety disorder: results of a double-blind, placebo-controlled study. J Clin Psychiatry 2003; 64:785–792.

19. Bouwer C, Stein DJ. Use of the selective serotonin reuptake inhibitor citalopram in the treatment of generalized social phobia. J Affect Disord 1998; 49:79–82.

20. Atmaca M, Kuloglu M, Tezcan E, Unal A. Efficacy of citalopram and moclobemide in patients with social phobia: some preliminary findings. Hum Psychopharmacol 2002; 17:401–405.

21. Black B, Uhde T, Tancer M. Fluoxetine for the treatment of social phobia. J Clin Psychopharmacol 1992; 12:293–295.

22. Van Ameringen M, Mancini C, Streiner DL. Fluoxetine efficacy in social phobia. J Clin Psychiatry 1993; 54:27–32.

23. Kobak KA, Greist JH, Jefferson JW, Katzelnick DJ. Fluoxetine in social phobia: a double-blind, placebo-controlled pilot study. J Clin Psychopharmacology 2002; 22:257–262.

24. Fava M, Judge R, Hoog SL, Nilsson ME, Koke SC. Fluoxetine versus sertraline and paroxetine in major depressive disorder: changes in weight with long-term treatment. J Clin Psychiatry 2000; 61:863–867.

25. Bandelow B, Behnke K, Lenoir S, Hendriks GJ, Alkin T, Dombrowski A, Goebel C. Sertraline versus paroxetine in the treatment of panic disorder: a multinational randomized double-blind 15 week study. Eur Neuropsychopharmacol 2002; 12:S364–S364.

26. Price JS, Waller PC, Wood SM, MacKay AV. A comparison of the post-marketing safety of four selective serotonin re-uptake inhibitors including the investigation of symptoms occurring on withdrawal. Br J Clin Pharmacol 1996; 42:757–763.

27. Stahl MM, Lindquist M, Pettersson M, Edwards IR, Sanderson JH, Taylor NF, Fletcher AP, Schou JS. Withdrawal reactions with selective serotonin re-uptake inhibitors as reported to the WHO system. Eur J Clin Pharmacol 1997; 53:163–169.

28. Harden CL. The co-morbidity of depression and epilepsy: epidemiology, etiology, and treatment. Neurology 2002; 59:S48–S55.
29. Liebowitz MR. Comparison of venlafaxine XR and paroxetine in the short-term treatment of social anxiety disorder. 2003.
30. Stein MB, Mangano R. Long-term treatment of generalized social anxiety disorder with venlafaxine XR. Annual Meeting, Anxiety Disorders Association of America, Toronto, Canada 2003.
31. Altamura AC, Pioli R, Vitto M, Mannu P. Venlafaxine in social phobia: a study in selective serotonin reuptake inhibitor non-responders. Int Clin Psychopharmacol 1999; 14:239–245.
32. Kelsey JE. Venlafaxine in social phobia. Psychopharmacol Bull 1995; 31:767–771.
33. IMCTGMSP. The International Multicenter Clinical Trial Group on Moclobemide in Social Phobia. Moclobemide in social phobia. A double-blind, placebo-controlled clinical study. Eur Arch Psychiatry Clin Neurosci 1997; 247:71–80.
34. Stein DJ, Cameron A, Amrein R, Montgomery SA. Moclobemide is effective and well tolerated in the long-term pharmacotherapy of social anxiety disorder with or without comorbid anxiety disorder. Int Clin Psychopharmacol 2002; 17:161–170.
35. Versiani M, Nardi AE, Mundim FD, Alves AB, Liebowitz MR, Amrein R. Pharmacotherapy of social phobia. A controlled study with moclobemide and phenelzine. Br J Psychiatry 1992; 161:353–360.
36. Schneier FR, Goetz D, Campeas R, Fallon B, Marshall R, Liebowitz MR. Placebo-controlled trial of moclobemide in social phobia. Br J Psychiatry 1998; 172:70–77.
37. Noyes R, Jr., Moroz G, Davidson JR, Liebowitz MR, Davidson A, Siegel J, Bell J, Cain JW, Curlik SM, Kent TA, et al. Moclobemide in social phobia: a controlled dose-response trial. J Clin Psychopharmacol 1997; 17:247–254.
38. Bisserbe J-C, Lépine J-P. Moclobemide in social phobia: a pilot open study. J Clin Neuropharmacol 1994; 17(suppl 1):s88–s94.
39. van der Linden GJ, Stein DJ, van Balkom AJ. The efficacy of the selective serotonin reuptake inhibitors for social anxiety disorder (social phobia): a meta-analysis of randomized controlled trials. Int Clin Psychopharmacol 2000; 15(suppl 2):S15–S23.
40. van Vliet I, Den Boer J, Westenberg H. Psychopharmacological treatment of social phobia: clinical and biochemical effects of brofaromine, a selective MAO-A inhibitor. Eur Neuropsychopharmacol 1992; 2:21–29.
41. Fahlen T, Nilsson HL, Borg K, Humble M, Pauli U. Social phobia: the clinical efficacy and tolerability of the monoamine oxidase-A and serotonin uptake inhibitor brofaromine. A double-blind placebo-controlled study. Acta Psychiatr Scand 1995; 92:351–358.
42. Lott M, Greist JH, Jefferson JW, Kobak KA, Katzelnick DJ, Katz RJ, Schaettle SC. Brofaromine for social phobia: a multicenter, placebo-controlled, double-blind study. J Clin Psychopharmacol 1997; 17:255–260.

43. Baker GB, Wong JT, Yeung JM, Coutts RT. Effects of the antidepressant phenelzine on brain levels of gamma-aminobutyric acid (GABA). J Affect Disord 1991; 21:207–211.

44. Versiani M, Mundim FD, Nardi AE, Liebowitz MR. Tranylcypromine in social phobia. J Clin Psychopharmacol 1988; 8:279–283.

45. Goddard AW, Brouette T, Almai A, Jetty P, Woods SW, Charney D. Early coadministration of clonazepam with sertraline for panic disorder. Arch Gen Psychiatry 2001; 58:681–686.

46. Munjack DJ, Baltazar PL, Bohn PB, Cabe DD, Appleton AA. Clonazepam in the treatment of social phobia: a pilot study. J Clin Psychiatry 1990; 51(suppl 5):35–40.

47. Davidson JRT, Potts N, Richichi E, Krishnan R, Ford SM, Smith R, Wilson WH. Treatment of social phobia with clonazepam and placebo. J Clin Psychopharmacol 1993; 13:423–428.

48. Davidson JR, Ford SM, Smith RD, Potts NL. Long-term treatment of social phobia with clonazepam. J Clin Psychiatry 1991; 52(suppl):16–20.

49. Connor KM, Davidson JR, Potts NL, Tupler LA, Miner CM, Malik ML, Book SW, Colket JT, Ferrell F. Discontinuation of clonazepam in the treatment of social phobia. J Clin Psychopharmacol 1998; 18:373–378.

50. Gelernter CS, Uhde TW, Cimbolic P, Arnkoff DB, Vittone BJ, Tancer ME, Bartko JJ. Cognitive-behavioral and pharmacological tretments of social phobia. Arch Gen Psychiatry 1991; 48:938–945.

51. Rickels K, Schweizer E, Case WG, Greenblatt DJ. Long-term therapeutic use of benzodiazepines. I. Effects of abrupt discontinuation [published erratum appears in Arch Gen Psychiatry 1991 Jan;48(1):51]. Arch Gen Psychiatry 1990; 47:899–907.

52. Rickels K. Benzodiazepines in the treatment of anxiety. Am J Psychother 1982; 36:358–370.

53. Feltner DE, Pollack MH, Davidson JRT. A placebo-controlled study of pregabalin in the treatment of social phobia (abstr). Anxiety Disorders of America's 20th Annual Conference, Washington, DC, 2000.

54. Simpson HB, Schneier FR, Campeas RB, Marshall RD, Fallon BA, Davies S, Klein DF, Liebowitz MR. Imipramine in the treatment of social phobia. J Clin Psychopharmacol 1998; 18:132–135.

55. van Vliet IM, den Boer JA, Westenberg HG, Pian KL. Clinical effects of buspirone in social phobia: a double-blind placebo-controlled study. J Clin Psychiatry 1997; 58:164–168.

56. Munjack DJ, Bruns J, Baltazar PL, Brown R, Leonard M, Nagy R, Koek R, Crocker B, Schafer S. A pilot study of buspirone in the treatment of social phobia. J Anxiety Disord 1991; 5:87–98.

57. Schneier FR, Saoud JB, Campeas R, Fallon BA, Hollander E, Coplan J, Liebowitz MR. Buspirone in social phobia. J Clin Psychopharmacol 1993; 13:251–256.

58. Clark DB, Agras WS. The assessment and treatment of performance anxiety in musicians. Am J Psychiatry 1991; 148:598–605.

59. James IM, Griffith DN, Pearson RM, Newbury P. Effect of oxprenolol on stage-fright in musicians. Lancet 1977; 2:952–954.
60. James IM, Burgoyne W, Savage IT. Effect of pindolol on stress-related disturbances of musical performance: preliminary communication. J R Soc Med 1983; 76:194–196.
61. James I, Savage I. Beneficial effect of nadolol on anxiety-induced disturbances of performance in musicians: a comparison with diazepam and placebo. Am Heart J 1984; 108:1150–1155.
62. Gorman JM, Liebowitz MR, Fyer AF, Campeas R, Klein DF. Treatment of social phobia with atenolol. J Clin Psychopharmacol 1985; 5:298–301.
63. Liebowitz MR, Gorman JM, Fyer AJ, Campeas R, Levin AP, Sandberg D, Hollander E, Papp L, Goetz D. Pharmacotherapy of social phobia: an interim report of a placebo- controlled comparison of phenelzine and atenolol. J Clin Psychiatry 1988; 49:252–257.
64. Turner SM, Beidel DC, Jacob RG. Social phobia: a comparison of behaviour therapy and atenolol. Journal of Consulting and Clinical Psychology 1994; 62:350–358.
65. Barnett SD, Kramer ML, Casat CD, Connor KM, Davidson JR. Efficacy of olanzapine in social anxiety disorder: a pilot study. J Psychopharmacol 2002; 16:365–368.
66. Van Ameringen M, Mancini C, Oakman J, Walker J, Kjernisted K, Chokka P, Johnston D. All serotonergic agents are created equal in social phobia. Nefazodone: a placebo controlled trial. 23rd Annual Conference of the Anxiety Disorders Association of America, Toronto, 2003.
67. Emmanuel NP, Brawman-Mintzer O, Morton WA, Book SW, Johnson MR, Lorberbaum JP, Ballenger JC, Lydiard RB. Bupropion-SR in treatment of social phobia. Depress Anxiety 2000; 12:111–113.
68. Simpson HB, Schneier FR, Marshall RD, Campeas RB, Vermes D, Silvestre J, Davies S, Liebowitz MR. Low dose selegiline (L-Deprenyl) in social phobia. Depress Anxiety 1998; 7:126–129.
69. Pande AC, Davidson JR, Jefferson JW, Janney CA, Katzelnick DJ, Weisler RH, Greist JH, Sutherland SM. Treatment of social phobia with gabapentin: a placebo-controlled study. J Clin Psychopharmacol 1999; 19:341–348.
70. Kinrys G, Pollack MH, Simon NM, Worthington JJ, Nardi AE, Versiani M. Valproic acid for the treatment of social anxiety disorder. Int Clin Psychopharmacol 2003; 18:169–172.
71. Goldstein S. Treatment of social phobia with clonidine. Biol Psychiatry 1987; 22:369–372.
72. Walker JR, Van Ameringen MA, Swinson R, Bowen RC, Chokka PR, Goldner E, Johnston DC, Lavallie YJ, Nandy S, Pecknold JC, et al. Prevention of relapse in generalized social phobia: results of a 24-week study in responders to 20 weeks of sertraline treatment. J Clin Psychopharmacol 2000; 20:636–644.
73. Stein DJ, Versiani M, Hair T, Kumar R. Efficacy of paroxetine for relapse prevention in social anxiety disorder: a 24-week study. Arch Gen Psychiatry 2002; 59:1111–1118.

74. Stein DJ, Stein MB, Goodwin W, Kumar R, Hunter B. The selective serotonin reuptake inhibitor paroxetine is effective in more generalized and in less generalized social anxiety disorder. Psychopharmacology (Berl) 2001; 158:267–272.

75. Stein MB, Sareen J, Hami S, Chao J. Pindolol potentiation of paroxetine for generalized social phobia: a double-blind, placebo-controlled, crossover study. Am J Psychiatry 2001; 158:1725–1727.

76. Van Ameringen M, Mancini C, Wilson C. Buspirone augmentation of selective serotonin reuptake inhibitors (SSRIs) in social phobia. J Affect Disord 1996; 39:115–121.

77. Ballenger JC, Davidson JRT, Lecrubier Y, Nutt DJ, Bobes J, Beidel DC, Ono Y, Westenberg HGM. Consensus statement on social anxiety disorder from the International Consensus Group on Depression and Anxiety. J Clin Psychiatry 1998; 59:54–60.

78. Austin MPV, Mitchell PB. Psychotropic medications in pregnant women: treatment dilemmas. Med J Austr 1998; 169:428–431.

79. Ericson A, Kallen B, Wiholm BE. Delivery outcome after the use of antidepressants in early pregnancy. Eur J Clin Pharmacol 1999; 55:503–508.

80. Misri S, Kostaras D, Kostaras X. The use of selective serotonin reuptake inhibitors during pregnancy and lactation: current knowledge. Can J Psychiatry 2000; 45:285–287.

81. Misri S, Burgmann A, Kostaras D. Are SSRIs safe for pregnant and breastfeeding women? Can Fam Physician 2000; 46:626–628.

82. Emslie G, Judge R. Tricyclic antidepressants and selective serotonin reuptake inhibitors: use during pregnancy, in children/adolescents and in the elderly. Acta Psychiatr Scand 2000; 101:26–34.

83. Altshuler LL, Cohen LS, Moline ML, Kahn DA, Carpenter D, Docherty JP. The Expert Consensus Guideline Series. Treatment of depression in women. Postgrad Med 2001:1–107.

84. Ward RK, Zamorski MA. Benefits and risks of psychiatric medications during pregnancy. Am Fam Physician 2002; 66:629–636.

85. Wisner KL, Gelenberg AJ, Leonard H, Zarin D, Frank E. Pharmacologic treatment of depression during pregnancy. JAMA 1999; 282:1264–1269.

86. Nordeng H, Lindemann R, Perminov KV, Reikvam A. Neonatal withdrawal syndrome after in utero exposure to selective serotonin reuptake inhibitors. Acta Paediatr 2001; 90:288–291.

87. Goldstein DJ, Sundell K. A review of the safety of selective serotonin reuptake inhibitors during pregnancy. Hum Psychopharmacol Clin Exp 1999; 14:319–324.

88. Laegreid L, Olegard R, Conradi N, Hagberg G, Wahlstrom J, Abrahamsson L. Congenital malformations and maternal consumption of benzodiazepines: a case-control study. Dev Med Child Neurol 1990; 32:432–441.

89. Iqbal MM, Sobhan T, Ryals T. Effects of commonly used benzodiazepines on the fetus, the neonate, and the nursing infant. Psychiatr Serv 2002; 53:39–49.

90. Simpson K, Noble S. Fluoxetine—a review of its use in women's health. CNS Drugs 2000; 14:301–328.

91. Spigset O, Hagg S. Excretion of psychotropic drugs into breast milk—pharmacokinetic overview and therapeutic implications. CNS Drugs 1998; 9:111–134.

92. Hendrick V, Altshuler L, Wertheimer A, Dunn WA. Venlafaxine and breast-feeding. Am J Psychiatry 2001; 158:2089–2090.

93. Chavira DA, Stein MB. Combined psychoeducation and treatment with selective serotonin reuptake inhibitors for youth with generalized social anxiety disorder. J Child Adolesc Psychopharmacol 2002; 12:47–54.

94. Randall CL, Johnson MR, Thevos AK, Sonne SC, Thomas SE, Willard SL, Brady KT, Davidson JR. Paroxetine for social anxiety and alcohol use in dual-diagnosed patients. Depress Anxiety 2001; 14:255–262.

95. Stein MB, Fyer AJ, Davidson JR, Pollack MH, Wiita B. Fluvoxamine treatment of social phobia (social anxiety disorder): a double-blind, placebo-controlled study. Am J Psychiatry 1999; 156:756–760.

96. Kobak KA, Greist JH, Jefferson JW, Katzelnick DJ. Fluoxetine in social phobia: a double-blind, placebo-controlled pilot study. J Clin Psychopharmacol 2002; 22:257–262.

97. Heimberg RG, Liebowitz MR, Hope DA, Schneier FR, Holt CS, Welkowitz LA, Juster HR, Campeas R, Bruch MA, Cloitre M, et al. Cognitive behavioral group therapy vs phenelzine therapy for social phobia: 12-week outcome. Arch Gen Psychiatry 1998; 55:1133–1141.

98. Falloon IRH, Lloyd GG, Harpin RE. The treatment of social phobia. J Nerv Ment Dis 1981; 169:180–184.

99. Liebowitz MR, Mangano RM. Venlafaxine XR in generalized social anxiety disorder. Poster, CINP Congress, Montreal, 2002.

100. Liebowitz M, Allgulander C, Mangano M. Comparison of Venlafaxine XR and Paroxetine in the Short-Term Treatment of SAD (abstr). American Psychiatric Association Congress, San Francisco, CA, 2003.

101. Reich J, Yates W. A pilot study of treatment of social phobia with alprazolam. Am J Psychiatry 1988; 145:590–594.

102. Reiter SR, Pollack MH, Rosenbaum JF, Cohen LS. Clonazepam for the treatment of social phobia. J Clin Psychiatry 1990; 51:470–472.

103. DeVane CL, Ware MR, Emmanuel NP, Brawman-Mintzer O, Morton WA, Villarreal G, Lydiard RB. Evaluation of the efficacy, safety and physiological effects of fluvoxamine in social phobia. Int Clin Psychopharmacol 1999; 14:345–351.

104. Liebowitz MR, Fyer AJ, Gorman JM, Campeas R, Levin A. Phenelzine in social phobia. J Clin Psychopharmacol 1986; 6:93–98.

18

The Relationship Between Psychotherapy and Pharmacotherapy for Social Anxiety Disorder

Talia I. Zaider and Richard G. Heimberg
Temple University,
Philadelphia, Pennsylvania, U.S.A.

I. INTRODUCTION

Social anxiety disorder, also known as social phobia, is a chronic and disabling condition known to affect between 13 and 16% of the population (1,2). In the National Comorbidity Survey, it was the third most common mental disorder and the most prevalent of the anxiety disorders (1). Individuals afflicted with this disorder, particularly those with the generalized subtype, experience considerable impairment across multiple areas of their lives, including work, school, daily activities, and family and social relationships (3). Over the last several decades, we have seen an impressive growth of research activity devoted to the development and testing of treatments for this disorder. As a result, our knowledge about how best to intervene has advanced significantly. Individuals struggling with what was once referred to as the "neglected anxiety disorder" (4) now have available to them multiple treatment options with demonstrated efficacy.

The two forms of treatment that have met consistent success in treating social anxiety disorder are pharmacotherapy and the cognitive-behavioral therapies (CBT), although there is also preliminary support for the use of other therapies in this population (5,6). Therapies that fall under the rubric of CBT may include relaxation and social skills training but most often involve guided, systematic exposure to feared situations and cognitive restructuring techniques. More detailed descriptions of these treatment approaches can be found in several comprehensive reviews (7,8) (this volume, chapter by Holaway and Heimberg). Individuals with social anxiety disorder who are treated with CBT, either in individual or group format, enjoy substantial reductions in both the severity and functional interference of their symptoms. Changes resulting from CBT consistently exceed those associated with placebo or wait-list control conditions. Additionally, improvements appear to endure well beyond the acute phase of treatment (9).

Pharmacological interventions for social anxiety disorder have similarly gained substantial empirical support. Serotonin reuptake inhibitors (SSRIs), serotonin-noradrenaline reuptake inhibitors (SNRIs), irreversible and reversible monoamine oxidase inhibitors (MAOIs/RIMAs), and high potency benzodiazepines are among the drug treatments that have been tested with some success for social anxiety disorder (this volume, chapter by Bandelow and Stein). As a class, SSRIs such as paroxetine, sertraline and fluvoxamine have all demonstrated superiority to placebo control groups and have proven to be viable and well-tolerated options for the treatment of social anxiety disorder (11–14).

Although we now have treatment strategies that work well for many patients, questions remain about how to use these strategies in order to maximize and prolong treatment response in this population. A particularly important challenge to researchers in this area is to better understand the compatibility and relative efficacy of psychological and pharmacological therapies. Indeed, there is little information to guide clinicians in the selection and sequencing of these two treatment approaches. In this chapter, we address these issues by reviewing the current status of research in this area and exploring the relationship between psychological and pharmacological treatments for social anxiety disorder.

II. COMPARING THE EFFICACY OF CBT AND PHARMACOTHERAPY FOR SOCIAL ANXIETY DISORDER

To date, only a handful of studies have directly compared CBT with pharmacological treatments for social anxiety disorder, and the question of which approach is most effective remains difficult to answer. Methodological limitations in several studies make it difficult to interpret findings in this body of research. For example, in a study by Gelernter and colleagues, comparable gains were made by patients receiving group CBT, phenelzine, alprazolam, and pill placebo (15). Outcome assessment was limited to self-report, and exposure exercises were included in every treatment condition (including placebo), making it difficult to isolate the active ingredients in the medication and placebo conditions. A recent study comparing CBT with clonazepam, a high-potency benzodiazepine, faced a similar limitation (16). Here too, medication administration was accompanied by instruction for self-exposure to anxiety-provoking situations. In this study, CBT and clonazepam yielded similar outcomes with regard to posttreatment remission of symptoms, percentage of dropouts during treatment, and scores on a number of self-report and clinician-rated measures (16). Unfortunately, no control group was included in this trial, leaving us unable to conclude whether within-treatment differences in this sample are greater than might be expected given the passage of time or other nonspecific factors. Three additional studies that examined the relative efficacy of CBT and pharmacotherapy used medications that did not perform better than placebo in controlled trials, making them poor candidates for comparison with CBT (17–19).

Metaanalyses can be particularly useful in providing a quantitative summary of research findings in this area. Gould and colleagues conducted a metaanalytic review of the literature on the efficacy of medication and psychotherapy treatments for social anxiety disorder (5). They calculated effect sizes (ESs), derived from validated self-report questionnaires, across 24 trials that examined either CBT or pharmacological treatments for social anxiety disorder. They selected studies on the basis of certain criteria, including the presence of a control group (e.g., wait-list or pill placebo) and the use of a clinically diagnosed sample. Interestingly, they found no significant differences in effect sizes between CBT and pharmacological treatments (ESs on measures of social anxiety were 0.74 and 0.62, respectively), nor were there significant differences in mean attrition rates (10% for CBT versus 13.7% for medication treatments). The largest effect sizes were found for groups of patients treated with either exposure or exposure with cognitive restructuring as well as for patients treated with SSRIs. Treatment groups receiving an SSRI had the lowest dropout rates (1.5%), perhaps because these medications are well tolerated and easily managed. Gould and colleagues concluded that psychotherapy and pharmacotherapy appear to be equally effective for the short-term treatment of social anxiety disorder. However, they raise the caveat that CBT may have had the advantage of being compared more often to a wait-list control group, presumably a "weaker" control group than pill placebo, which may have resulted in inflated effect sizes (20).

A recent metaanalytic review conducted by Fedoroff and Taylor revealed a slightly different pattern of findings (21). Unlike Gould and colleagues, Fedoroff and Taylor included uncontrolled studies but excluded studies in which medication treatments were accompanied by directed exposure exercises. Additionally, outcome was evaluated using a combination of self-report and clinician-rated measures that broadly assessed the severity of social anxiety symptoms. The authors argued that the use of broad rather than specific (e.g., public speaking only) severity measures allowed for a more accurate reflection of treatment efficacy and made findings more relevant to the types of patients typically presenting to clinical practice (that is, with more generalized concerns). Their review evaluated the efficacy of three classes of pharmacological agents (i.e., MAOIs, SSRIs, and high-potency benzodiazepines), and four types of cognitive-behavioral interventions for social anxiety disorder.

Consistent with reports by Gould and colleagues, Fedoroff and Taylor found no significant differences in attrition rates across treatments, indicating that CBT and medication treatments were equally well tolerated (21). However, pharmacotherapies, particularly benzodiazepines, tended to be more effective than CBTs in reducing pretreatment to posttreatment severity of symptoms. Although SSRIs were as effective as benzodiazepines, this class of medications produced effect sizes that were no different than those of CBT. Unfortunately, the durability of treatment gains was not compared across treatments due to the scarcity of drug studies that included a follow-up assessment. Nevertheless, the available data showed that CBTs maintained moderate effect sizes after follow-up periods of up to 6 months. The authors concluded that pharmacotherapies appear to be most effective for the acute treatment of social anxiety disorder and suggested that there may be some utility in supplementing medications with CBT either during or after discontinuation of drug treatments.

One issue emerging from both reviews is that there are few data available on the comparative long-term efficacy of CBT and medication for social anxiety disorder. Are the benefits conferred by these interventions maintained after treatment has been completed? Follow-up assessments present an opportunity to learn about the extended effects of treatment, some of which may not appear until well after the treatment has terminated. Studies evaluating drug efficacy are especially lacking in follow-up data, and among studies that include a follow-up assessment, there is often insufficient information about the extent of active treatment-seeking behavior or the types of life events that may occur during the follow-up period. There is some evidence to suggest that symptoms recur after medication is discontinued

(22). CBT, however, has been associated with maintenance of gains during posttreatment follow-up periods (9).

One of the few studies that included a direct comparison of the long-term efficacy of medication and CBT for social anxiety disorder was a large, multisite study conducted by Heimberg and colleagues (23). This study compared cognitive-behavioral group therapy (CBGT) with the MAOI phenelzine sulfate during acute, maintenance, and follow-up phases. Two additional treatment conditions served as control groups: 1) a pill placebo and 2) educational-supportive group psychotherapy, a nonspecific group intervention with credibility comparable to CBGT but excluding the active cognitive-behavioral strategies of CBGT. Exposure instructions were exclusive to the CBGT condition. Patients responding to a 12-week acute phase of active treatment were enrolled in 6 months of maintenance treatment, followed by a 6-month follow-up period.

Consistent with previous findings, there were no significant differences between CBGT and phenelzine in response rate. CBGT and phenelzine were both superior to the control groups with regard to percentage of patients classified as responders (58 and 65%, respectively, intent-to-treat analyses). Only 33% of patients receiving placebo and 27% of those in the educational support group were classified as responders. Posttreatment scores on the Liebowitz Social Anxiety Scale (LSAS) (24) and some other dimensional measures favored phenelzine over CBGT, although both treatments performed better than the control groups. Moreover, a closer examination of patients' progress during the course of treatment revealed differences in patterns of response. Most patients classified as responders to phenelzine met response criteria after 6 weeks. CBGT, however, was associated with a more gradual course of improvement, which is consistent with a treatment that involves cultivating and practicing new skills.

Additional differences between phenelzine and CBGT were revealed when patients were assessed 6 months after treatment discontinuation (25). By the end of the 6-month follow-up assessment, 50% of patients receiving phenelzine had relapsed, compared to only 17% of patients receiving CBGT. Considered together, these data tell us that phenelzine may produce somewhat greater immediate improvements but that CBGT confers greater protection against relapse. However, both appear to be efficacious treatments for social anxiety disorder.

III. COMBINING CBT AND PHARMACOTHERAPY FOR SOCIAL ANXIETY DISORDER

Recently, there has been great interest in the potential utility of combining medication and psychotherapy treatments for social anxiety disorder.

Although the notion of combining two efficacious treatments is initially appealing, there are few empirical data to support this practice. Several possible outcomes should be considered. One possibility is that the combination of CBT and medication will have additive or synergistic effects. In this scenario, administering CBT with medication may result in greater therapeutic "punch," such that the outcome of combined treatment is better than that achieved by either intervention alone. This might occur if the presence of one treatment enhances the efficacy of the other. For example, medication might reduce severe discomfort, such that the patient is better able to engage with the therapist, has better moment-to-moment access to the tools and concepts learned in therapy, and is more willing to participate in exposure to feared social situations. Similarly, certain aspects of CBT (e.g., psychoeducation, working alliance with the therapist) can potentially facilitate compliance with the medication regimen.

A second possibility is that one treatment may detract from the efficacy of the other. For example, if the patient is experiencing little anxiety due to the effects of medication, he or she might be less motivated to complete homework assignments or participate in exposure exercises. Hope and colleagues (26) noted that heightened anxiety helps to facilitate cognitive restructuring during exposure exercises, allowing the patient to gain awareness of and subsequently challenge maladaptive beliefs that are activated during exposure to the feared situation. A third possible outcome is that combined treatment offers no added benefit over either treatment alone.

Although the number of studies investigating the efficacy of CBT combined with pharmacotherapy is steadily growing, this body of research is still in its infancy. Two of the studies that examined combination treatments employed classes of medications that did not surpass placebo in controlled studies (17,27). In their metaanalysis, Gould and colleagues (5) reported an overall effect size of 0.49 for combination treatments, which, although based on only two identified studies, was comparable to effect sizes for CBT and pharmacotherapy administered alone. Mean attrition rates were also comparable across combined and single treatments.

Blomhoff and colleagues recently conducted a randomized, double-blind trial in which participants received 24 weeks of the SSRI sertraline or pill placebo, each of which was combined with either physician-assisted exposure therapy or "general medical care" (GMC; non-directive encouragement and support) (12). Exposure therapy consisted of eight 15- to 20-minute sessions administered during the first 12 weeks. This study was unique in that participants were treated in a primary care setting by physicians who were specifically trained to administer a 12-week exposure therapy. The primary measure of outcome was the number of partial and full responders in each condition as determined by the clinician-administered

Clinical Global Impression scale (CGI-SP) and the patient-rated Social Phobia Scale (SPS). At the final assessment point (week 24), there were significantly more responders in the sertraline-GMC and sertraline-exposure conditions than in the placebo-GMC condition (full response rates were 40.2, 45.5, and 23.9%, respectively). At week 24, there was a non-significant trend toward greater efficacy of exposure (full response rate of 33.0%) compared with pill placebo. Given that exposure therapy was discontinued at week 12, outcome assessed at this point may provide a better measure of acute response to exposure therapy. In fact, during the second half of the study (weeks 12 to 24), it was assumed that exposure-only participants would continue to engage in exposure exercises on their own, although no compliance data were reported. Indeed, at week 12, exposure therapy administered alone was associated with significant improvement (i.e., partial or full response) compared to placebo, with no significant differences between this and other active treatments (12). Taken together, these findings suggest that sertraline, both alone and in combination with exposure therapy, is an effective treatment for generalized social anxiety disorder. The combined treatment was not clearly superior to sertraline alone, although it demonstrated greater efficiency. That is, compared to other active treatments, a larger number of patients in the combined condition met response criteria sooner (as early as week 8), and high response rates were maintained at all subsequent time points. The fact that the exposure therapy was administered mostly by nonspecialist clinicians with limited training may have limited its potential, both alone and in combination with sertraline. It is possible that the combined treatment would have had stronger effects if the duration and breadth of the exposure component was increased.

When the same sample was assessed at 1-year follow-up, all four groups showed significant improvement in CGI and SPS scores from baseline (28). However, during the follow-up period itself (weeks 24 to 52), patients who had received exposure therapy (without sertraline) showed *additional* improvement on symptom and severity scores after treatment was discontinued, whereas those who had received sertraline—with or without exposure—did not show any additional improvement during the follow-up period. In fact, those who received sertraline alone or in combination with exposure showed a tendency toward deterioration on several measures, although this finding was only significant relative to placebo on one of the secondary outcome measures.

The authors conclude that exposure therapy may yield a better long-term outcome when administered alone than with sertraline and that sertraline may be associated with relapse after discontinuation (28). This would suggest that sertraline may have detracted from the efficacy of exposure in the combination treatment, one of the three possible combination outcomes described above. However, closer examination of the data from these studies suggests an alternative interpretation. In an editorial commentary, Bandelow (29) pointed out that Haug and colleagues do not report follow-up analyses on the primary outcome measure from the acute study (i.e., number of partial/full responders as determined by scores on the CGI and SPS). Moreover, although they report significant within-group changes between baseline and follow-up, they do not indicate whether gains from baseline differed between groups or between active treatments and placebo. When the mean changes reported in the acute study (weeks 0 to 24) are added to those reported in the follow-up study (weeks 24 to 52), one finds that all four study groups made nearly identical gains. Bandelow (29) notes that the exposure therapy group appears to "catch up" to the sertraline and combination groups during the follow-up period rather than conferring additional long-term benefit. Indeed, the gains associated with exposure therapy during follow-up were not significantly different than gains made by the placebo group. Haug and colleagues (28) acknowledge that the placebo group was associated with an unusually positive response, perhaps because this condition included therapeutic support and encouragement.

Taken together, the acute and follow-up analyses suggest that a key difference between the combination treatment and sertraline or exposure therapy administered alone may be the rate at which response is achieved. Although individuals in all treatment groups eventually achieved similar gains, the combination treatment was associated with earlier treatment response relative to the other groups. Heimberg and colleagues (23) similarly found that phenelzine was associated with earlier response than CBGT, which demonstrated a more gradual course of improvement. These findings suggest that future research in this area should focus on understanding the patterns of response and relapse that characterize different treatment combinations. Inclusion of multiple assessment points and an adequate follow-up period are essential to making this type of analysis possible.

A recently completed study by Heimberg and Liebowitz similarly examined the utility of combined treatment for social anxiety disorder. Patients were treated with either CBGT, phenelzine, CBGT combined with phenelzine, or pill placebo. In this study, the psychotherapy component of the combined treatment was a previously tested 12-week program of psychoeducation, self-monitoring, cognitive restructuring and exposure activity, and was administered by experienced and certified therapists. Preliminary data from this study suggest modest benefit for the combined treatment after 12 weeks, although data from the full sample or regarding maintenance or relapse are not yet available. Another investigation that has just been completed by Davidson and Foa compared the efficacy of group CBT, fluoxetine, CBT combined with fluoxetine, CBT combined with placebo, and placebo alone. Preliminary unpublished results suggest the superiority of all active treatments over placebo, but there is no clear suggestion that combined treatment will be superior to either modality administered separately.

IV. CLINICAL CONSIDERATIONS IN THE DELIVERY OF COMBINED TREATMENTS FOR SOCIAL ANXIETY DISORDER

Much remains unknown about the compatibility of CBT and medication in the treatment of social anxiety disorder. On average, neither treatment modality, alone or in combination, has a clear advantage over the other. Moreover, it is becoming increasingly apparent that similar psychological and biological outcomes may be achieved by both medication and psychotherapy treatments. For example, Furmark and colleagues recently characterized neurofunctional changes associated with response to CBGT and the SSRI citalopram (30). Both CBGT and citalopram resulted in significant pre- to posttreatment changes in neural patterns, as represented by reduced activity in the amygdala, hippocampus, and other nearby regions of the brain during a public speaking task. This effect was not observed in the waitlist control condition. CBT has been shown to result in significant decreases in physiological arousal (e.g., heart rate) during exposure to anxiety-provoking situations (8). Likewise, pharmacological treatments for social anxiety disorder have been shown to produce changes in anxiety-related cognitions and social avoidance, despite the fact that these processes are not explicitly targeted during drug administration. Otto and Safren noted that by attenuating negative affect and anxious arousal, medication may facilitate reengagement in previously avoided situations (31). They further propose that medication offers the particular advantage of requiring less in-the-moment effort than is required by the application of relaxation or cognitive restructuring techniques, thereby allowing the individual to focus his or her attention on relevant situational cues (31). Given the potential similarities in performance and mechanisms of action between CBT and pharmacotherapy, what are some considerations that might bear on the choice and administration of these treatments?

Our understanding of factors that differentially predict pharmacotherapy and psychotherapy response among individuals with social anxiety disorder is limited. This is, in part, a result of the fact that studies vary in the extent to which they examine demographic and clinical moderators of treatment outcome and the degree to which comorbid or axis II conditions are excluded from or formally assessed in clinical trials (5). Demographic characteristics have not consistently predicted treatment response for either

CBT, pharmacotherapy, or their combination. For example, in the meta-analysis conducted by Gould and colleagues, the male-to-female ratio in study samples was not associated with differences in the efficacy of active treatment conditions (5). Similarly, Fedoroff and Taylor reported that characteristics such as age, duration of social anxiety disorder, and sex distribution were not predictive of effect sizes across psychological and pharmacological treatment conditions (21). Otto and colleagues found that neither gender nor the degree of comorbid depression and anxiety predicted response to clonazepam or CBGT (16). One study did report that relapse rates were significantly higher among women than men regardless of the treatment they received (CBGT or phenelzine). However, among respond-ers, there were no main effects of sex or sex by treatment interactions at maintenance or follow-up assessment points (25). Another characteristic often examined as a potential moderator of treatment outcome is subtype of social anxiety disorder (32,33). Some research suggests that response to CBT is reduced in patients with the generalized subtype of social anxiety disorder (34). Other evidence suggests that individuals with generalized social anxiety disorder show rates of improvement similar to those achieved by individuals with nongeneralized social anxiety disorder. However, those with the gen-eralized subtype are consistently more impaired before and after treatment with either medication or psychotherapy (33).

What are some considerations relevant to combination treatments? A closer look at some of the processes that facilitate change in CBT reveals a number of complications that may arise when combining medication and psychotherapy for the treatment of social anxiety disorder. One issue of potential concern is the effect of combined treatment on the beliefs that patients develop about the changes that they experience in treatment. Patients who attribute improvements to their medication, viewed as an external source of change, and deny the contribution of their own efforts (e.g., increased engagement in social activities), may have reduced invest-ment in CBT. Moreover, externalized attributions may impede the patient's ability to develop a strong sense of self-efficacy, that is, the perceived ability to competently master anxiety-provoking situations without reliance on medication. Self-efficacy, although sometimes referred to in terms of per-ceived social skills, has been shown to be a strong predictor of response to CBT (35). A study of agoraphobic patients who received a combination of 8 weeks of alprazolam and exposure or relaxation therapy showed evidence for the importance of these attributional processes. During phases of drug tapering and follow-up, patients who attributed their improvement primarily to the alprazolam were significantly more likely to relapse and experience withdrawal symptoms than patients who attributed their improvement primarily to their own efforts (36).

Another issue that merits attention is the potential interference of medication use with exposure exercises. In order to examine how this might happen, it is useful to first consider the mechanism by which exposure works. The use of exposure to treat anxiety disorders has been traditionally based on the notion that repeated engagement in feared situations facilitates habituation to anxiety-provoking stimuli and leads to eventual extinction of learned fear associations. The suggestion that successful exposure treatment obliterates the original learned associations has been disputed by Bouton and others (31,37), who argue that exposure does not lead to "unlearning" but rather generates new learning. This is indeed consistent with the goals of the cognitive-behavioral approach, which uses exposures to facilitate reinterpretation of threatening stimuli (8). Bouton explains that following repeated exposure, a stimulus (e.g., public speaking situation) that is initially associated with a fear response comes to acquire a more ambiguous meaning that competes with the original learned association but does not entirely replace it (37). Furthermore, according to Bouton, the degree to which the fear response is retrieved by subsequent presentation of the same stimulus depends largely on the context in which the stimulus appears as well as the context in which extinction of the response occurred. *Context* refers to anything from location and time to interoceptive cues, such as may arise from a drug or a specific affective state. Interestingly, there is evidence from animal research that the successful extinction of learned responses appears to be more context-dependent than conditioning of the same response (38). The difficulty this presents for combined treatment is that if exposure activity occurs in the context of pharmacologically reduced anxious arousal, the generalizability of any new learning may be limited to similar contexts, such that relapse may occur when medication is discontinued.

These implications are consistent with other theoretical perspectives as well. According to emotional processing theory, an information-processing model of anxiety disorders put forth by Foa and Kozak (39), when an individual with an anxiety disorder faces a feared situation, a composite of responses known as a "fear structure" is activated and serves to facilitate avoidant or adaptive behavior. According to Foa and Kozak, activation of this fear structure is one of the conditions required for therapeutic change to occur (39). By reducing anxiety, medication may impede the activation of the fear structure, thereby limiting the degree to which any corrective information can be integrated and processed during an exposure exercise. Otto further suggests that the patient who experiences heightened anxiety during exposure exercises may show more resilience when faced with a posttreatment resurgence of anxiety and may therefore be better protected against relapse than the patient who experienced little anxiety during treatment (40). It is also possible that different classes of medications may interact differently with CBT. For example, Heimberg and Becker (8) suggest that patients who become dependent on benzodiazepines may be less likely to tolerate anxiety during exposure exercises, may be inclined to rely on extra doses of their medication during therapy, and may be particularly vulnerable to relapse. Although other medications may less problematic in combination with CBT, the risk that clients will attribute their progress during therapy to medication rather than to their own efforts remains a potential concern with all classes of medication.

V. SUMMARY AND FUTURE DIRECTIONS

Medication and CBT are the most widely investigated treatments for social anxiety disorder. What does the prescribing clinician need to know in order to best serve patients affected by this disorder? For the acute treatment of the disorder, it appears that neither treatment modality has a clear advantage over the other, that both are efficacious for most patients, and that the simultaneous combination of medication with CBT does not necessarily confer synergistic effects relative to either treatment administered alone, although it may be associated with earlier treatment response. Moreover, there is reason to exercise caution in adding medication to CBT, since the mechanisms of action implicated in CBT may be disrupted when medication is introduced as an active ingredient. There is empirical evidence indicating that CBT is a treatment with enduring success. There are limited data suggesting that pharmacotherapy is associated with substantial immediate improvement but greater risk for relapse once treatment is discontinued.

Perhaps of primary concern is the fact that many patients who receive CBT or pharmacotherapy either remain symptomatic following treatment and/or relapse following treatment discontinuation. Relapse rates following medication discontinuation have ranged from 30 to 60% in studies of sertraline, paroxetine, and phenelzine (25,41–43), with lower rates (e.g., 17%) reported for CBT (25). The current challenge to researchers in this area is to determine how to maximize augmentation of treatment gains and protect against relapse. Increased understanding of the unique strengths of each treatment modality has led researchers to explore variations in the sequencing of medication and CBT. Specifically, there has been recent interest in using CBT both to assist patients with the tapering and discontinuation of medication and to provide therapeutic tools that can be used well after treatment has ended to combat social anxiety symptoms. This strategy has been successfully employed to enhance and prolong treatment gains among patients treated for depression and panic disorder (44–46). For example, following discontinuation of alprazolam, half of the patients who discontinued medication without CBT experienced relapses, whereas none of the patients who received CBT during the period of drug taper relapsed (47). The role of CBT in facilitating discontinuation of medication and preventing relapse was further supported in long-term follow-up studies of patients who had received combined treatments for panic disorder (48,49). Whether this strategy proves useful for patients with social anxiety disorder remains to be determined. A multisite study by Heimberg and Liebowitz is currently under way to examine whether CBT confers protection against relapse in patients with generalized social anxiety disorder who respond to an acute trial of treatment of paroxetine. It is also worth considering whether medication can provide further symptom relief among individuals who remain symptomatic after a trial of CBT.

Although progress has been made in this area, we still know very little about how, when, for whom, and in what order to combine these treatment modalities. In their discussion of combined treatments for panic disorder, Spiegel and Bruce (50) suggest that successful delivery of combined treatments requires careful consideration of the particular reasons for which treatment is being offered. For example, does the individual need immediate relief from severe anxiety in order to meet with a therapist? Is medication needed to prevent attrition or enhance compliance with CBT? Has the individual recently discontinued medication? Or are there reasons for which medication is contraindicated? Such questions should ultimately guide both researchers and clinicians in developing optimal treatment strategies for individuals with social anxiety disorder.

REFERENCES

1. Kessler RC, McGonagle KA, Zhao S, Nelson CB, Hughes M, Eshleman S, Wittchen HU, Kendler KS. Lifetime and 12-month prevalence of DSM-III-R psychiatric disorders in the United States: results from the National Comorbidity Survey. Arch Gen Psychiatry 1994; 51:8–19.
2. Wacker HR, Mullejans R, Klein KH, Battegay R. Identification of cases of anxiety disorders and affective disorders in the community according to the ICD-10 and DSM-III-R using the Composite International Diagnostic Interview (CIDI). International J Methods Psych Res 1992; 2:91–100.
3. Schneier FR, Heckelman LR, Garfinkel R, Campeas AR, Fallon BA, Gitow A, Street L, Del Bene D, Liebowitz MR. Functional impairment in social phobia. J Clin Psychiatry 1994; 55:322–331.
4. Liebowitz MR, Gorman JM, Fyer AJ, Klein DF. Social phobia: review of a neglected anxiety disorder. Arch Gen Psychiatry 1985;42:729–36.
5. Gould RA, Buckminster S, Pollack MH, Otto MW, Yap L. Cognitive-behavioral and pharmacological treatment for social phobia: a meta-analysis. Clin Psychol Sci Pract 1997; 4:291–306.

6. Lipsitz JD, Markowitz JC, Cherry S, Fyer AJ. Open trial of interpersonal psychotherapy for the treatment of social phobia. Am J Psychiatry 1999; 156:1814–1816.
7. Heimberg RG. Cognitive-behavioral therapy for social anxiety disorder: current status and future directions. Biol Psychiatry 2002; 51:101–108.
8. Heimberg RG, Becker RE. Cognitive-Behavioral Group Therapy for Social Phobia: Basic Mechanisms and Clinical Applications. New York: Guilford Press, 2002.
9. Heimberg RG, Salzman D, Holt CS, Blendell K. Cognitive behavioral group treatment of social phobia: effectiveness at 5-year follow-up. Cogn Ther Res 1993; 17:325–339.
10. Scott E, Heimberg RG. Social phobia: an update on treatment. Psychiatr Ann 2000; 30:678–686.
11. Stein MB, Fyer AJ, Davidson JT, Pollack MH, Wiita B. Fluvoxamine treatment of social phobia (social anxiety disorder): a double-blind, placebo-controlled study. Am J Psychiatry 1999; 156:756–760.
12. Blomhoff S, Haug TT, Hellstrøm K, Holme I, Humble M, Madsbu HP, Wold JE. Randomised controlled general practice trial of sertraline, exposure therapy and combined treatment in generalized social phobia. Br J Psychiatry 2001; 179:23–30.
13. Van Ameringen M, Lane RM, Walker JR, Bowen RC, Chokka PR, Goldner EM, Johnston DG, Lavallee YJ, Nandy S, Pecknold JC, Hadrava V, Swinson RP. Sertraline treatment of generalized social phobia: a 20-week, double-blind, placebo-controlled study. Am J Psychiatry 2001; 158:275–281.
14. Stein MB, Liebowitz MR, Lydiard B, Pitts CD, Bushnell W, Gergel I. Paroxetine treatment of generalized social phobia (social anxiety disorder): a randomized controlled trial. JAMA 1998; 280:708–713.
15. Gelernter CS, Uhde TW, Cimbolic P, Arnkoff DB, Vittone BJ, Tancer ME, Bartko JJ. Cognitive-behavioral and pharmacological treatments of social phobia: a controlled study. Arch Gen Psychiatry 1991; 48:938–945.
16. Otto MW, Pollack MH, Gould RA, Worthington JJ, McArdle ET, Rosenbaum JF, Heimberg RG. A comparison of the efficacy of clonazepam and cognitive-behavioral therapy for the treatment of social phobia. J Anxiety Disord 2000; 14:345–358.
17. Clark DB, Agras WS. The assessment and treatment of performance anxiety in musicians. Am J Psychiatry 1991; 148:598–605.
18. Turner SM, Beidel DC, Jacob RG. Social phobia: a comparison of behavior therapy and atenolol. J Consult Clin Psychol 1994; 62:350–358.
19. Clark DM, Ehlers A, McManus F, Hackmann A, Fennell M, Campbell H, Flower T, Davenport C, Louis B. Cognitive therapy vs fluoxetine in generalized social phobia: a randomized placebo controlled trial. J Consult Clin Psychol 2003; 71:1058–1067.
20. Gould RA, Johnson MW. Comparative effectiveness of cognitive-behavioral treatment and pharmacotherapy for social phobia: meta-analytic outcome.

In: Hofmann SG, DiBartolo PM, eds. From Social Anxiety to Social Phobia: Multiple Perspectives. Needham Heights, MA: Allyn & Bacon, 2001:379–390.

21. Fedoroff IC, Taylor, S. Psychological and pharmacological treatments of social phobia: a meta-analysis. J Clin Psychopharmacol 2001; 21:311–324.

22. Davidson JRT, Tupler LA, Potts NLS. Treatment of social phobia with ben-zodiazepines. J Clin Psychiatry 1994; 55:28–32.

23. Heimberg RG, Liebowitz MR, Hope DA, Schneier FR, Holt CS, Welkowitz LA, Juster HR, Campeas R, Bruch MA, Cloitre M, Fallon B, Klein DF. Cognitive behavioral group therapy versus phenelzine therapy in social phobia: 12-week outcome. Arch Gen Psychiatry 1998; 55:1133–1141.

24. Liebowitz MR. Social phobia. Mod Probl Pharmacopsychiatry 1987; 22:141–173.

25. Liebowitz MR, Heimberg RG, Schneier FR, Hope DA, Davies S, Holt CS, Goetz D, Juster HR, Lin S, Bruch MA, Marshall RD, Klein DF. Cognitive-behavioral group therapy versus phenelzine in social phobia: long-term out-come. Depress Anxiety 1999; 10:89–98.

26. Hope DA, Heimberg RG, Bruch MA. Dismantling cognitive-behavioral group therapy for social phobia. Behav Res Ther 1995; 33:637–650.

27. Falloon IR, Lloyd GG, Harpin RE. The treatment of social phobia: real-life rehearsal with nonprofessional therapists. J Nerv Ment Dis 1981; 169:180–184.

28. Haug TT, Blomhoff S, Hellström K, Holme I, Humble M, Madsbu HP, Wold JE. Exposure therapy and sertraline in social phobia: 1-year follow-up of a randomised controlled trial. Br J Psychiatry 2003; 182:312–318.

29. Bandelow B, Haug TT. Sertraline and exposure therapy in social phobia. Br J Psychiatry 2004; 184:271–272.

30. Furmark T, Tillfors M, Marteinsdottir I, Fischer H, Pissiota A, Langstrom B, Fredrikson M. Common changes in cerebral blood flow in patients with social phobia treated with citalopram or cognitive behavioral group therapy. Arch Gen Psychiatry 2002; 59:425–433.

31. Otto MW, Safren SA. Mechanisms of action in the treatment of social phobia. In: Hofmann SG, DiBartolo PM, eds. From Social Anxiety to Social Phobia: Multiple Perspectives. Needham Heights, MA: Allyn & Bacon, 2001:391–407.

32. Hope DA, Herbert JD, White C. Diagnostic subtype, avoidant personality disorder, and efficacy of cognitive-behavioral group therapy for social phobia. Cogn Ther Res 1995; 19:399–417.

33. Brown EJ, Heimberg RG, Juster HR. Social phobia subtype and avoidant personality disorder: effect on severity of social phobia, impairment and out-come of cognitive behavioral treatment. Behav Ther 1995; 26:467–486.

34. Chambless Dl, Tran GQ, Glass CR. Predictors of response to cognitive-behavioral group therapy for social phobia. J Anxiety Disord 1997; 11:221–240.

35. Hofmann SG. Treatment of social phobia: potential mediators and moderators. Clin Psychol Sci Pract 2000; 7:3–16.

36. Basoglu M, Marks IM, Kilic C, Brewin CR, Swinson RP. Alprazolam and exposure for panic disorder with agoraphobia: attribution of improvement

to medication predicts subsequent relapse. Br J Psychiatry 1994; 164:652–659.

37. Bouton ME. Context, ambiguity, and unlearning: sources of relapse after behavioral extinction. Biol Psychiatry 2002; 52:976–986.

38. Bouton ME, King DA. Effect of context on performance to conditioned stimuli with mixed histories of reinforcement and nonreinforcement. J Exp Psychol Anim Behav Processes 1986; 12:4–15.

39. Foa EB, Kozak MJ. Emotional processing of fear: exposure to corrective information. Psychol Bull 1986; 99:20–35.

40. Otto MW. Learning and "unlearning" fears: preparedness, neural pathways, and patients. Biol Psychiatry 2002; 52:917–920.

41. Stein MB, Chartier MJ, Hazen AL, Kroft CDL, Chale RA, Cote D, Walker JR. Paroxetine in the treatment of generalized social phobia: open-label treatment and double-blind placebo-controlled discontinuation. J Clin Psychopharmacol 1996; 16:218–222.

42. Stein DJ, Veriani M, Hair T, Kumar R. Efficacy of paroxetine for relapse prevention in social anxiety disorder. Arch Gen Psychiatry 2002; 59:1111–1118.

43. Walker JR, van Ameringen MA, Swinson R, Bowen RC, Chokka PR, Goldner E, Johnston DC, Lavallie YJ, Nandy S, Packnold JC, Hadrava V, Lane RM. Prevention of relapse in generalized social phobia: results of a 24-week study in responders to 20 weeks of sertraline treatment. J Clin Psychopharmacol 2000; 20: 636–644.

44. Fava GA, Grandi S, Zielezny M, Canestrari R, Morphy MA. Cognitive behavioral treatment of residual symptoms in primary major depressive disorder. Am J Psychiatry 1994; 151:1295–1299.

45. Fava GA, Grandi S, Zielezny M, Rafanelli C, Canestrari R. Four-year outcome for cognitive-behavioral treatment of residual symptoms in major depression. Am J Psychiatry 1996; 153:945–947.

46. Otto MW, Pollack MH, Sachs GS, Reiter SR, Meltzer-Brody S, Rosenbaum JF. Discontinuation of benzodiazepine treatment: efficacy of cognitive-behavioral therapy for patients with panic disorder. Am J Psychiatry 1993; 150:1485–1490.

47. Spiegel DA, Bruce TJ, Gregg SF, Nuzzarello A. Does cognitive behavior therapy assist slow-taper alprazolam discontinuation in panic disorder? Am J Psychiatry 1994; 151:876–881.

48. Bruce TJ, Spiegel DA, Hegel MT. Cognitive-behavioral therapy helps prevent relapse and recurrence of panic disorder following alprazolam discontinuation: a long-term follow-up of the Peoria and Dartmouth studies. J Consult Clin Psychol 1999; 67:151–156.

49. Hegel MT, Ravaris CL, Ahles TA. Combined cognitive-behavioral and time-limited alprazolam treatment of panic disorder. Behav Ther 1994; 25:183–195.

50. Spiegel DA, Bruce TJ. Benzodiazepines and exposure-based cognitive behavior therapies for panic disorder: conclusions from combined treatment trials. Am J Psychiatry 1997; 154:773–781.

19

Treatment of Social Anxiety Disorder in Children

Deborah C. Beidel, Robin Yeganeh,
Courtney Ferrell, and Candice Alfano
University of Maryland,
College Park, Maryland, U.S.A.

I. INTRODUCTION

Social anxiety disorder (social phobia) is "a marked and persistent fear of one or more social performances in which the person is exposed to unfamiliar people or to possible scrutiny by others" (Ref. 1, p. 417). Over the past 10 years, there has been increasing interest in the occurrence of this disorder among children and adolescents. Most of these studies have focused on its psychopathology, and—as reviewed elsewhere in ths volume—the resultant data clearly document the pervasive and serious nature of social anxiety disorder in children as well as its immediate and long-term consequences. Thus the need for effective interventions is evident, and data examining both pharmacological and psychosocial interventions are beginning to emerge. In this chapter, the current status of both pharmacological and psychosocial interventions for children with social anxiety disorder is reviewed.

II. OVERALL TREATMENT CONSIDERATIONS

The literature on efficacious treatments for childhood social anxiety disorder is limited when compared to that for adults with this disorder (2,3). Recent studies within the anxiety literature have reported the efficacy of cognitive behavioral therapy as well as exposure and social skills training for children (4,5) and adolescents (6–8). Particularly in the last few years, controlled pharmacological trials have been added to literature that previously consisted of case studies or open trials (3). An important recent trend is that both pharmacological and psychosocial trials are moving away from including socially anxious children among large samples of children with various types of anxiety disorders toward samples composed entirely of children with social anxiety disorder. Finally, comparative trials (psychosocial versus pharmacological interventions) are under way, as are treatment studies examining new types of treatment modalities and approaches. In the following section, the empirical evidence for both pharmacological and psychosocial interventions for children with social anxiety disorder is examined.

III. PHARMACOLOGICAL TREATMENT

As noted previously (9), prior to the fourth edition of the *Diagnostic and Statistical Manual of Mental Disorders* (DSM-IV), children with social anxiety were given various diagnoses, including social phobia, avoidant disorder of childhood, overanxious disorder, and selective mutism. Early pharmacological trials of children with these disorders provided some of the first data regarding the treatment of children with social anxiety concerns. Below, data on pharmacological treatments for children with these related disorders are reviewed, followed by studies of children meeting DSM criteria for social anxiety disorder (SAD).

A. Samples of Children with Conditions That Resemble Social Anxiety Disorder

In one of the first pharmacological trials, 20 children (ages 8 to 16) with overanxious disorder or avoidant disorder of childhood were treated in a 6-week open trial of alprazolam (10). Six children (30%) given doses ranging from 0.5 to 1.5 mg daily appeared to demonstrate moderate clinical improvement. A follow-up 4-week double-blind placebo-controlled trial (11) examined 30 children (ages 8 to 16 years; mean age 12.6 years) with either overanxious disorder ($n = 21$) or avoidant disorder ($n = 9$). The average daily dose was 1.57 mg (range 0.5 to 3.5 mg) and alprazolam appeared superior to placebo on clinical global ratings of anxiety at day 28. However, there were no significant group differences on the Clinical Global Impression

Scale of Improvement (CGI-I) at posttreatment. Furthermore, following tapering (day 42), there was a nonsignificant trend for patients in the alprazolam group to relapse, whereas the placebo group continued to improve. Thus, the positive outcome reported in the initial open trial was not replicated in the double-blind study. These negative results, coupled with potentially serious side effects and other dose-related complications, have led to the recommendation that benzodiazepines be considered only after all other medications have failed (3,12–14).

The majority of published clinical trials for children with SAD have evaluated selective serotonin reuptake inhibitors (SSRIs), now considered first-line agents for childhood anxiety disorders and related conditions because of their high tolerance levels, minimal side effects, and the lack of a need for blood level monitoring (3,12,13). Common SSRIs include fluvoxamine (Luvox), fluoxetine (Prozac), sertraline (Zoloft), and paroxetine (Paxil). More recently, citalopram (Celexa) has been examined. In general, no side effects or minimal side effects—such as headaches, nausea, drowsiness, insomnia, jitteriness, and stomachaches—have been reported (13). For example, these agents have been used for the treatment of selective mutism. Although the relationship of selective mutism to SAD in children is not yet clear, most children with selective mutism also meet diagnostic criteria for social anxiety disorder (15,16). Thus, the treatment of selective mutism with SSRIs is of relevance for understanding the pharmacological treatment of children with SAD.

Two trials (one open and one double-blind) have examined the use of fluoxetine with selectively mute children. In a 9-week open trial (16), 21 children (ages 5 to 14 years, mean age 8.2 years) were treated for selective mutism. The children also were comorbid for either avoidant disorder of childhood ($n = 18$) or social phobia ($n = 3$). The average daily dose of fluoxetine was 28.1 mg/day. Seventy-eight percent of the children had decreased anxiety and increased speech at posttreatment. Although encouraging, these findings are limited because of the nonblinded nature of the outcome ratings used. Using a 12-week double-blind research design (15), 15 selectively mute children (ages 6 to 12 years) comorbid for either social phobia or avoidant disorder were randomly assigned to fluoxetine (average dose 21.4 mg/day) or placebo. At posttreatment, parental Clinical Global Impression (CGI) ratings showed significant improvement for those treated with fluoxetine, but there were no group differences using clinician or teacher ratings. It is important to note that the overall treatment effects were viewed as modest and most of the fluoxetine patients were still symptomatic at posttreatment. Thus, in contrast to the very promising results of the open clinical trial, this placebo-controlled trial resulted in only minimal support for the use of fluoxetine in the treatment of selective mutism.

B. Samples of Children with Anxiety Disorders Including Those with Social Anxiety Disorder

In one of the first studies to examine the efficacy of SSRIs for anxiety disorders in children, Birmaher et al. (17) treated 21 children and adolescents ages 11 to 17 years (mean age 14 years) with fluoxetine (mean dosage 25.7 mg/day). Children were diagnosed with overanxious disorder, avoidant disorder, or social phobia. Outcome data using retrospective chart review (based on reports from attending nurses and patients' mothers), indicated that 81% of the children exhibited marked improvement in anxiety symptoms after 6 to 8 weeks of treatment.

In another open trial (18), 16 outpatient children (ages 9 to 18 years), with various anxiety disorders and considered nonresponsive to psychotherapy, were treated with fluoxetine (mean doses for children and adolescents were 24 and 40 mg/day, respectively). Outcome was rated by parental and clinician report, the latter including change scores on the CGI Severity (CGI-S) scale. Similar to the results of Birmaher et al. (17), treatment gains were realized at 6 to 9 weeks, and lower doses were efficacious for children who had only one anxiety disorder. Eighty percent of those with social phobia (8 out of 10) were judged to be clinically improved. Similar percentages were reported for other diagnostic groups. Even though judged to be clinically improved, 62.5% of the entire sample still met criteria for an anxiety disorder at posttreatment, indicating a continuing degree of impairment.

In a multicenter controlled trial known as the Rupp Anxiety Trial, 128 children with separation anxiety disorder, SAD, or generalized anxiety disorder ages 6 to 17 years were randomly assigned to either 8 weeks of fluvoxamine or placebo (19). The average fluvoxamine dose was 300 mg/day. Both groups also received supportive psychotherapy. Outcome (based on anxious symptomatology and clinical impairment) was assessed by parent and self report and by clinician ratings. Using the Pediatric Anxiety Rating Scale, fluvoxamine was superior to placebo in the reduction of anxiety symptoms. Furthermore, 76% (48 of 63) of children in the fluvoxamine group showed marked clinical improvement as measured by the CGI-I in comparison to 29% (19 of 65) of the placebo group. Significant between-group differences were detected by week 3, and these increased through week 6. Following 6 weeks of treatment, group differences were maintained but no further improvement was noted for either group.

In a separate publication (20), an examination of potential moderators and mediators of treatment outcome revealed a significant interaction effect for SAD and type of treatment. Among those treated with fluoxetine, there was no difference in response rate for children with a primary or secondary diagnosis of SAD versus children without a diagnosis of SAD (79 versus

71%, respectively). In contrast, the placebo response rate was 25% for children with a primary or secondary diagnosis of social phobia versus 40% for children without this diagnosis. These results suggest that fluvoxamine is efficacious when a diagnosis of SAD is present, although it is unclear how the presence of comorbid disorders may affect treatment response. Furthermore, the results indicate that children with a diagnosis of SAD may be less responsive to placebo than children with other types of anxiety disorders.

In an open-label 6-month extension of the RUPP anxiety study (21), 94% of those children and adolescents who initially responded to fluvoxamine maintained their improvement. Overall, the outcome of the RUPP anxiety trial appears quite promising. Nonetheless, as indicated by the authors, the results must be interpreted cautiously because, although this was a double-blind study, treating clinicians (not independent evaluators) rated both clinical outcome and adverse events. Thus, knowledge of side effects may have created some degree of bias regarding outcome ratings. Finally, a large majority of the sample was diagnosed with more than one of the three anxiety disorders, and the outcome was not examined separately for children with SAD.

Most recently, Birmaher et al. (22) conducted a randomized, placebo-controlled trial of fluoxetine for 74 children (ages 7 to 17) and adolescents with anxiety disorders including generalized anxiety disorder, separation anxiety disorder, and/or SAD (54% had a diagnosis of SAD). Children were randomized to either fluoxetine or placebo. At week one, 10 mg/day of fluoxetine was administered. If tolerated, the dose was titrated to 20 mg/day, which was maintained for the rest of the 12-week trial. At posttreatment, 61% of the fluoxetine group and 35% of the placebo group were rated as much or very much improved according to the treating clinician's CGI-I ratings. Consistent with the results of the RUPP study, children with SAD who were treated with fluoxetine had a significantly better clinical outcome (76% were rated as much or very much improved on the CGI-I) than those treated with placebo (21%). Furthermore, the treatment effect for children with SAD was significantly greater than the treatment effect for patients with anxiety disorders other than SAD. Similar results were not found when group comparisons were made based on other diagnostic categories [i.e., children with generalized anxiety disorder (GAD) versus children without GAD or children with separation anxiety disorder versus children without separation anxiety disorder]. Furthermore, functional outcome in this trial was defined as a score of 70 or higher on the Children's Global Assessment Scale (scores range from 0 to 100). The percentage of socially anxious children who scored above that cutoff was significantly higher for those treated with fluoxetine than for those treated with placebo (45.5 versus 10%, respectively). No significant differences in functional outcome were reported between treated and untreated groups of children with generalized anxiety disorder or separation anxiety disorder. However, as noted by the authors, even with this improvement, at least 50% of the sample remained symptomatic (defined as still having at least three symptoms of anxiety at posttreatment). Of note, 70% of these children had two anxiety disorders and 26% had three anxiety disorders. Thus, the efficacy of fluoxetine specifically for children with SAD alone remains unclear.

C. Treatment of Children with Social Anxiety Disorder

In a sample composed entirely of children with SAD, Compton et al. (23) administered sertraline to children and adolescents ages 10 to 17 (mean age 13.6 years). All children had four 1-hour sessions of cognitive-behavioral therapy prior to the pharmacological trial, however, no subject made significant improvement following the brief CBT intervention. The trial was 8 weeks in length and the mean daily dosage at 8 weeks was 123.21 mg/day. Treatment outcome was assessed based on 1) CGI-S ratings assigned by an independent evaluator, 2) scores on the Social Phobia and Anxiety Inventory for Children (SPAI-C) (24), and 3) ratings of distress when the children were engaged in two behavioral tasks—an 8-minute speech and a one-on-one conversation with a confederate. Responders were those children who had a CGI-I rating of much or very much improved and a CGI-S rating of normal or borderline ill. Partial responders had a rating of at least much improved but were still judged to be mildly to extremely ill. Nonresponders were those who had an improvement score of less than much improved and a severity rating of mildly to severely ill. At posttreatment, 36% of the children were treatment responders and 29% were partial responders. Children's scores on the SPAI-C improved significantly from pre- to posttreatment, and posttreatment scores were in the range reported by children never diagnosed with SAD. Ratings of distress on the behavioral tasks likewise showed significant improvement. Side effects were characterized as mild or moderate and all were controlled by decreasing the dosage as necessary. The results of this trial are very promising, although—as noted by the authors—the study is limited by the small number of patients, the lack of a placebo control group, no randomization, and the possible carryover effects of the brief CBT trial. Interestingly, the authors noted that at the debriefing, several patients attributed their improvement to the combination of the two interventions rather than to either one alone. A follow-up investigation using a double-blind placebo-controlled trial is worthy of investigation.

In summary, there currently is some promising evidence that SSRIs are effective for the treatment of childhood anxiety disorders. SSRIs may also be appropriate specifically for those with SAD, although at this time the majority of the evidence is indirect and limited to small sample sizes. Furthermore, pharmacological trials to date have not included long-term follow-up assessment or, in most cases, have not assessed outcome in terms of the specifics of social functioning. Of course, some of these same issues pertain to the studies of psychosocial trials discussed below.

IV. PSYCHOSOCIAL TREATMENT

The status of the psychosocial treatment literature for children with SAD is somewhat ahead of the pharmacological treatment literature. That is, although the initial studies included children with SAD among a group of patients with various types of anxiety disorders (24–30), there are now several randomized studies using samples consisting solely of children and adolescents with SAD. Studies using samples of children with various anxiety disorders are reviewed first, followed by those consisting solely of children with SAD.

A. Psychosocial Treatment Studies for Mixed Samples of Childhood Anxiety Disorders

Kendall's Coping Cat program was one of the first manualized CBT programs to be examined in controlled trials of children with various types of anxiety disorders. Coping Cat is a 16-week treatment program that includes psychoeducation, modifying negative cognition in anxiety-provoking situations, developing a plan to cope with anxiety, actual exposure to distressful situations, and self-reinforcement. In the initial publication (28), 27 children ages 9 to 13 (including a few children with avoidant disorder) treated with the Coping Cat program were compared to 20 children in a wait-list control group. At posttreatment, the CBT group was significantly improved across a variety of measures when compared to the wait-list control group. Treatment gains were maintained 3.35 years later (32). In a replication study using the same treatment design (29) and a sample including a few children with avoidant disorder, 53% of the CBT group no longer met diagnostic criteria at posttreatment, compared to 6% of the wait-list control group. Although the specific outcomes were not presented, there were reportedly no differences across diagnostic groups. A more recent study examined administration of the Coping Cat program in a group versus individual format (27). The outcome was quite positive regardless of the manner of intervention. However, children's social functioning (e.g., social anxiety, friendships, and social activities) did not improve at posttreatment, suggesting that a different or more comprehensive intervention may be needed to address the unique aspects of SAD.

Using Kendall's CBT intervention, others (26) have examined the additive effects of a family intervention component (CBT+FAM) that included training in reinforcement/contingency management strategies, teaching parents coping techniques to deal with their own emotionality, and communication and problem-solving skills. Using a sample of 79 children that included 27% with SAD, CBT and CBT+FAM were both efficacious when compared to a wait-list control. However, CBT+FAM was significantly superior to CBT alone; 84% of children in the CBT+FAM were diagnosis-free at posttreatment, compared to 57% in the CBT group. Among the children with SAD, 61.5% were diagnosis-free at posttreatment, with results maintained up to 6 years later (33); specifically, 10 out of 11 children originally diagnosed with social phobia did not meet diagnostic criteria at follow-up. Barrett (25) also conducted a comparative study of CBT and CBT+FAM administered in a group format (GCBT and GCBT+FAM, respectively). Both interventions were equally effective when compared to the control group. Only children in the GCBT+ FAM group continued to improve over the 12-month follow-up. However, because only 7% of the sample had a primary diagnosis of SAD, it is unclear if these positive results would be replicated with a larger sample of socially anxious children. Finally, in an extension of this CBT intervention, the FRIENDS program (34) which combines traditional CBT interventions (exposure, cognitive strategies, relaxation, and contingency management) with a family-skills component (cognitive restructuring for parents, partner support training, and encouragement to build social networks), with emphasis on the establishment of new friendships and specialized training for children in making internal attributions about their accomplishments. In this sample, 14% of the children had a primary diagnosis of social phobia. At the end of the 10-session treatment program, 69% of the children in the FRIENDS condition were without a diagnosis of an anxiety disorder, compared to 6% of the control group. Results were maintained at 1-year follow-up.

Two studies by Silverman and colleagues (30,31) also examined group (GCBT) and individual CBT for children, ages 6 to 16, with various anxiety disorders. In the first study (30), 15 (27%) of 56 children had a primary diagnosis of SAD. GCBT included 12 weeks of gradual exposure, parent-child contingency management, and cognitive self-control training. At posttreatment, 64% of the GCBT group no longer met criteria for their primary diagnosis, compared to 13% of controls. Furthermore, gains were maintained at 3-, 6-, and 12-month follow-up. In a second study, Silverman and colleagues (31) compared individual exposure-based CBT (ICBT) components to an active control condition. Children ($n = 81$) with various phobic conditions and their parents were randomly assigned to: 1) a contingency management treatment condition consisting of reinforcement and extinction strategies; 2) a self-control treatment condition consisting of self-evaluation and self-regulatory skills; or 3) an active control condition consisting of educational support. The treatment program was 10 weeks in length and all three conditions significantly decreased children's phobic symptoms. Treatment gains were maintained at follow-up. However, because only 10% of the sample had a primary diagnosis of social anxiety disorder, results were not reported separately by that diagnosis.

Manassis et al. (35) compared GCBT and ICBT for children with various anxiety disorders. The intervention (Coping Bear Workbook) was an adaptation of Kendall's Coping Cat program. Seventy-eight children (ages 8 to 12) were randomly assigned to either group or individual treatment, and both interventions included a parental component. However, only 5 of the participants had a primary diagnosis of SAD; thus, the relevance of the primary outcome for children with this disorder is unclear. Both forms of CBT were equally effective. Interestingly, those high in self-reported social anxiety who received ICBT were significantly more improved on a self-report measure of anxiety than those high in social anxiety treated with GCBT.

In a final study, Rapee et al. (36) administered GCBT to children (ages 7 to 16) with various anxiety disorders. Approximately 29% of the children had social phobia/avoidant disorder. The treatment program consisted of 9 sessions over 11 weeks and parents were included in all phases of the intervention. While the intervention for children included typical CBT strategies, parents were simultaneously trained in child management skills. The intervention resulted in significant improvement across a broad range of child and parent measures when compared to the wait-list control group, and results were maintained at 1 year follow-up. A subset of children continued to make improvements during the follow-up period.

These studies are included in this review because children with SAD made up part of the samples. However, the small numbers/percentage of children with SAD is noteworthy, and the results should be interpreted cautiously. For example, other than the diagnostic interviews, only one (27) included specific measures of social anxiety symptoms or functioning. Thus it is unclear if these interventions decrease general arousal or address the unique aspects of childhood SAD. Additionally, except for Silverman et al. (31), interventions have been compared only to a wait-list control group, which is a less stringent comparison than using placebo or active control condition. In summary, although these studies provide information about the treatment of anxiety in children, they have not specifically addressed SAD.

B. Psychosocial Treatment Studies of Children with Social Anxiety Disorder

The first CBT program designed specifically for adolescents with SAD (37) was a group intervention, Group Cognitive-Behavioral Treatment for Adolescents (GCBT-A). The 3-month treatment program consists of psychoeducation, skill building (such as social skills, problem-solving, and assertiveness training), cognitive restructuring, behavioral exposure, and parental involvement. In the initial investigation, 5 adolescents (ages 13 to 17) with social anxiety disorder were treated with GCBT-A. At posttreatment, social phobia symptoms had decreased to subclinical levels in 80% of the adolescents. The results of this investigation were promising and larger, controlled trials followed.

Hayward et al. (8) randomized 35 female adolescents (mean age 15 years) with SAD to GCBT-A (without parental involvement) or a no-treatment control group. After treatment, 45% of the GCBT-A group no longer met diagnostic criteria for SAD, compared to only 4% of the no-treatment group. However, as noted by the authors, considerable residual social phobia symptoms remained at posttreatment as indicated by the adolescents' scores on the Social Phobia Anxiety Inventory (SPAI) (38). At 1-year follow-up, there were no significant group differences in the frequency of SAD diagnoses or SPAI score. It is unclear why these follow-up results were less favorable than those reported for adult populations utilizing a similar treatment protocol (2) or the initial single-case design (37). However, some of the adolescents had comorbid depressive symptoms, and this may have attenuated treatment outcome.

One important issue in the area of anxiety disorders, including social anxiety disorder in children, is the potential role of cognitions in their etiology, maintenance, and treatment. Many of the interventions developed to treat anxiety disorders in children are adapted from those developed for adults and many but not all of these adult interventions include a cognitive component. However, there currently is insufficient evidence that negative cognitions play a major role in the clinical presentation of SAD in children, at least in preadolescent children (39). Thus it is not clear that interventions need to include specific components designed to eliminate negative cognitions. Alternatively, although few current interventions specifically include social skills training, the documented lack of social skills in children with SAD suggests that this may be a necessary component of psychosocial interventions (40,41).

With these issues in mind, Beidel and colleagues (4) recently developed and compared the effectiveness of a multicomponent behavioral treatment for childhood social phobia, Social Effectiveness Therapy for Children

(SET-C), to an active, nonspecific intervention (Testbusters). The sample of 67 children, ages 8 to 12 years, were randomly assigned to one of the two groups. SET-C includes 12 weeks of group social skills training, peer-generalization experiences, and individual in vivo exposure. One session per week was devoted to group social skills training and a peer generalization session. The second weekly session focuses on individualized in vivo exposure. The comparison intervention, Testbusters, is a study-skills and test-taking strategy program designed to reduce test-taking anxiety and promote good study habits. It has strong face validity given that many children with social phobia endorse anxiety in testing situations. At posttreatment, 67% of the SET-C group no longer met criteria for SAD, compared to 5% in the Testbusters group. Across the various treatment measures, those in the SET-C group were less anxious, less avoidant of social situations, more skillful in their social interactions, and engaged in more social discourse as reported by children, parents, and independent evaluators at posttreatment. At 6-month follow-up, those treated with SET-C showed continued improvement; 85% no longer meeting criteria for SAD. These results are particularly encouraging because, unlike the designs of previous investigations, SET-C was compared to an active, nonspecific control treatment and not a wait-list control. Additionally, unlike the studies cited above (7,37), this investigation used a sample of preadolescent rather than adolescent children. Yet it remains unclear whether SET-C would be equally effective for adolescents with SAD, although such a study is currently under way (see Sec. VII, below).

A 5-year follow-up of the efficacy of SET-C is halfway complete. Twenty-seven of the children treated with SET-C (mean age at follow-up, 14.9 years) have completed a 3-year follow-up (31); the results thus far indicate that all treatment gains are maintained and in some cases even enhanced. For example, among the 9 children treated with SET-C who still met diagnostic criteria at posttreatment (i.e., nonresponders), 44% were judged to be responders 3 years later. Conversely, among those who were judged responders at posttreatment, less than 20% were considered to have relapsed 3 years later. These same variables will be examined at the 5-year follow-up point.

In one of the first non-American studies for adolescents with SAD (42,43), 59 Spanish adolescents ages 15 to 17 were randomly assigned to a psychosocial intervention that included distinct elements of traditional cognitive therapy (Therapy for Adolescents with Generalized Social Phobia) (42), CBGT-A, a version of SET-C for adolescents, or a wait list control. At posttreatment, all active interventions were significantly superior to the control group; at follow-up, there were few differences among the three active interventions in terms of decreases in social phobia symptoms, social skills, and self-esteem. Although the number of adolescents randomized to each condition was somewhat small, these results are promising and suggest that the interventions are effective across cultures.

The effectiveness of a CBT program that included social skills training, relaxation techniques, social problem solving, positive self-instruction, cognitive challenging, and exposure to social situations (CBT) was examined in children with SAD, ages 7 to 14 (5). The children were randomly assigned either to group CBT with parental involvement (CBT-PI), group CBT with no parental involvement (CBT-PNI), or a wait-list control group. Parental involvement focused on teaching proper modeling and reinforcement of children's newly acquired social skills and encouragement of participation in outside social activities. Following treatment, parental reports indicated that 87.5% of the CBT-PI group and 58% of the CBT-PNI group no longer met diagnostic criteria for SAD, compared to 7% of the wait-list control. Similar rates of outcome were reported when child report was used. Differences between the two CBT groups were not statistically significant. Treatment effects were maintained at 6- and 12-month follow-up, and both active treatment conditions were associated with improved social skills from pretreatment to 12-month follow-up (based on parent report). Although the interventions did not appear to affect the children's total number of peer interactions, parental reports of competence with peers, or independent observer ratings of assertiveness during behavioral observation from pre- to posttreatment, an interval longer than 12 weeks may be necessary in order to detect this magnitude of change.

V. COMBINATION AND COMPARATIVE TREATMENTS

Most recently, clinical trials are utilizing comparative and combination treatment designs. Chavira and Stein (44) examined the combination of psychoeducation and citalopram for 12 children and adolescents (ages 8 to 17) with generalized SAD. The mean age of the sample was 13.4 years and the mean dosage of citalopram was 35 mg/day. Over the 12-week pharmacological trial, children and parents also attended eight 15- to 20-minute psychoeducational sessions conducted by a clinical psychologist. The program consisted of an initial session of psychoeducation, two sessions of instruction in the construction of anxiety hierarchies, three sessions constructing graduated exposure tasks, and teaching of basic social skills and cognitive challenges. The final session was a review of progress and relapse prevention. At posttreatment, 10 of the 12 children (83.3%) were judged as improved: 41.7% as much improved and 41.7% as very much improved. Significant improvement was also found on several self-report measures of social anxiety, depression, and parents' ratings of social skills. However, even though scores were significantly decreased at posttreatment, the children were still somewhat impaired (according to the Social Phobia and Anxiety Inventory for Children) (24). These results are promising, but—as with other open-label trials using small sample sizes—they require replication with a larger sample and a randomized, placebo-controlled design.

Two multicenter trials are currently under way. In a large 4-year multicenter trial for the treatment of anxiety disorders in youth (Albano, personal communication, 3/31/03), 318 children (ages 7 to 16) with either generalized anxiety disorder, SAD, or separation anxiety disorder will be randomized to either fluvoxamine, CBT (Coping Cat program), the combination of fluvoxamine and CBT, or pill placebo. This will be a 12-week acute trial, followed by a 6-month treatment maintenance period for responders to the three active interventions. This will be the largest study of the treatment of childhood anxiety disorders to date, but it is unclear how many children with SAD will be included in the final sample.

A second ongoing two-site trial is comparing fluoxetine, SET-C, and pill placebo for the treatment of 250 children and adolescents (ages 7 to 16) with SAD (45). The goals of this 4-year project are to further evaluate the efficacy of SET-C across an expanded age range of children and adolescents, to determine the efficacy of fluoxetine for youth with social phobia, to compare fluoxetine to a pill placebo control and to SET-C, and to determine the long-term (1-year) durability of both active interventions. This study will be the first to compare a pharmacological and psychosocial intervention specifically for children with SAD.

VI. RECENT INNOVATIONS IN PSYCHOSOCIAL TREATMENTS

Masia and colleagues (8) investigated a 14-session group-treatment program for six adolescents with SAD. Conducted in the adolescents' actual school setting, this intervention included social skills training and in vivo exposure sessions. There was significant improvement on clinician severity ratings of SAD, but the adolescents' self-report of social fears did not decrease significantly. Based on these pilot data, there is now an ongoing randomized controlled trial (46) to further demonstrate the utility of this intervention and its provision in a school setting. To date, 35 children have been randomly assigned to either the active intervention or a wait-list control group. Treatment is conducted in groups and consists of psychoeducation, training in realistic thinking, social skills training, exposure, and relapse prevention. In addition, there are two brief individual meetings, two meetings with the adolescent's teacher, two sessions with the adolescent's parent, and four social activities that include the use of peer assistants. The preliminary results indicate that the intervention is quite effective in comparison to the wait-list control group, with significant improvement across clinician and self-report measures.

In a very recent innovation, Fung et al. (47) described the successful treatment of a 7-year-old child with selective mutism using an Internet web-based version of CBT. The program includes a child workbook as well as parent/teacher manuals that focus on psychoeducation. The training format followed that used in other CBT programs based on the Coping Cat program. The first eight sessions were devoted to training and the last six to practice of the skills. In this second phase, the child has the opportunity to record short messages via the computer that can be replayed by the therapist during the following treatment session. The use of recording and playback in the presence of the therapist was aimed at desensitization of social fears. In other words, it provided an opportunity for others to hear the child speak without the child having to actually produce the speech. Such desensitization procedures are often used by behavior therapists when treating children with selective mutism (although the use of a computer is a novel and perhaps extremely engaging variation on this strategy). Pre- and posttreatment ratings of anxiety by the child, parent, and teacher indicated some improvement, as did the selective mutism questionnaire. The results of this case description are interesting and, given the refractory nature of selective mutism, suggest that larger-scale interventions are warranted.

VII. SUMMARY AND FUTURE DIRECTIONS

Both pharmacological and psychosocial interventions for youth with SAD are beginning to emerge. However, the study of efficacious pharmacological and psychosocial treatments with childhood anxiety disorders is still limited at this time. There has been even less research examining pharmacotherapy and behavioral therapy/CBT using samples composed solely of children with SAD. With respect to open trials of medication, anxious children showed improvement on both SSRIs and benzodiazepines, and several controlled trials now confirm that the SSRIs are effective for children with anxiety disorders. Similarly, although more of the psychosocial treatment trials are controlled through the use of a wait-list control group, the majority of these studies have used samples of children with various types of anxiety disorders. The next challenge for pharmacological and psychosocial treatment trials however, is to demonstrate that these interventions are effective (and superior to placebo) for children with SAD (rather than examining efficacy across diagnostically different groups of children). For example, the few data available suggest that, in comparison to disorders such as GAD, SAD may be one of the few conditions where SSRIs actually may be significantly superior to placebo (22,20). Similarly, although CBT interventions appear to be effective in reducing general anxiety, they may not be as effective in addressing the specific deficits of children with SAD (27,30). Furthermore, even though current treatment outcomes indicate statistically significant improvement at posttreatment, many of these trials note that clinically significant symptoms remain at posttreatment and follow-up. Therefore the question that remains is whether additional treatment sessions would produce an even more positive outcome or whether an alternative treatment strategy is necessary.

One challenge for both types of interventions is that many children are diagnosed with more than one anxiety disorder. Although this often results in difficulty determining a primary diagnosis, there now are several studies that suggest that the existence of these comorbid conditions does not affect treatment outcome, at least with respect to psychosocial interventions (48,49). However, trials limited to children with a primary diagnosis of SAD along with measures that assess specific symptoms of this disorder and social functioning would make a significant contribution to the literature. There are few measures currently available to assess social functioning, although daily diary methods that assess number of social interactions, for example, would be an important first step.

Another area in need of further investigation is the relative contribution of specific treatment components in allowing greater efficiency in the delivery of these services. Currently, we do not know which component(s) are necessary or sufficient, although based on meta-analyses conducted with adult outcome studies, exposure in some form would appear to be the key ingredient (50). At this point, it appears unclear if parental involvement in the actual treatment sessions is necessary, although it is abundantly clear that parental cooperation in ensuring completion of homework assignments is necessary. Given the amount of time that children spend at school, school cooperation could be another crucial ingredient, although more data are necessary before drawing strong conclusions. Finally, little attention has been given to developmental considerations with regard to understanding the utility of specific psychosocial treatment components. Most studies include youth between the ages of 7 and 17, with few attempts to address developmental issues with respect to intervention or assessment of treatment outcome. Given the major developmental changes that occur across this age range, future studies may need to focus on restricted age ranges or examine outcomes separately for different developmental subgroups. Finally, long-term outcome data for psychosocial treatment are beginning to emerge and additional studies are under way. Pharmacological treatment trials lag behind in this regard, but hopefully such data will be forthcoming.

ACKNOWLEDGMENT

This chapter was supported in part by NIMH Grants MH53703 and MH60332 to the first author.

REFERENCES

1. American Psychiatric Association. Diagnostic and Statistical Manual of Mental Disorders, 4th ed. Washington, DC: APA, 1994.
2. Heimberg RG, Dodge CS, Hope DA, Kennedy CR, Zollo R, Becker RE. Cognitive-behavioral group treatment for social phobia: comparison to a credible placebo control. Cogn Ther Res 1990; 14: 1–23.
3. Pine DS, Grun JBS. Anxiety disorders. In: Walsh TB, ed. Child Psychopharmacology. Vol. 17. Washington, DC: American Psychiatric Press, 1998: 115–144.
4. Beidel DC, Turner SM, Morris TL. Behavioral treatment of childhood social phobia. J Consult Clin Psychol 2000; 68: 1072–1080.
5. Spence SH, Donovan C, Brechman-Toussaint M. The treatment of childhood social phobia: the effectiveness of a social skills training-based, cognitive-behavioral intervention, with and without parental involvement. J Child Psychol Psychiatry 2000; 41: 713–726.
6. Albano MA. Treatment of social phobia in adolescents: cognitive behavioral programs focused on intervention and prevention. J Cogn Psychother 2000; 14: 67–76.
7. Hayward C, Varady S, Albano AM, Thienemann M, Henderson L, Schatzberg AF. Cognitive-behavioral group therapy for social phobia in female adolescents: results of a pilot study. J Am Acad Child Adolesc Psychiatry 2000; 39: 721–726.
8. Masia CL, Klein RG, Storch EA, Corda B. School-based behavioral treatment for social anxiety disorder in adolescents: results of a pilot study. J Am Acad Child Adolesc Psychiatry 2001; 40: 780–786.
9. Beidel DC, Ferrell C, Alfano CA, Yeganeh R. The treatment of childhood social anxiety disorder. Psychiat Clin North Am 2001; 24:831–846.
10. Simeon JG, Ferguson HB. Alprazolam effects in children with anxiety disorders. Can J Psychiatry 1997; 32: 570–574.
11. Simeon JG, Ferguson HB, Knott V, Roberts N, Gauthier B, Dubois C, Wiggins D. Clinical, cognitive, and neurophysiological effects of alprazolam in children and adolescents with overanxious and avoidant disorders. J Am Acad Child Adolesc Psychiatry 1992; 31: 29–33.
12. Kratochvil C, Kutcher S, Reiter S, March JS. Pharmacotherapy of pediatric anxiety disorders. In: Russ SW, Ollendick TH, eds. Handbook of Psychotherapies with Children and Families. New York: Kluwer Academic, 1999:345–366.
13. Velosa JF, Riddle MA. Pharmacologic treatment of anxiety disorders in children and adolescents. Psychopharmacology 2000; 9:119–133.

14. Wilens TE, Spencer TJ, Frazier J, Biederman J. Child and adolescent psychopharmacology. In: Ollendick T, Hersen M, eds. Handbook of Child Psychopathology. New York: Plenum Press, 1998: 603–636.

15. Black B, Uhde TW. Treatment of elective mutism with fluoxetine: a double-blind placebo-controlled study. J Am Acad Child Adolesc Psychiatry 1994; 33: 1000–1006.

16. Dummit ES, Klein RG, Tancer NK, Asche B, Martin J. Fluoxetine treatment of children with selective mutism: an open trial. J Am Acad Child Adolesc Psychiatry 1996; 35: 615–621.

17. Birmaher B, Waterman GS, Ryan N, Cully M, Balach L, Ingram J, Brodsky M. Fluoxetine for childhood anxiety disorders. J Am Acad Child Adolesc Psychiatry 1994; 33: 993–998.

18. Fairbanks JM, Pine DS, Tancer NK, Dummit ES, Kentgen LM, Martin J, Asche BK, Klein RG. Open fluoxetine treatment of mixed anxiety disorder in children and adolescents. J Child Adolesc Psychopharmacol 1997; 7: 17–29.

19. RUPP Anxiety Study Group. Fluvoxamine treatment of anxiety disorders in children and adolescents. N Engl J Med 2001; 344: 1279–1285.

20. RUPP Anxiety Study Group. Searching for mediators and mediators of pharmacological treatment effects in children and adolescents with anxiety disorders. J Am Acad Child Adolesc Psychiatry 2003; 42: 13–21.

21. RUPP Anxiety Study Group. Treatment of pediatric anxiety disorders: an open-label extension of the Research Units on Pediatric Psychopharmacology Anxiety Study. J Child Adolesc Psychopharmacol 2002; 12: 175–188.

22. Birmaher B, Axelson DA, Monk K, Kalas C, Clark DB, Ehmann M, Bridge J, Heo J, Brent DA. Fluoxetine for the treatment of childhood anxiety disorders. J Am Acad Child Adolesc Psychiatry 2003; 42: 415–423.

23. Compton SC, Grant PJ, Chrisman AK, Gammon PJ, Brown VLO, March JS. Sertraline in children and adolescents with social anxiety disorder: an open trial. J Am Acad Child Adolesc Psychiatry 2001; 40: 564–571.

24. Beidel DC, Turner SM, Morris TL. A new inventory to assess childhood social anxiety and phobia: the Social Phobia and Anxiety Inventory for Children. Psychol Assess 1995; 7: 73–79.

25. Barrett PM. Evaluation of cognitive-behavioral group treatments for childhood anxiety disorders. J Clin Child Psychol 1998; 27: 459–468.

26. Barrett PM, Dadds MR, Rapee RM. Family treatment of childhood anxiety: a controlled trial. J Consult Clin Psychol 1996; 64: 333–342.

27. Flannery-Schroeder EC, Kendall PC. Group and individual cognitive-behavioral treatments for youth with anxiety disorders: a randomized clinical trial. Cogn Ther Res 2000; 24: 251–278.

28. Kendall PC. Treating anxiety disorders in children: results of a randomized clinical trial. J Consult Clin Psychol 1994; 62: 100–110.

29. Kendall PC, Flannery-Schroeder E, Panichelli-Mindel S, Southam-Gerow M, Henin A, Warman M. Therapy for youths with anxiety disorders: a second randomized clinical trial. J Consult Clin Psychol 1997; 65: 366–380.

30. Silverman WK, Kurtines WM, Ginsburg GS, Weems CF, Lumpkin PW, Carmichael DH. Treating anxiety disorders in children with group cognitive-behavioral therapy: a randomized clinical trial. J Consult Clin Psychol 1999; 67: 995–1003.
31. Silverman WK, Kurtines WM, Ginsburg GS, Weems CF, Rabian B, Serafini LT. Contingency management, self-control, and education support in the treatment of childhood phobic disorders: a randomized clinical trial. J Consult Clin Psychol 1999; 67: 675–687.
32. Kendall PC, Southam-Gerow MA. Long-term follow-up of a cognitive-behavioral therapy for anxious youth. J Consult Clin Psychol 1996; 62:724–730.
33. Barrett PM, Duffy AL, Dadds MR, Rapee RM. Cognitive-behavioral treatment of anxiety disorders in children: long-term (6 year) follow-up. J Consult Clin Psychol 1996; 69: 135–141.
34. Shortt AL, Barrett PM, Fox TL. Evaluating the FRIENDS program: a cognitive-behavioral group treatment for anxious children and their parents. J Clin Child Psychol 2001; 30: 525–535.
35. Manassis K, Mendlowitz SL, Scapillato D, Avery D, Fiksenbaum L, Freire M, Monga S, Owens M. Group and individual cognitive-behavioral therapy for childhood anxiety disorders: a randomized trial. J Am Acad Child Adolesc Psychiatry 2002; 41: 1423–1430.
36. Rapee RM. Group treatment of children with anxiety disorders: outcome and predictors of treatment response. Aust J Psychol 2000; 52:125–129.
37. Albano AM, Marten PA, Holt CS, Heimberg RG, Barlow DH. Cognitive-behavioral group treatment for social phobia in adolescents: a preliminary study. J Nerv Ment Dis 1995; 183: 649–656.
38. Turner SM, Beidel DC, Dancu CV, Stanley MA. An empirically derived inventory to measure social fears and anxiety: the social phobia and anxiety inventory. Psychol Assess 1989; 1: 35–40.
39. Alfano C, Beidel DC, Turner SM. Considering cognition in childhood anxiety disorders: conceptual, methodological and developmental considerations. Clin Psych Rev 2002; 22: 1209–1238.
40. Beidel DC, Turner SM, Morris TL. Psychopathology of childhood social phobia. J Am Acad Child Adolesc Psychiatry 1999; 38: 643–650.
41. Spence SH, Donovan C, Brechman-Toussaint M. Social skills, social outcomes, and cognitive features of childhood social phobia. J Abnorm Psychol 1999: 108: 211–221.
42. Olivares J, Garcia-Lopez LJ, Beidel DC, Turner SM, Albano AM, Hidalgo MD. Results at long-term among three psychological treatments for adolescents with generalized social phobia (I): statistical significance. Psicol Conduct 2002; 10: 147–164.
43. Olivares J, Garcia-Lopez LJ, Turner SM, Beidel DC, Albano AM, Sanchez-Meca J. Results at long-term among three psychological treatments for adolescents with generalized social phobia (II): clinical significance and effect size. Psicol Conduct 2002; 10: 371–385.

44. Chavira DA, Stein MB. Combined psychoeducation and treatment with selective serotonin reuptake inhibitors for youth with generalized social anxiety disorder. J Child Adolesc Psychopharmacol 2002; 12: 47–54.
45. Beidel DC, Turner SM, Sallee FR. Treatment of childhood social phobia. Unpublished manuscript. College Park, MD: University of Maryland, 2000.
46. Masia-Warner C, Klein R, Dent H, Albano AM, Guardin M. School-based intervention or social anxiety disorder: results of a wait-list control trial. Presented at the Anxiety Disorders Association of American Annual Convention, Toronto, Ontario, March 25–28, 2003.
47. Fung DSS, Manassis K, Kenny A, Fiksenbaum L. Web based CBT for selective mutism. J Am Acad Child Adolesc Psychiatry 2002; 41: 112–113.
48. Kendall PC, Brady EU, Verduin TL. Comorbidity in childhood anxiety disorders and treatment outcome. J Am Acad Child Adolesc Psychiatry 2001; 40: 787–794.
49. Rapee RM. The influence of comrbidity on treatment outcome for children and adolescents with anxiety disorders. Behav Res Ther 2003; 41: 105–112.
50. Beidel DC, Turner SM. Shy children, phobic adults: the nature and treatment of social phobia. Washington, DC: American Psychological Association, 1998.

20

Social Anxiety Disorder: Future Directions

Dan J. Stein

University of Stellenbosch,
Cape Town, South Africa
and University of Florida,
Gainesville, Florida, U.S.A.

Borwin Bandelow

University of Göttingen,
Göttingen, Germany

This volume has covered the phenomenology, pathogenesis, pharmacotherapy, and psychotherapy of social anxiety disorder (SAD). In this chapter we summarize key points that have particular relevance for the clinician and provide an algorithm for the management of SAD; we also consider future directions for the field. There have been significant recent advances in the field of SAD, but there are also important gaps that can and should be addressed during the next several years.

I. PHENOMENOLOGY OF SOCIAL ANXIETY DISORDER

Data reviewed in this volume demonstrate convincingly that SAD is highly prevalent, chronic, disabling, and costly (this volume, chapter by Blanco et al.; this volume, chapter by Baldwin and Buis). SAD is the most prevalent of the major anxiety disorders, and because it frequently begins quite early in life (this volume, chapter by Morris), associated impairment affects multiple areas of functioning. Furthermore, SAD frequently precedes comorbid mood and substance use disorders (this volume, chapter by Fehm and Wittchen). Nevertheless, SAD remains underdiagnosed and undertreated, particularly in primary care settings.

A key step for the future is to better understand the gap between the need for intervention and its relative rarity. Does this simply represent a lack of information, or are there more complex processes at play? These potentially include stigmatization of psychiatric symptoms, patients' symptoms themselves interfering with treatment-seeking, or physicians' personal familiarity with normal social anxiety impeding recognition of excessive social anxiety. Clearly additional resources are needed to help inform physicians and the public about SAD, to enhance screening for the disorder, and to increase the ratio of treated to untreated individuals.

One difficulty in diagnosing and understanding SAD lies in its heterogeneity (this volume, chapter by Berman and Schneier). Currently, it can also be argued that it is useful to conceptualize a range of different social anxiety spectrum disorders (this volume, chapter by Muller et al.). In the future, we can expect better delineations of the subtypes and spectrums of SAD; this may allow for advances in both the psychobiology and management of these conditions. Cross-cultural data (this volume, chapter by Seedat and Nagata) may provide useful hypotheses for conducting such studies.

Another key issue is to determine whether early and robust intervention for SAD is able to reduce the prevalence and impact of comorbidity. Although long-term prospective studies are resource intensive, information yielded from such work can be extremely informative (1). Relevant information can also be gleaned from other avenues, including careful analysis of epidemiological data (2). Existing data support the value of early treatment, but additional work is needed to determine fully how best to prevent comorbidity.

II. PATHOGENESIS OF SOCIAL ANXIETY DISORDER

It seems clear that several factors contribute to the pathogenesis of SAD, including genetic susceptibility (this volume, chapter by Stein et al.), environmental factors (this volume, chapter by Bandelow et al.), and cognitive variables (this volume, chapter by Roth). Functional imaging has played a particularly important role in delineating the neurocircuitry of SAD and in showing that both pharmacotherapy and psychotherapy are able to normalize activity in specific brain regions (this volume, chapter by Fredrikson and Furmark). Given recent advances in the field, we can look forward to integration of different findings in the future.

One important area of potential integration is research on the relevant endophenotypes involved in SAD. We know that behavioral inhibition (BI), for example, is an inherited trait that poses a susceptibility risk for later development of SAD (3). There is some evidence that particular genes may be associated with BI, and further work in this area is needed. We also know that certain genetic variants (4) and BIs (5) are associated with increased activation of the amygdala during functional imaging of the processing of facial expressions. Further extension of this work will likely be useful.

By understanding in more detail the neurobiology of the endophenotypes relevant to SAD, we may, for example, be able to better predict the outcomes of treatment for SAD. We already know that specific pharmacotherapies and psychotherapies are able to normalize activity in discrete neuronal circuits in SAD and to decrease SAD symptoms. In the future we can expect that genetic and pharmacogenetic data, structural and functional imaging data (including radioligand work), and treatment outcomes will be increasingly integrated (6) (this volume, chapter by van Ameringen and Mancini).

The further development of animal models will also be key to progress in SAD. Given the importance of social interactions for primates, some may be skeptical of the validity of rodent models. Nevertheless, it can be argued that mechanisms involved in evaluating and responding to social hierarchies in a range of species are crucially relevant to SAD (this volume, chapter by Mathew and Coplan). Certainly such mechanisms have a long evolutionary history and may also provide a valuable perspective on the adaptive value of social anxiety (7).

III. PHARMACOTHERAPY OF SOCIAL ANXIETY DISORDER

The early impression that monoamine oxidase inhibitors (MAOIs) were useful in SAD, but that tricyclic antidepressants were relatively ineffective was important not only in advancing the management of this condition but also in attracting the attention of researchers to the neuropsychopharmacology of SAD (this volume, chapter by Bandelow and Stein). Nevertheless, the classical MAOIs have important practical disadvantages and in recent years have been primarily used as a treatment of last resort.

In contrast, a number of selective serotonin reuptake inhibitors (SSRIs) and the selective noradrenaline serotonin reuptake inhibitor (SNSRI) venlafaxine are clearly not only effective for SAD but also well tolerated. Several of these agents are now approved by the U.S. Food and Drug Administration and by the European Agency for the Evaluation of Medicinal Products. Furthermore, there is growing evidence that long-term treatment with these medications is successful in maintaining treatment response. The introduction of these agents for the management of SAD represents another important step forward for the field.

Certain benzodiazepines also appear useful for SAD. Nevertheless, given the problematic adverse event profile of these agents and the fact that they are not effective for a number of disorders that are commonly co-morbid with SAD, they are now less likely to be recommended in consensus treatment guidelines as first-line agents (8,9). There are also theoretical concerns about their negative effects on exposure treatments (10), although this is an issue that is not fully resolved (11).

Although the reversible MAOI moclobemide is effective in some SAD studies, there have been concerns that its effect size is smaller than that of other agents (12) (this volume, Bandelow and Stein). Nevertheless, there are few head-to-head studies of the SSRIs with moclobemide, and the latter agent has a particularly advantageous adverse-event profile. Thus it may be a useful option for some patients in those countries where it is on the market.

There remain multiple gaps in our knowledge base. In particular, there are few data on the pharmacotherapy of SAD in children and adolescents (this volume, chapter by Beidel et al.), of SAD with comorbid disorders (13,14), and of SAD in primary care settings (15). Recent work has focused primarily on generalized SAD, and there is a need for additional attention to less generalized and discrete SAD (16). The value of combining anti-depressants with benzodiazepines at the start of treatment has received little attention (30). Furthermore, the pharmacotherapy of treatment-refractory SAD has also received relatively little attention (17).

Novel agents also deserve attention. Pregabalin, for example, may be a useful alternative to currently used antidepressants; it has a novel mechanism of action (binding to the alpha$_2$ subunit of voltage-dependent calcium channels) that does not resemble the mechanisms of action of currently used anxiolytic drugs. Thus it may offer the advantages of benzodiazepines in terms of fast onset of action and lack of initial jitteriness but without the disadvantage of withdrawal on discontinuation. NK1 (Neurokinin 1) antagonists are also under study for the treatment SAD, although to date no NK1 antagonist has shown efficacy in controlled studies of anxiety disorders. Other novel anxiolytic medications, such as CRH (corticotrophin-releasing hormone) antagonists, also deserve attention.

The methodology of pharmacotherapy trials for SAD is an issue that also deserves increased attention. Although the Liebowitz Social Anxiety Scale (LSAS) is commonly used, there is little consensus on what percentage reduction represents a clinical response, what score represents remission, or the relevance of the decreased score on different LSAS factors. Developments in trials for other psychiatric indications—including omission of placebo run-in, inclusion of a comparator arm, assessment of early treatment response, and use of more sophisticated statistical analyses—need to be applied to the field of SAD (18–20).

IV. PSYCHOTHERAPY

Cognitive-behavioral psychotherapy (CBT) is the best-studied of the psychotherapies for SAD and is clearly effective. There is evidence that CBT is at least as effective as pharmacotherapy and may be more effective in the long-term (this volume, chapter by Holaway and Heimberg). There is some evidence for the value of combining different modalities—pharmacotherapy may be especially useful to achieve short-term gains, whereas psychotherapy may be useful in allowing discontinuation of medication—although the data on this issue are not entirely consistent (this volume, chapter by Zaider and Heimberg).

Further work needs to be done, to establish the key therapeutic elements of CBT. There is some evidence that exposure is key (21). The development of a streamlined CBT that is effective for a broad range of patients over both short and long term will be helpful in convincing general practitioners and other primary care clinicians of the feasibility and effectiveness of this intervention in their settings. There is also a need to extend CBT studies in younger subjects (this volume, chapter by Beidel et al.).

Furthermore, in our view, more needs to be done to link the theoretical constructs of CBT with advances in the cognitive-affective neuroscience of SAD. For example, as we understand more about the inseparability of cognitive and affective processes at a brain level, we may need to revise some of the theoretical framework of cognitive therapy. Functional imaging provides new tools for delineating the complex cognitive-affective parallel processes that underpin normal and pathological social anxiety, and our prediction is that this will ultimately lead to a revision of the relatively linear models that are relied on in contemporary CBT.

Self-help manuals are often prescribed for SAD. These are increasingly available over the Internet (unfortunately, the number of bad websites may exceed the number of good ones). Such resources may be particularly useful in areas where there is a lack of trained psychotherapists or when symptoms interfere with patients' ability to seek help in the first place. Nevertheless, these kinds of treatment modalities deserve more formal evaluation. The therapeutic relationship remains a powerful tool for change (this volume, chapter by Busch and Milrod), and may be particularly useful in allowing an exploration of the patient's own explanatory model of SAD as well as in addressing associated shame.

In other areas of anxiety disorder, consumer advocacy plays an important role in directing the attention of professionals and the public (22).

Our anecdotal experience is that it is relatively harder to achieve good consumer advocacy for SAD, perhaps partly because sufferers from this disorder, even when much improved, are uncomfortable with taking a highly visible public role. There is a need for more work in this area; consumer advocates have contributed to advancing awareness of specific kinds of social anxiety disorder [such as shy bladder or paruresis (23)] and could potentially do more.

Finally, more attention needs to be paid to the possibility of the prevention of SAD. Behaviorally inhibited children of people with SAD, for example, are at relatively high risk of developing SAD. It is therefore important to study school-based interventions for such individuals. A certain degree of social anxiety is certainly advantageous, and may be particularly so in certain cultures (this volume, chapter by Seedat and Nagata); but the prevention of pathological social anxiety would have major benefits.

V. ALGORITHM FOR THE TREATMENT OF SAD

A number of guidelines addressing the treatment of SAD have recently been published (8,9,24). Treatment algorithms run the risk of oversimplifying complex medical decision making; certainly they cannot be applied without clinical judgment. Nevertheless, algorithms are useful insofar as they summarize the relevant considerations in medical decision making, integrate the current empirical data, serve as teaching tools, and point to gaps where future research is required (25).

The first step in the treatment of SAD is correct diagnosis and identification of target symptoms for treatment. Fortunately the symptoms of SAD are fairly easy to recognize, so that the most important part of making the diagnosis is to screen patients for these symptoms (this volume, chapter by Lipsitz and Liebowitz). Comorbid disorders also need to be evaluated, particularly mood, anxiety, and substance use disorders. It is helpful to evaluate symptom severity using a standardized scale, such as the LSAS. Associated symptoms, such as disability, also require careful assessment.

Both pharmacotherapy and psychotherapy are effective for the treatment of SAD. The decision as to which to use first therefore depends on individual factors, such as patient preference, existence of comorbid disorders, previous response to treatment, and availability of appropriate clinicians. As noted earlier, there remains debate about the value of combining pharmacotherapy and psychotherapy (this volume, chapter by Zaider and Heimberg). Nevertheless, there are some data supporting such a strategy (26), and there is a theoretical argument that pharmacotherapy may be especially useful to achieve short-term gains, whereas psychotherapy may be useful in allowing discontinuation of medication.

Within the pharmacotherapies, the SSRIs and the SNSRIs are the treatments of choice. There have been few head-to-head trials between these agents, and they are currently considered equally effective (this volume, chapter by Bandelow and Stein). Thus choice should be based on considerations such as previous response, family history of response, and adverse-event profile. Treatment trials should be at least 10 to 12 weeks in duration, as around 27% of nonresponders at week 8 can become responders at week 12 (24). Although the dose-response curve of SSRIs is relatively flat, individual patients may do better at higher doses.

The first-line psychotherapy of SAD is CBT. This can be applied in individual or group settings, although the former is often more practicable in the clinical setting. Information about SAD and about exposure techniques may be a valuable resource for encouraging and strengthening CBT techniques. In some cases (e.g., younger patients), it may be particularly important to involve family members in the psychotherapy. It may be especially useful to consider CBT when discontinuing pharmacotherapy.

Current guidelines emphasize the importance of treating SAD symptoms to remission, addressing comorbid symptoms, and adequate duration of treatment. Treatment should be continued for at least 12 to 24 months after remission. There is growing evidence that both pharmacotherapy and psychotherapy are able to maintain response, whereas premature discontinuation of treatment increases the risk of relapse. Patients understandably often want to discontinue treatment as soon as possible, so appropriate psychoeducation is needed to fully present the options. Understanding patients' models of their social anxiety is crucial in negotiating a shared treatment plan.

In refractory cases, it may be useful to switch to a different medication or modality of treatment. Thus, for example, there is some evidence that venlafaxine may be effective when a SSRI has failed (27). It may also be useful to augment SSRIs with buspirone (29). although there are no positive controlled studies. There are also no trials that directly compare switching with augmentation strategies, but a rule of thumb may be to switch when a first drug is ineffective and to augment when a second drug is partially effective or even when a third is ineffective. Irreversible MAOIs remains a valuable option for patients who do not respond to more modern agents (28).

VI. CONCLUSION

There have been major advances in understanding SAD in recent years. We know a great deal about its epidemiology, are able to diagnose it reliably and assess it rigorously, and have effective and well-tolerated pharmacotherapies and psychotherapies. It is important to convey these advances to primary care practitioners, the general public, and policy makers in order to make an impact on the relatively low SAD treatment rates.

In addition, we can predict significant additional advances in the years to come. In particular, we can expect to see better delineation of the relevant endophenotypes, advances in and integration of genetics and imaging data, and more data on currently less well studied aspects of treatment, including management of the treatment-refractory patient. Such advances will surely lead to a better prognosis for patients.

REFERENCES

1. Yonkers KA, Dyck IR, Keller MB. An eight-year longitudinal comparison of clinical course and characteristics of social phobia among men and women. Psychiatr Serv 2001;52:637–643.
2. Goodwin RM, Gorman JM. Psychopharmacologic treatment of generalized anxiety disorder and the risk of major depression. Am J Psychiatry 2002;159: 1935–1937.
3. Kagan J, Reznick JS, Gibbons J. Biological basis of childhood shyness. Science 1988;240:167–171.
4. Hariri AR, Mattay VS, Tessitore A, et al. Serotonin transporter genetic variation and the response of the human amygdala. Science 2002;297:400–403.
5. Schwartz CE, Wright C, I, Shin LM, et al. Inhibited and uninhibited infants "grown up": adult amygdalar response to novelty. Science 2003;5627:1952–1953.
6. Lerer B, Macciardi F. Pharmacogenetics of antidepressant and mood-stabilizing drugs a review of candidate-gene studies and future research directions. Int J Neuropsychopharmacol 2002;5:255–275.
7. Stein DJ, Bouwer C. A neuro-evolutionary approach to the anxiety disorders. J Anxiety Disord 1997;11:409–429.
8. Ballenger JC, Davidson JA, Lecrubier Y, et al. Consensus statement on social anxiety disorder from the international consensus group on depression and anxiety. J Clin Psychiatry 1998;59(suppl 8):54–60.
9. Bandelow B, Zohar J, Hollander E, et al. World Federation of Societies of Biological Psychiatry (WFSBP) guidelines for the pharmacological treatment of anxiety, obsessive-compulsive and posttraumatic stress disorders. World J Biol Psychiatry 2002;3:171–199.
10. Wilhelm FH, Roth WT. Acute and delayed effects of alprazolam on flight phobics during exposure. Behav Res Ther 1997;35:831–841.
11. Wardle J. Behaviour therapy and benzodiazepines: allies or antagonists? Br J Psychiatry 1990;156:163–168.
12. van der Linden GJH, Stein DJ, van Balkom AJLM. The efficacy of the selective serotonin reuptake inhibitors for social anxiety disorder (social phobia): A meta-analysis of randomized controlled trials. Int Clin Psychopharmacol 2000;15(suppl 2):15–24.

13. Randall CL, Johnson MR, Thevos AK, et al. Paroxetine for social anxiety and alcohol use in dual-diagnosed patients. Depress Anxiety 2001;14:255–262.

14. Stein DJ, Cameron A, Amrein R, et al. Moclobemide is effective and well tolerated in the long-term pharmacotherapy of social anxiety disorder with or without comorbid anxiety disorder. Int Clin Psychopharmacol 2002;17:161–170.

15. Blomhoff S, Haug TT, Hellström K, et al. Randomised controlled general practice trial of sertraline, exposure therapy and combined treatment in generalised social phobia. Br J Psychiatry 2001;179:23–30.

16. Stein DJ, Stein MB, Goodwin W, et al. The selective serotonin reuptake inhibitor paroxetine is effective in more generalized and less generalized social anxiety disorder. Psychopharmacology 2001;158:267–272.

17. Stein MB, Sareen J, Hami S, et al. Pindolol potentiation of paroxetine for generalized social phobia: a double-blind, placebo-controllled, crossover study. Am J Psychiatry 2001;158:1725–1727.

18. Bandelow B, Brunner E, Beinroth D, et al. Application of a new statistical approach to evaluate a clinical trial with panic disorder patients. Eur Arch Psychiatr Clin Neurosci 1999;249:21–27.

19. Montgomery SA, Bech P, Blier P, et al. Selecting methodologies for the evaluation of differences in time to response between antidepressants. J Clin Psychiatry 2002;63:694–699.

20. Oosterbaan DB, van Balkom AJ, Spinhoven P, et al. The placebo response in social phobia. J Psychopharmacol 2001;15:199–203.

21. Hope DA, Heimberg RG, Bruch MA. Dismantling cognitive-behavioral group therapy for social phobia. Behav Res Ther 1995;33:637–650.

22. Stein DJ, Wessels C, Zungu-Dirwayi N, et al. Value and effectiveness of consumer advocacy groups: a survey of the anxiety disorders support group in South Africa. Depression Anxiety 2001;13:105–107.

23. Vythilingum B, Stein DJ, Soifer S. Is "shy bladder syndrome" a subtype of social anxiety disorder? A survey of people with paruresis. Depress Anxiety 2002;16:84–87.

24. Stein DJ, Kasper S, Matsunaga H, et al. Pharmacotherapy of social anxiety disorder: an algorithm for primary care—2001. Primary Care Psychiatry 2001; 7:107–110.

25. Fawcett J, Stein DJ, Jobson KO. Textbook of Treatment Algorithms in Psychopharmacology. Chichester, UK: Wiley, 1999.

26. Gelernter CS, Uhde TW, Cimbolic P, et al. Cognitive-behavioral and pharmacological treatments of social phobia: a controlled study. Arch Gen Psychiatry 1991;48:938–945.

27. Altamura AC, Pioli R, Vitto M, et al. Venlafaxine in social phobia: a study in selective serotonin reuptake non-responders. Int Clin Psychopharmacol 1999;14:239–245.

28. Aarre TF. Phenelzine efficacy in refractory social anxiety disorder: A case series. Nord J Psychiatry 2003;57:313–315.

29. van Ameringen M, Mancini C, Wilson C. Buspirone augmentation of selective serotonin reuptake inhibitors (SSRIs) in social phobia. J Affect Disord 1996; 39:115–121.
30. Seedat S, Stein MB. Double-blind, placebo-controlled assessment of combined clonazepam with paroxetine compared with paroxetine monotherapy for generalized social anxiety disorder. J Clin Psychiatry 2004;65(2):244–248.

Appendix

Information for Patients

SOCIAL ANXIETY DISORDER (SOCIAL PHOBIA)

What is social anxiety disorder? Do you experience intense anxiety when meeting or talking to other people? Do you avoid speaking in front of others, dining with co-workers, or dating for fear of embarrassment? Do you sweat or tremble at the thought of meeting your teacher, your boss, or other authority figures? If so, you may be suffering from social anxiety disorder (SAD), also known as social phobia.

People with social anxiety disorder often experience significant emotional distress in the following situations:

- Being the center of attention
- Being introduced to other people
- Meeting strangers
- Making "small talk" at parties
- Meeting people in authority
- Going to a job interview
- Being teased or criticized
- Being watched while working
- Using a public rest room

From: *Social Anxiety Disorder*, Editors: Borwin Bandelow, M.D., Ph.D. & Dan J. Stein, M.D., Ph.D.

- Eating out
- Writing in the presence of other people, as when signing a form
- Talking on the phone

Social anxiety disorder is characterized by overwhelming anxiety and excessive self-consciousness in everyday social situations. People with social anxiety disorder suffer from intense fear of being observed and judged negatively by others. They worry that they might act in a way that is clumsy, embarrassing, or humiliating. In their own minds, they greatly exagerrate the seriousness of small mistakes they make.

If you suffer from this anxiety disorder, you tend to think that other people are very competent in social situations but that you are not.

While many people with social anxiety disorder recognize that their fear of being around people may be excessive or unreasonable, they are unable to overcome it. They often worry for days or weeks in advance of a dreaded situation. Even if they manage to confront what they fear, they usually feel very anxious beforehand and are intensely uncomfortable throughout. Afterwards, the unpleasant feelings may linger, as they worry about how they may have been judged or what others may have thought or observed about them. They spend days brooding over what they should have said or done in these situations.

What are the signs and symptoms of social anxiety disorder?

The bodily symptoms that accompany social anxiety may include:

- Intense fear
- Racing heart or "palpitations"
- Sweating
- Turning red or blushing
- Dry throat and mouth
- Difficulty swallowing

From: *Social Anxiety Disorder*, Editors: Borwin Bandelow, M.D., Ph.D. & Dan J. Stein, M.D., Ph.D.

- Shaky legs or hands
- Muscle twitches
- A quivering voice, stammering, or even a speech-block

To make matters worse, outward symptoms—such as blushing, sweating, or a trembling voice—can make you worry that others can see that you are worried or uncertain, so you may become even more anxious.

Is social anxiety disorder the same as shyness?

Although social anxiety disorder is often thought of as simple shyness, the two are not the same. In people with social anxiety disorder, there is a large discrepancy between their desire to be accepted, liked, or loved on the one hand and their inability to achieve this goal on the other. Almost everyone experiences some social anxiety now and then. However, in contrast to shy people, people with social anxiety disorder tend to avoid social situations. The disorder may therefore severely limit their quality of life, in some cases causing them to avoid participating in school, making friends, or taking advantage of important opportunities at work.

What other illnesses co-occur with social anxiety disorder?

Some people with social anxiety disorder may also suffer from depression or other anxiety disorders, such as panic disorder and obsessive-compulsive disorder.

Which other illnesses can be mistaken for social anxiety disorder?

- The anxiety symptoms described earlier may also occur in other anxiety disorders, such as panic disorder or generalized anxiety disorder.
- A fear of going to public places may also occur in agoraphobia.
- A tendency to avoid meeting with friends or acquaintances may also be a symptom of depression.
- The fear of being watched by other people may occur in psychoses.

From: *Social Anxiety Disorder*, Editors: Borwin Bandelow, M.D., Ph.D. & Dan J. Stein, M.D., Ph.D.

What is the course of social anxiety disorder?	Social anxiety disorder often begins in childhood or early adolescence and rarely develops after age 25. Without treatment, it may become a lifelong condition.

However, it is important to know that the anxiety people with SAD may feel in social situations is not necessarily "just the way they are." No matter how long people have lived with such symptoms, social anxiety does not have to be part of their personalities or lives. Social anxiety disorder can be treated, no matter how or why it develops.

How common is social anxiety disorder?

Social anxiety disorder is a much more common problem than past estimates have led us to believe. Millions of people all over the world suffer from this devastating and traumatic problem every day of their lives. According to recent epidemiological studies, social anxiety disorder was the third most common psychiatric disorder. About 3 to 4% of the population experience social anxiety disorder in any given year. This disorder occurs in women twice as often as in men, although a higher proportion of men seeks help for this disorder.

What are the consequences of social anxiety disorder?

- To help cope with fears, people with social anxiety disorder may avoid anxiety-causing situations, arranging their lives around the symptoms. As a result, social anxiety disorder may significantly diminish their quality of life and hinder family, working, and social relationships.
- Social anxiety disorder can stop people from doing their best at school or work. Often, individuals with this disorder will work in low-paid low-skill jobs even though they are capable of doing more rewarding work.
- People with social anxiety disorder may become depressed about the effect this condition is having on their lives and may even develop suicidal thoughts.

From: *Social Anxiety Disorder*, Editors: Borwin Bandelow, M.D., Ph.D. & Dan J. Stein, M.D., Ph.D.

- As a consequence of finding it difficult to meet or dating other people, those with social anxiety disorder may find it hard to find a partner, marry, and have children.
- Some people with social anxiety disorder may use alcohol or illegal drugs as a way to self-medicate to help them get through social situations. Although alcohol or drugs may seem to help initially, they eventually become another problem in the lives of individuals with social anxiety disorder.
- People with social anxiety disorder may even find it difficult to approach a doctor to seek medical help.

What causes social anxiety disorder?

Although no one has discovered a single cause of social anxiety disorder, studies suggest that both biological and psychological factors may play a role.

- A person may be more likely to develop social anxiety disorder if a close family member also has it. There is evidence that a proneness to develop social anxiety is hereditary.
- There is also a theory that people may acquire social fears from having observed socially anxious behavior in parents or other close relatives, a process called observational learning or social modeling. The family environment one grows up in may also affect the way one thinks about oneself and how one deals with social contacts.
- Some researchers have investigated the influence of early traumatic experiences in childhood on the development of social anxiety disorder.
- According to one theory, social anxiety may stem from embarrassing or humiliating social events in the past, but this does not appear the case for everyone with social anxiety disorder.

From: *Social Anxiety Disorder*, Editors: Borwin Bandelow, M.D., Ph.D. & Dan J. Stein, M.D., Ph.D.

- One line of research is investigating a biochemical basis for the disorder. One theory is that social anxiety disorder may be related to an imbalance of a chemical called serotonin, which transports signals between nerve cells in the brain. Interestingly, a similar imbalance is associated with other mood and anxiety disorders. Also, many drugs that improve serotonin neurotransmission in the brain are effective in social anxiety disorder. Moreover, dysfunctions of other neurotransmitters, such as dopamine, have been associated with social anxiety disorder.

Why do many people with social anxiety disorder not seek treatment?

Sometimes people suffering from social anxiety disorder think they are the only ones in the whole world who have these terrible symptoms. Therefore they think that they must hide their secret, and they find it difficult or embarrassing to approach a doctor in order to seek professional help.

What treatments are available for social anxiety disorder?

Both medication and behavior therapy have proven successful in treating social anxiety disorder. Medication treatment includes several classes of medications that have shown to have markedly beneficial effects for many people with social anxiety disorder. Cognitive behavioral therapy (CBT) is also a successful method for decreasing anxiety and avoidance in social situations. A combination of medication and CBT may be most effective. A clinician can help choose the most appropriate course of action.

Which medications help those with social anxiety disorder?

In recent years, some medications have been found that can effectively treat social anxiety disorder and that are well tolerated.

Some of these medications are among the antidepressant drugs and can also treat depressive symptoms. The selective serotonin reuptake inhibitors

From: *Social Anxiety Disorder*, Editors: Borwin Bandelow, M.D., Ph.D. & Dan J. Stein, M.D., Ph.D.

(SSRIs) and serotonin and noradrenaline reuptake inhibitors (SNRIs) are considered the first-line treatment for social anxiety disorder. Monoamine oxidase inhibitors (MAOIs) are very effective in treating social anxiety disorder, but they are considered second-line treatments due to the possibility of side effects and interactions with food and other drugs. Modern MAOIs have fewer side effects.

Benzodiazepines, a class of sedating drugs, have also been used in social anxiety disorder, but their long-term use remains controversial. Some people may find it difficult to discontinue these agents.

Other promising treatments may be available in the near future.

Your doctor will inform you about possible side effects or precautions to consider in taking psycho-pharmacological drugs.

Are there herbal or other natural medications that help in treating social anxiety disorder?

There is no evidence that any herbal or other natural medication can effectively treat social anxiety disorder.

Which kind of psychotherapy helps in social anxiety disorder?

Many psychotherapeutic methods exist, but cognitive-behavioral therapy (CBT) is the only modality that has been shown to work effectively. CBT teaches people with social anxiety disorder to react differently to the situations that trigger their anxiety symptoms. The therapist helps the patient confront his or her negative feelings about social situations and the fear about being judged or scrutinized by others.

Patients learn how certain thinking patterns worsen the symptoms of social anxiety disorder and how to

From: *Social Anxiety Disorder*, Editors: Borwin Bandelow, M.D., Ph.D. & Dan J. Stein, M.D., Ph.D.

change their thinking so that symptoms begin to lessen. Another central component of this treatment is exposure therapy, in which patients are confronted with anxiety-provoking situations. Social skills training is also a component of cognitive therapy. Patients are shown how to make eye contact, speak louder as well as more slowly and clearly, greet people, ask others for favors, and respond to criticism. The principle is that knowing what to say and do in social situations will ease anxiety.

**What can
I do myself?**

Psychological therapies and medications are very helpful in treating social anxiety disorder, but people can also do much on their own.

- Most importantly, know that you can overcome social anxiety disorder.
- It doesn't help if people tell you that you don't have a problem or that you are "just shy." If social anxiety disorder remains untreated, other complications can arise.
- Never try to avoid social situations. People with social anxiety disorder should actively try to find and identify social situations in which they can rehearse social skills. They should keep a goal in mind, whether it's to speak to a group of people, ask someone for a date, go to a party, or make new friends.
- Many people who have joined social anxiety disorder support groups or have spoken to others with the same problem find this a very helpful and positive experience. Because of the very nature of social anxiety disorder, this may be difficult, but it's always a good idea to try it anyway.

From: *Social Anxiety Disorder*, Editors: Borwin Bandelow, M.D., Ph.D. & Dan J. Stein, M.D., Ph.D.

Subject Index